Biotech's

# DICTIONARY *Of* Genomics

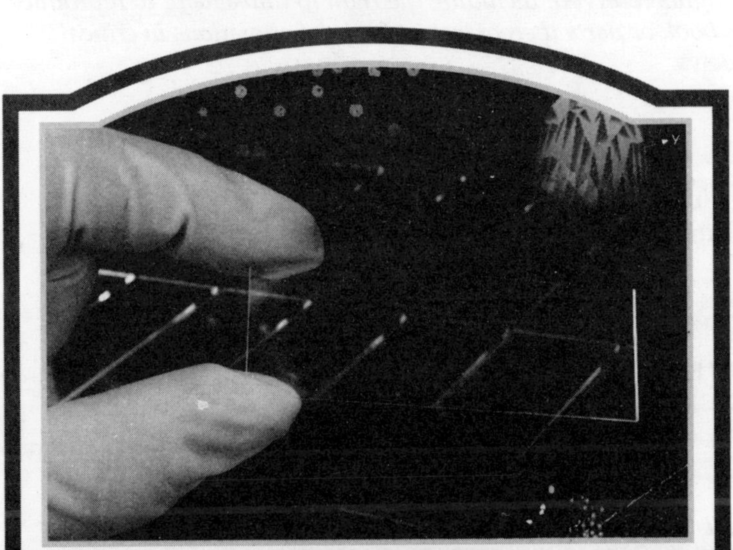

*Compiled & Edited by*
*Dinesh Arora*

BIOTECH

2007

BIOTECH BOOKS
DELHI - 110035

Biotech's

# DICTIONARY Of Genomics

*Compiled & Edited by*
*Dinesh Arora*



First Indian Edition 2007


ISBN 81-7622-181-3

***Published by*** : BIOTECH BOOKS
1123/74, Tri Nagar,
Delhi - 110 035
Phone: 27382765
e-mail: biotechbooks@yahoo.co.in

***Showroom*** : 4762-63/23, Ansari Road, Darya Ganj,
New Delhi - 110 002
Phone: 23245578, 23244987

***Printed at*** : Chawla Offset Printers
New Delhi - 110 052

PRINTED IN INDIA

# Preface

Genomics is the study of an organism's genome and the use of the genes. It deals with the systematic use of genome information, associated with other data, to provide answers in biology, medicine, and industry. Genomics has the potential of offering new therapeutic methods for the treatment of some diseases, as well as new diagnostic methods. Other applications are in the food and agriculture sectors. The major tools and methods related to genomics are bioinformatics, genetic analysis, measurement of gene expression, and determination of gene function. The first genome to be sequenced in its entirety was that of bacteriophage in 1980. The first free-living organism to be sequenced was that of Haemophilus influenzae in 1995, and since then genomes are being sequenced at a rapid pace. A rough draft of the human genome was completed by the Human Genome Project in early 2001 amid much fanfare.

If a particular DNA sequence or pattern is present among many members of a clade, that sequence is said to have been conserved among the species. Evolutionary conservation of a DNA sequence may imply that it confers a relative selective advantage to the organisms that possess it. Conservation also suggests that sequence has functional significance. It may be a protein coding sequence or regulatory region. Experimental investigation of some of these sequences has shown that some are transcribed into small RNA molecules, although the functions of these RNAs were not immediately apparent.

The identification of similar sequences (including many genes) in two distantly related organisms, but not in other members of one of the clades, has led to the theory that these sequences were acquired by horizontal gene transfer. This phenomenon is most prominent in bacteria, although it also seems that genes were transferred from Archaea to Eubacteria. It has also been noticed that bacterial genes exist in eukaryotic nuclear genomes and that these genes generally encode mitochondrial and plastid proteins, giving support to the endosymbiotic theory of the origin of these organelles. This theory holds that the mitochondria and chloroplast organelles found in many animal and plant genomes were originally free-living bacteria that were absorbed by an ancestral eukaryote, and that subsequently became an integral part of the eukaryotic cell.

This dictionary provides definition regarding the new and rapidly changing subject of genomics, a rapidly exploding field exploring the complete genome sequence of a variety of organisms. With its emphasis on computational analysis, high-through-put technologies, and identification of biological networks, this dictionary covers comparative genomics, structural genomics, phylogenomics, and pharmacogenomics. This dictionary is useful for professionals in the field of biology and genomics.

- **16s rrna, ribosomes**
  This is covered in more detail in the lab. Ribosomes are cellular organelles that are the site of protein synthesis. They comprise various protein molecules as well as associated RNA molecules (known as ribosomal RNA or rRNA). 16S rRNA is one of the three RNA molecules associated with the ribosomes of procaryotes. 16S signifies its size.

- **3' - end**
  The end of a polynucleotide with a free (or phosphorylated) 3' - hydroxyl group.

- **5' - end**
  The end of a polynucleotide with a free (or phosphorylated or capped) 5' - hydroxyl group; transcription/translation begins at this end.

- **a (aminoacyl) site**
  The site on the ribosome occupied by an aminoacyl-tRNA just prior to peptide bond formation.

- **a form DNA**
  The form of DNA at high humidity; it has tilted base pairs and more base pairs per turn than does B DNA.

- **abdomen**
  The part of the body that contains the stomach, small intestine, colon, rectum, liver, spleen, pancreas, kidneys, appendix, gallbladder, and bladder.

- **abdominal muscles**
  The large group of muscles that assists in the regular breathing movement and supports the muscles of the spine while lifting and keeps other abdominal organs and intestines in place.

- **abdominoplasty**
  Plastic surgery repair of the muscles of the abdominal wall.

- **abduction**
  The act of turning outward; the movement of part from the axis (midline) of the body.

- **aberration**
  An anomaly- a change from the normal or ordinary.

- **ablation**
  Elimination or removal.

- **abnormality**
  A change from the normal or ordinary.

- **abortive transduction**
  The failure of a transducing DNA segment to be incorporated into the recipient chromosome.

- **abr**
  Auditory Brainstem Response.

- **abruptio placenta**
  Premature detachment of a normally situated placenta.

- **absent**
  Not present- missing or not existing.

- **absorption**
  Process by which nutrients are absorbed through the lining of the intestinal tract into capillaries and into the bloodstream. Nutrients must be absorbed to affect the body.

- **acalculous**
  Without the presence of stones, gallstones in this instance.

- **acceptor splice site**
  The boundary between the 3' end of an intron and the 5' end of the adjacent exon.

- **accessory pathways**
  Additional and abnormal electrical-impulse conducting tissues in the heart.

- **accessory spleen**
  Normal spleen tissue in an abnormal anatomical location.

- **acentric chromosome**
  A chromosome having no centromere.

- **acentric fragment**
  A chromosomal piece without a centromere.

- **acetabulum**
  The socket in the hip into which the head of the femur (thigh bone) fits.

- **acetone**
  A chemical formed in the blood when the body uses fat instead of glucose (sugar) for energy. If acetone forms, it usually means that the cells do not have enough insulin, or cannot use the insulin that is in the blood, to use glucose for energy. Acetone passes through the body into the urine. Someone with a lot of acetone in the body can have breath that smells fruity and is called "acetone breath.

- **acetylation**
  The introduction of an acetyl group into a molecule; often used by the body to help eliminate substances by the liver.

- **achilles tendon**
  One of the longest tendons in the body, it attaches the calf muscles to the heel bone.

- **acholasia of esophagus**
  Inability to relax muscles of the upper digestive tract, specifically where the esophagus enters the stomach.

- **achondroplasia**
  The most common and well known form of short limbed dwarfism characterized by a normal trunk size with disproportionally short arms and legs, and a disproportionally large head; autosomal dominant condition.

- **acidosis**
  Too much acid in the body. For a person with diabetes, this can lead to diabetic ketoacidosis.

- **acquired mutations**
  gene changes that arise within individual cells and accumulate

throughout a person's lifetime; also called somatic mutations.

- **acrocentric**
  Term used to describe a chromosome where the centromere is near one end and the short arm usually consists of satellite material.

- **acrodysostosis acquired mutations**
  Gene changes that arise within individual cells and accumulate throughout a person's lifetime; also called somatic mutations.

- **activation energy (deltag)**
  Energy needed to initiate a chemical reaction.

- **active site**
  The part of a protein that must be maintained in a specific shape if the protein is to be functional, for example, the part to which the substrate binds in an enzyme. The part of an enzyme where the actual enzymatic function is performed.

- **acute**
  Intense and of short duration, usually said of a disease. Marked by sudden onset, sharp rise, and lasting a short time, demanding urgent attention.

- **acute cerebellar ataxia of childhood**
  Syndrome characterized by severe gait ataxia,usually follows innoculation or viral infection; usually resolves in months.

- **acute phase proteins**
  A number of proteins involved in innate immunity produced in reaction to infection which include C-reactive protein, mannose binding protein and serum amyloid P component.

- **adaptation**
  In the evolutionary sense, some heritable feature of an individual's phenotype that improves its chances of survival and reproduction in the existing environment.

- **adaptive landscape**
  The surface plotted in a three-dimensional graph; with all possible combinations of allele frequencies for different loci plotted in the plane; and mean fitness for each combination plotted in the third dimension.

- **adaptive peak**
  A high point (perhaps one of several) on an adaptive landscape; selection tends to drive the genotype composition of the population toward a combination corresponding to an adaptive peak.

- **additive genetic effects**
  When the combined effects of alleles at different loci are equal to the sum of their individual effects.

- **additive genetic variance**
  Genetic variance associated with the average effects of substituting one allele for another.

• **additive model**

A mechanism of quantitative inheritance in which alleles at different loci either add a fixed amount to the phenotype or add nothing.

• **adduction**

A movement toward a median line or axis (midline) of the body.

• **adenine**

A nitrogenous base, one member of the base pair AT.

• **adenine, cytosine, guanine, thymine**

Nitrogen-containing bases that are part of nucleotides in DNA. They are often referred to by the letters A, C, G, and T. The sequences of these bases in a DNA molecule comprise the genetic code. Because of the structure of the bases, adenine can form two hydrogen bonds with thymine while cytosine can form three hydrogen bonds with guanine. A-T and C-G pairs are thus termed complementary, and this property of the bases is fundamental for allowing DNA to self-replicate.

• **adenoids**

Pharyngeal tonsil in the back wall of the nose, may cause snoring in children, and mouth breathing if enlarged.

• **adenoma**

An ordinarily benign neoplasm of epithelial tissue in which the tumor cells form glands or gland like structures in the stroma. These are usually well circumscribed, tending to compress rather than infiltrate or invade adjacent tissue.

• **adenosine**

The nucleoside containing adenine as its base.

• **adhesion**

A band of tissue, such as scar tissue, that sticks to other structures such as the abdominal wall.

• **adjacent segregation**

In a reciprocal translocation heterozygote during meiosis the segregation of a translocated and a normal chromosome together, giving unbalanced gametes with duplications and deficiencies leading to non-viable zygotes. Adjacent segregation is of two kinds depending on whether non-homologous (adjacent-1) or homologous (adjacent-2) centromeres segregate together. Adjacent-1 segregation is the usual type of adjacent segregation, adjacent-2 segregation is rare.

• **adnexa**

Ovaries, fallopian tubes and supporting structures.

• **adp**

Adenosine diphosphate; the low energy product produced when ATP releases energy to the cell.

- **adrenal**
  Pertaining to the adrenal or suprarenal glands located on top of the kidneys.

- **adrenal glands**
  A pair of small glands, one located on top of each kidney. The adrenal glands produce hormones (epinephrine, norepinephrine, and steroid hormones) that help control heart rate, blood pressure, the way the body uses food, and other vital functions.

- **adrenocortical**
  Pertaining to the suprarenal cortex.

- **adult-onset diabetes**
  Former term for noninsulin-dependent or type II diabetes. See also: Noninsulin-dependent diabetes mellitus.

- **advanced maternal age**
  Women over age 34 (age 35 at delivery) have a slightly increased risk for nondisjunction trisomy in the fetus.

- **adventitia**
  Outer layer of an organ.

- **aetiology**
  The science of the origin and development of disease.

- **affected**
  An individual who manifests symptoms of a particular condition; Individuals in a pedigree that exhibit the specific phenotype under study.

- **affected relative pair**
  Individuals related by blood, each of whom is affected with the same trait. Examples are affected sibling, cousin, and avuncular pairs.

- **afo**
  Ankle foot Orthodontic, a molded plastic insert worn in the shoes as a foot brace.

- **agenesis**
  Imperfect development or lack of development.

- **aggregation technique**
  A technique used in model organism studies in which embryos at the 8-cell stage of development are pushed together to yield a single embryo (used as an alternative to microinjection).

- **agonist**
  The muscle directly engaged in contraction.

- **albepharia**
  Absence or reduced size of eyelids at birth.

- **albinism**
  Lack of coloring of the skin, hair, and eyes due to an insufficient amount of the pigment melanin. Hereditary absence of pigment in an organism. Albino animals have no colour in their skin, hair and eyes. Albino plants lack chlorophyll.

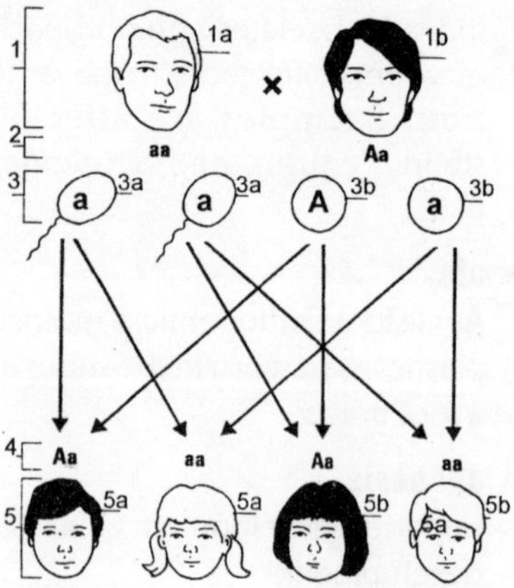


1 Parental phenotype
1a Albino
1b Carrier
2 Parental genotype
3 Gametes produced by meiosis
3a Sperm
3b Ovum
4 $F_1$ genotype
5 $F_1$ phenotype
5a Carrier
5b albino
5c carrier
5d albino

- **albino**

  A pigmentless white phenotype, determined by a mutation in a gene coding for a pigment-synthesizing enzyme.

- **albuminuria**

  More than normal amounts of a protein called albumin in the urine. Albuminuria may be a sign of kidney disease, a problem that can occur in people who have had diabetes for a long time.

- **alcoholism**

  A chronic and progressive condition characterized by the inability to control the consumption of alcohol.

- **alkylating agent**

  A chemical agent that can add alkyl groups (for example, ethyl or methyl groups) to another molecule; many mutagens act through alkylation.

- **allele**

  Alternative form of a genetic locus; a single allele for each locus is inherited from each parent (e.g., at a locus for eye color the allele might result in blue or brown eyes); One of many possible forms of a given gene. Different alleles produce variation in inherited characteristics such as hair and eye color. In an individual, one form of an allele may be expressed (dominant) while the other form may be masked (recessive).

- **allele frequency**

  Often called gene frequency. A measure of how common an allele is in a population; the proportion of all alleles at one gene locus that are of one specific type in a population.

- **allele specific oligonucleotide (aso)**

  A short synthetic DNA probe, less than 20 base pairs, that is used to detect a specific base pair mutation

- **allele-specific oligonucleotide testing**

  The detection of a specific mutation using a synthetic segment of DNA approximately 20 base pairs in length (an oligonucleotide) that binds to and hence identifies the complementary sequence in a DNA sample

- **allelic exclusion**
A process whereby only one immunoglobulin light chain and one heavy chain gene are transcribed in any one cell; the other genes are repressed.

- **allelic heterogeneity**
Different mutations in the same gene at the same chromosomal locus that cause a single phenotype.

- **allelic variant of unknown significance**
An alteration in the normal sequence of a gene, the significance of which is unclear until further study of the genotype and corresponding phenotype in a sufficiently large population; complete gene sequencing often identifies numerous (sometimes hundreds) allelic variants for a given gene

- **allogeneic**
Variation in alleles among members of the same species.

- **allograft**
A tissue graft between non-identical individuals.

- **allopatric speciation**
Speciation is the evolution of new species. Allopatric speciation refers to the evolution of two or more species from an ancestral species as a result of geographical separation:
  - The ancestral gene pool becomes split into two or more gene pools that are no longer connected by gene flow (the movement of genes between populations).
  - The resulting gene pools diverge from one another to establish new species.
  - Over many generations, the new forms become sufficiently distinct that were they to be brought together with each other, or the original parental population, they would be unable to interbreed successfully.

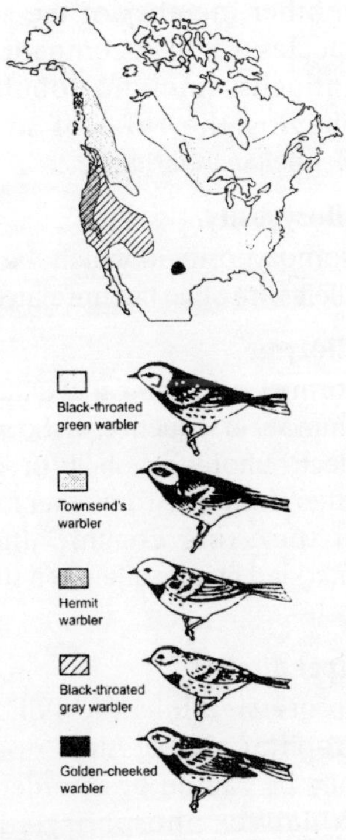

- **allopolyploid**
Polyploid produced by the hybridization of two species.

- **allosteric protein**
A protein whose shape is changed when it binds a particular molecule. In the new shape the protein's ability to react to a second molecule is altered.

- **allosteric transition**
A change from one conformation of a protein to another.

- **allotype**
The protein product (or the result of its activity) of an allele which may be detected as an antigen in another member of the same species.(eg histocompatibility antigens, immunoglobulins), obeying the rules of simple Mendelian inheritance.

- **allozygosity**
Homozygosity in which the two alleles are alike but unrelated.

- **allozyme**
Form of an enzyme that differs in amino acid sequence, as shown by electrophoretic mobility or some other property, from other forms of the same enzyme and is encoded by one allele at a single locus.

- **alper disease**
Progressive Infantile Poliodystrophy. Cases of Alper disease may be caused by disorders of oxidative phosphorylation, including mitochondrial DNA depletion syndromes.

- **alpha (α) thalassaemia**
Inherited disorder of haemoglobin involving underproduction of the α-globin chains occurring most commonly in persons from South-East Asia.

- **alpha-feto protein (afp)**
A protein made in the fetal liver which is disbursed within the amniotic fluid and from there into the mother's bloodstream via the placenta.

- **alpha-feto protein blood test**
It is performed on pregnant women to identify the presence of a particular protein which suggests a neural tube deletion in the fetus.

- **alternate paternity**
The situation in which the alleged father of a particular individual is not the biological father

- **alternate segregation**
At meiosis in a reciprocal translocation heterozygote, the passage (segregation) of both normal chromosomes to one pole and both translocated chromosomes to the other pole, giving genetically balanced gametes. Segregation of centromeres during meiosis in a reciprocal translocation heterozygote such that genetically balanced gametes are produced.

- **alternation of generations**
  The alternation of gametophyte and sporophyte stages in the life cycle of a plant.
- **alternative pathway**
  One of the two pathways of the activation of complement which, in this instance, involves cell membranes of microorganisms.
- **alternative splicing**
  A "cutting-and-pasting" process by which cells splice together elements of the same gene to make different proteins.That's how the human body manufactures more than 100,000 proteins from a set of about 30,000 genes.
- **altruism**
  A form of behaviour in which an individual risks lowering its fitness for the benefit of another.
- **alu family**
  A dispersed intermediately repetitive DNA sequence found in the human genome in about three hundred thousand copies. The sequence is about 300 bp long. The name Alu comes from the restriction endonuclease AluI that cleaves it.
- **alu repeat**
  Short repeated DNA sequences which appear to have homology with transposable elements in other organisms.
- **alu repetitive sequence**
  The most common dispersed repeated DNA sequence in the human genome accounting for 5% of human DNA. The name is derived from the fact that these sequences are cleaved by the restriction endonuclease Alu.
- **alveolar**
  Hollow; the socket within the jawbone in which the roots of the tooth are set.
- **alveolar ridges**
  The teeth-bearing surfaces of the gums.
- **alveoli**
  Microscopic air sacs in the lungs where gases are exchanged.
- **alveolus**
  A tooth socket.
- **alzheimer's disease**
  A disease that causes memory loss, personality changes, dementia and, ultimately, death. Not all cases are inherited, but genes have been found for familial forms of Alzheimer's disease.
- **am**
  The group of genetic variants associated with the IgA heavy chain.
- **amaurosis fugax**
  Temporary visual loss, in one eye, usually due to inadequate blood flow to the eye.
- **amber codon**
  The codon UAG, a nonsense codon.

- **amber suppressor**
  A mutant allele coding for a tRNA whose anticodon is altered in such a way that the suppressor tRNA inserts an amino acid at an amber codon in translation suppressing (preventing) termination.

- **ambiguous**
  Uncertain or doubtful.

- **ambulatory**
  Being able to move from place to place with or without assistive devices.

- **amenorrhea**
  Absence of menstruation.

- **amentia**
  General term for mental impairment which may be a result of congenital or developmental factors.

- **ames test**
  A widely used test to detect possible chemical carcinogens; based on mutagenicity in the bacterium Salmonella.

- **amino acid**
  Any of a class of 20 molecules that are combined to form proteins in living things. The sequence of amino acids in a protein and hence protein function are determined by the genetic code. A group of small molecules that join to form proteins, amino acids are often referred to as the building blocks of proteins. Although more than 100 amino acids occur naturally, only 20 are usually involved in the synthesis of protein — and humans can synthesize at least 100,000 different proteins. The 20 amino acids have the same backbone, but each has a separate side chain — known as an R-group — that distinguishes it from the others.

- **amino acid sequence**
  The linear order of the amino acids in a protein or peptide.

- **aminoacyl-trna**
  Transfer RNA (tRNA) molecule with its cognate amino acid attached.

- **aminoacyl-trna synthetase**
  enzyme that attaches an amino acid to its cognate tRNA(s).

- **amniocentesis**
  A prenatal diagnosis procedure to test for abnormalities typically performed near the 16th week of pregnancy (though sometimes as early as the 11th). A few milliliters of amniotic fluid (which contains fetal cells) is withdrawn by syringe and needle from the amniotic sac surrounding the fetus in the uterus. This method is used to determine the number and kind of chromosomes of the fetus and, when indicated, perform biochemical studies; A clinical procedure in which a few milliliters of amniotic fluid is withdrawn from the uterus. This fluid and the fetal cells that are

present in the fluid may be tested to detect various genetic conditions.

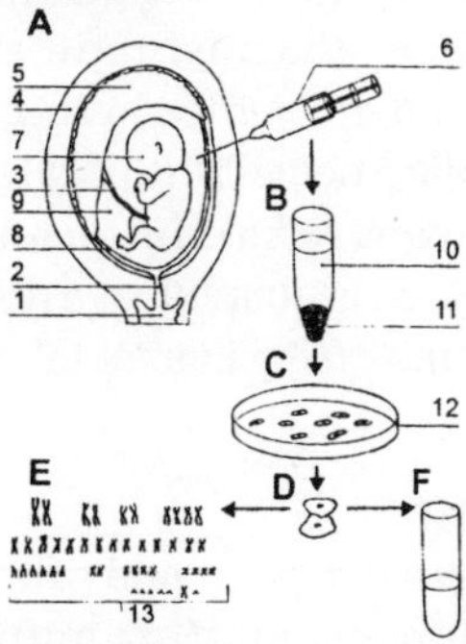


A Sample of amniotic fluid, including cells
B Amniotic fluid centrifuged
C Cells grown in nutrient solution
D Cultured cells
E Chromosomal analysis
1 Vagina
2 Cervix
3 Umbilical cord
4 Uterine wall
5 Placenta
6 Syringe
7 Fetus
8 Amnion
9 Amniotic fluid
10 Supernatant
11 Cells
12 Culture dish
13 Down's syndrome karyotype

- **amniocyte**

  Cells shed by the developing fetus and found in the surrounding amniotic fluid.

- **amnioscopy**

  A prenatal diagnostic procedure in which the fetus is seen by use of a fibro-optic light.

- **amniotic fluid**

  The fluid which, contained in the sac of membranes known as the amnion, surrounds the fetus and provides a shock absorber and a secondary vehicle for the exchange of body chemicals with the mother.

- **amniotic sac**

  Membranes which contain the fetus and the amniotic fluid. The amniotic sac and the amniotic fluid are often refereed to as the "bag of waters."

- **amniotomy**

  The intentional rupturing of the amniotic sac to induce labor.

- **amorph**

  A mutant showing the complete lack of some normal substance or structure.

- **amp**

  Adenosine monophosphate.

- **amphidiploid**

  An allopolyploid; a polyploid formed from the union of two separate chromosome sets and their subsequent doubling. An organism produced by hybridization of two species followed by chromosome doubling. An allotetraploid that appears to be a normal diploid.

- **amplification**

  An increase in the number of copies of a specific DNA fragment; can be in vivo or in vitro.

- **amplification of dna**

  The production of many DNA copies from one or a few copies.

- **ampulla of vater**

  The location at which the common bile duct and pancreatic duct deliver their contents into the duodenum.

- **amylase**

  A digestive enzyme made by the pancreas and salivary glands.

• **amyloidosis**
A rare condition in which certain blood cells produce an abnormal protein that deposits in the tissues. If the deposits are in the heart, heart failure can result.

• **amyoplasia**
A condition where there is a congenital rigidity of the joints.

• **amyotrophic lateral sclerosis**
An inherited, fatal degenerative nerve disorder; also known as Lou Gehrig's disease.

• **amyotrophy**
A type of diabetic neuropathy that causes muscle weakness and wasting.

• **anagenesis**
The evolutionary process whereby one species evolves into another without any splitting of the phylogenetic tree.

• **analysis of the entire coding region: mutation scanning**
A process by which a segment of DNA is screened via one of a variety of methods to identify variant gene region(s). Variant regions are further analyzed (by sequence analysis or mutation analysis) to identify the sequence alteration.

• **analysis of the entire coding region: sequence analysis**
Process by which the nucleotide sequence is determined for a segment of DNA.

• **analyte**
A complex biological component of an enzymatic reaction; a substance that is typically measured in a Biochemical/ Metabolic specialty laboratory that is absent, reduced in quantity, or increased in quantity, as a result of an abnormality in a metabolic pathway

• **anaphase**
The stage of meiosis and mitosis in which sister chromatids (meiosisII) or homologous chromosomes (mitosis and meiosisI) are separated by spindle fibers. An intermediate stage of nuclear division during which chromosomes or chromatids are pulled to the poles of the spindle.

• **anaphase lag**
Loss of a chromosome as it moves to the pole of the cell during anaphase which can lead to monosomy.

• **anaphylactic shock**
Reaction by an individual suffering a severe reaction to a substance to which they are allergic.

• **anastomosis**
A natural, pathological (traumatic or disease-produced) or surgical join between two hollow or tubular organs, as in parts of the bowel.

• **androgen**
The generic term for an agent, usually a hormone like

androsterone, or testosterone, that stimulates activity of the accessory male sex organs, encourages development of male sex characteristics, or prevents changes in the latter that follow castration. Steroids are natural androgens. Synonym: testoid.

- **anemia**

The condition of having less than the normal number of red blood cells or hemoglobin in the blood. The oxygen-transporting units are, therefore, insufficient. Patients can feel tired, fatigue easily, appear pale, develop palpitations, and become short of breath. There are many causes of anemia, including bleeding, abnormal hemoglobin formation (such as in sickle cell anemia), iron, B12 (pernicious anemia), or folate deficiency, rupture of red blood cells (hemolytic anemia), and bone marrow diseases.

- **aneuploid**

The total number or chromosomes in a cell if not an exact multiple of the haploid number of 23. The most common aneupolid numbers are 45 (Turner syndrome) and 47 (Down syndrome).

- **aneuploid cell**

A cell having a chromosome number that differs from the normal chromosome number for the species by a small number of chromosomes.

- **aneuploidy**

The occurrence of one or more extra or missing chromosomes leading to an unbalanced chromosome complement, or, any chromosome number that is not an exact multiple of the haploid number

- **aneurism**

A swelling in the wall of the artery.

- **aneuvysion assay**

A prenatal diagnostics assay that analyzes chromosome 13, 18, 21, X and Y for abnormal copy numbers in fetal (amniotic fluid) cells. Utilizing Vysis Fluoresence In Situ Hybridization (FISH) technology, the assay provides test results in 24 to 48 hours. While designed for use as an adjunct to standard cytogenetic analysis of fetal cells, the assay can be used alone in medically urgent situations.

- **angelman syndrome**

A condition characterized by severe mental deficiency, developmental delay and growth deficiency, puppet-like gait and frequent laughter unconnected to emotions of happiness.

- **angiogram**

A picture or map of the blood vessels in a particular area of the body, usually produced by injecting a special dye into the blood vessels and taking x-ray pictures.

- **angioma**
  An unusual growth made up of blood or lymphatic vessels, forming a benign tumor; a hemangioma (blood vessels) or lymphangioma (lymphatic vessels). In VHL, angiomas are made up of blood vessels and so are technically hemangiomas.

- **angioplasty**
  Method for dilating narrowed or blocked part of a blood vessel.

- **angiosperm**
  Plant whose seeds are enclosed within an ovary. Flowering plants.

- **animal breeding**
  The practical application of genetic analysis for development of lines of domestic animals suited to human purposes.

- **aniridia**
  Absence of the iris or under-developed iris.

- **ankylosed**
  Immobile, as a joint that is less mobile due to changes in it or surrounding tissues.

- **anneal, melt, extend**
  These are the three status indicators that appear during PCR. In the context of PCR, annealing refers to the cooling phase following a melting phase. During the melting phase, DNA's double strands separate. During the annealing phase, single strands that are complementary come together to reform double strands (this process is called hybridizing). During PCR, instead of the two original strands coming together, a primer molecule, which is present in a much higher concentration than the DNA, will bind to the single strand DNA. Then, during the extend phase, DNA polymerase extends the 3' end of the primer molecule, making a copy of the DNA.

- **annealing**
  Spontaneous alignment of two complementary single polynucleotide (RNA, or DNA, or RNA and DNA) strands to form a double helix.

- **annotation**
  Adding pertinent information such as gene coded for, amino acid sequence, or other commentary to the database entry of raw sequence of DNA bases.

- **anomalad**
  A syndrome where the characteristics vary from the normal.

- **anomaly**
  Birth defect; abnormality; variation from the normal .

- **anophthalmia**
  A developmental defect characterized by absence of the eyes (rare).

- **anoplasty**
  Surgical procedure to correct malformations of the anus.

- **anopthalma**
Congenital absence of one or both eyes.

- **anoxia**
A lack of oxygen in body tissues.

- **antenatal**
Before birth; also called prenatal.

- **anterior**
In front, or towards the front.

- **anterior fontanelle**
The soft spot towards the front of the top of an infant's head, representing the incomplete joining of the component skull-bones and providing a clinical method of assessment of degree of dehydration or pressure of fluid within the brain (as in meningitis).

- **anterior horn cells**
Nerve cells in spine and connected to muscles. When damaged muscles become partially or wholly paralysed.

- **anterior information**
Information previously known which leads to the prior probability.

- **anteversion**
An organ that is leaning forward is anteverted.

- **anteverted**
Turned forwards, from their normal downwards direction in this case of the nostrils.

- **antibody**
A protein produced by the immune system that helps the body fight a particular disease or develop an immunity to it. The human body is capable of generating more than a trillion different antibodies; A serum protein which is formed in response to an antigenic stimulus and reacts specifically with that antigen; A protein produced by a B lymphocyte that protects the organism against an antigen. A protein (immunoglobulin) molecule, produced by the immune system, that recognizes a particular foreign antigen and binds to it; if the antigen is on the surface of a cell, this binding leads to cell aggregation and subsequent destruction; An antibody binds to the specific antigen that has stimulated the immune system. Once bound, the antigen can be destroyed by other cells of the immune system.

- **anticipation**
Each generation of offspring has increased severity of a genetic disorder; e.g., a grandchild may have earlier onset and more severe symptoms than the parent, who had earlier onset than the grandparent.

- **anticoding strand**
The DNA strand that forms the template for both the transcribed mRNA and the coding DNA strand.

- **anticodon**
  The three-base sequence in tRNA complementary to a codon on mRNA. A nucleotide triplet in a tRNA molecule that aligns with a particular codon in mRNA under the influence of the ribosome, so that the amino acid carried by the tRNA is added to a growing protein chain.

- **antigen**
  A molecule whose shape triggers the production of antibodies (immunoglobulins) that will bind to the antigen. A foreign substance capable of triggering an immune response in an organism.

- **antigen binding fragment (fab)**
  The fragment of the antibody molecule produced by papain digestion responsible for antigen binding.

- **antimorph**
  A mutant expressing some agent that antagonizes a normal gene product.

- **antimutator mutation**
  Mutation of DNA polymerase that decreases the overall mutation rate.

- **anti-oncogene**
  A gene that prevents malignant (cancerous) growth and whose absence, by mutation, results in malignancy (eg retinoblastoma).

- **antiparallel**
  A term used to describe the opposite orientations of the two strands of a DNA double helix; the 5' end of one strand aligns with the 3' end of the other strand.

- **antisense**
  Nucleic acid that has a sequence exactly opposite to an mRNA molecule made by the body; binds to the mRNA molecule to prevent a protein from being made.

- **antisense oligonucleotide.**
  A short oligonucleotide synthesized to bind to a particular RNA or DNA sequence to block its expression.

- **antisense rna**
  RNA product of mic (mRNA-interfering complementary RNA) genes that regulates another gene by base pairing with and thus preventing translation from its mRNA.

- **antiterminator protein**
  A protein that, when bound at its normal attachment sites in DNA, lets RNA polymerase read through normal terminator sequences (eg the N- and Q-gene products of phage lambda).

- **antrioventricular canal defect**
  A large hole in the center of the heart where the upper and lower heart chambers meet,the individual valves aren't formed normally but are instead a single large valve crossing the hole.

- **anus**
  Outlet of the rectum, through which fecal waste passes.

- **aorta**
  Largest artery in the body; it carries blood from the heart's left ventricle and distributes it throughout the body.

- **aortic aneurysm**
  Localised ballooning of the aorta, potentially causing pressure on adjacent structures and liability to rupture.

- **aortic insufficiency**
  Failure of the aortic valve to prevent backflow of oxygen-rich blood from aorta to left ventricle, resulting in dilatation, hypertrophy and ultimately failure of the pumping mechanism.

- **aortic valve**
  Valve located where the aorta meets the left ventricle of the heart. It allows the blood to flow from the heart into the aorta and prevents back flow.

- **ap endonuclease**
  Endonuclease that initiates excision repair at apurinic and apyrimidinic sites on DNA.

- **ap site**
  Apurinic or apyrimidinic site resulting from the loss of a purine or pyrimidine residue from the DNA.

- **apert syndrome**
  A condition caused by the premature closure of the sutures of the skull bones, resulting in an altered head shape, with webbed fingers and toes. Autosomal dominant.

- **apgar score**
  An evaluation of a newborn's physical condition after birth that enables professionals to quickly identify the infant at risk. It is the sum of ratings (0, 1, & 2) on five criteria; Appearance or coloring, Pulse (heart rate), Grimace (responsiveness to stimuli), Activity (muscle tone), and Respiration. (The first letter in each word combines to make the acronym APGAR.) Ratings are taken at one minute and again at five minutes after birth.

- **aphasia**
  Impaired or absent language function, usually referring to speech; which results from an injury to brain structures usually in the dominant hemisphere (the side of the brain that controls language function is usually the side opposite to the handedness of the person and is referred to as the dominant hemisphere by definition).

- **aphasic**
  Defect or loss of power to produce or understand spoken or written speech.

- **apical ectodermal ridge**
  Area of ectoderm in the developing limb bud which produces growth factors.

- **aplasia**
Complete or partial failure of an organ or tissue to grow.

- **aplastic**
Lack of development of a tissue or an organ.

- **aplastic anemia**
Deficiency of all of the formed elements of the blood (red and white blood cells and platelets) due to a failure of bone marrow production.

- **apnea**
Cessation of breathing.

- **apneic**
Referring to apnea, the absence of spontaneous or automatic breathing.

- **apneic spells**
Periods of cessation of spontaneous breathing, characteristic of prematurity and newborn brain-damage.

- **apolipoproteins**
A number of different proteins which are involved in lipid transportation in the circulation.

- **apoptosis**
Programmed cell death, the body's normal method of disposing of damaged, unwanted, or unneeded cells.

- **appendix**
Vestigial tubular pouch of cecum.

- **apraxia**
Inability to perform purposeful voluntary movements, the nature and mechanism of which are understood in the absence of motor or sensory impairment.

- **aqueous humor**
A fluid that lies between the lens and cornea of the eye.

- **arachnodactyly**
A condition characterized by abnormally long and slender fingers and toes.(The name comes from Arachnids, or spiders, as the fingers or toes are long and "spider-like").

- **arachnoiditis**
Inflammation of the middle (arachnoid mater) of 3 linings of the spinal cord and the subarachnoid space containing the cerebrospinal fluid.

- **archaea**
A family of microorganisms that evolved separately from bacteria, plants, and animals.Some live in extreme environments, such as thermal vents deep in the ocean.

- **arrayed library**
Individual primary recombinant clones (hosted in phage, cosmid, YAC, or other vector) that are placed in two-dimensional arrays in microtiter dishes. Each primary clone can be identified by the identity of the plate and the clone location (row and column) on that plate. Arrayed libraries of clones can be used for many applications, including screening

for a specific gene or genomic region of interest.

- **arrhincephaly**
  Congenital absence or underdevelopment of one or both of the olfactory lobes of the brain and lack of development of the corresponding external olfactory organs.

- **arrhythmia**
  Abnormal rate or rhythm of the heartbeat.

- **arteriole**
  A tiny branch of an artery.

- **arteriosclerosis**
  A group of diseases in which the walls of the arteries get thick and hard. In one type of arteriosclerosis, fat builds up inside the walls and slows the blood flow. These diseases often occur in people who have had diabetes for a long time.

- **artery**
  A large blood vessel that carries blood high in oxygen content away from the heart to other parts of the body. Arteries are thicker and have walls that are stronger and more elastic than the walls of veins.

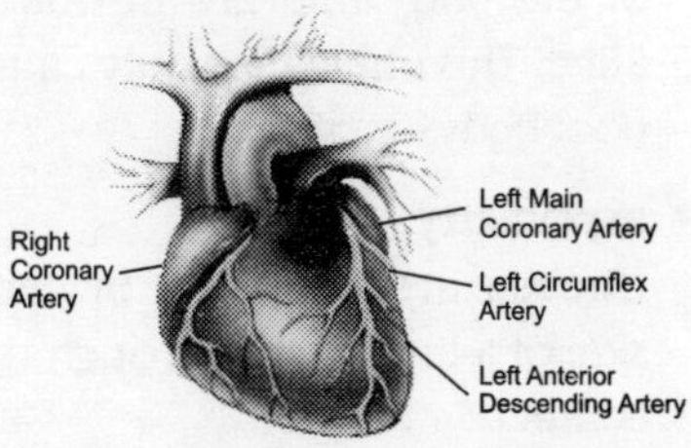


- **arthropathy**
  Any disease or condition affecting a joint.

- **artificial insemination**
  Placement of sperm into the female reproductive tract. The mixing of male and female gametes by artificial means.

- **artificial insemination by donor (aid)**
  Use of semen from a male donor as a reproductive option for couples at high risk of transmitting a genetic disorder.

- **ascending aorta**
  The first part of the major trunk carrying oxygen-risk blood from the heart to the rest of the body.

- **ascending colon**
  The first part of the large intestine.

- **ascertainment**
  The selection of individuals for inclusion in a genetic study (severity, age of onset, certain features of the trait).

- **ascites**
  An accumulation of body fluid with large amounts of protein or electrolytes.

- **ascospore**
  A sexual spore from certain fungus species in which spores are found in a sac called an ascus. Haploid spores found in the asci of Ascomycete fungi.

- **ascus**
  In fungi, a sac that encloses a tetrad or an octad of ascospores. The sac in Ascomycete fungi that holds the ascospores.

- **asd**
  Congenital heart defect (hole in the wall between atria of heart).

- **ashkenazi jewish**
  The Eastern European Jewish population primarily from Germany, Poland, and Russia, as opposed to the Sephardic Jewish population primarily from Spain, parts of France, Italy, and North Africa

- **asphyxia**
  Severe oxygen deficiency leading to loss of consciousness or death.

- **aspiration**
  Removal of fluids by suction from cavities such as the nose, throat or lungs; also, the inhalation into the lungs of fluids, such as water in drowning or stomach contents in vomiting.

- **aspiration pneumonia**
  Inflammation of the lungs caused from inhalation of a foreign material.

- **assembly**
  Putting sequenced fragments of DNA into their correct chromosomal positions.

- **assignment test**
  A test that determines whether a locus is on a specific human chromosome by observation of the concordance of the locus and the specific chromosome in a panel of human-mouse hybrid cell lines containing only one or a few of the normal set (22 autosomes, X and Y) of human chromosomes.

- **association**
  In a specific population, the occurrence together of 2 or more different phenotypes more often than expected by chance.

- **assortative mating**
  The mating of individuals with similar phenotypes.

- **asthma**
  A condition in which difficult breathing is usually accompanied by wheezing.

- **astigmatism**
  A refractive problem that occurs when the surface of the cornea is uneven or structurally defective, preventing the light rays from converging at a point.

- **asymmetrical**
  Lack of symmetry, i.e., lack of similarity between corresponding parts or organs on opposite sides of the body that are normally alike. This imbalance may cause poor body functioning.

- **asymmetry**
  Unequal in size or shape on each side of a line drawn through the center of an object.

- **asymptomatic**
  The patient is not experiencing discomfort or other symptoms; no clear sign of disease present.

- **ataxia**
  A condition wherein the individual experiences extreme difficulties in controlling fine and gross motor movements and balance Resulting from damage to the cerebellum.

- **ataxia-telangiectasia**
  A disease (loss of muscle control, and reddening of the skin) in human beings caused by a defect in DNA repair mechanisms induced by ionising radiation (X-rays, beta and alpha particles, gamma rays).

- **atelectasis**
  An abnormal condition where the lung or part of the lung collapses.

- **atherosclerosis**
  One of many diseases in which fat builds up in the large- and medium-sized arteries. This buildup of fat may slow down or stop blood flow. This disease can happen to people who have had diabetes for a long time.

- **athetoid, athetosis**
  Uncontrolable weaving or purposeless motions of the body or arms or legs as in Cerebral Palsy.

- **athetosis**
  1. A condition characterized by constant, contorted twisting motions in the wrists and fingers.
  2. Slow, smooth movements; mostly involving muscles of the arms and legs.

- **atonia**
  A condition evidenced by lack of muscle tone.

- **atp**
  Adenosine triphosphate; cellular energy is stored in the third phosphate bond. ATP is formed from ADP and phosphate in the process known as oxidative phosphorylation.

- **atresia**
  A birth defect in which a normal body opening, passage, or canal is absent, usually requiring surgical repair soon after birth.

- **atrial**
  Referring to the two thin walled cavities of the heart.

- **atrioventricular**
  Between the atria and ventricles.

- **atrioventricular block**
  Block of the electrical signal between the atria and ventricles; can vary in severity from first, second or third degree (complete heart block).

- **atrioventricular node**
  Also called AV node: cluster of cells between the atria and ventricles that slows the electrical current of the heart as it passes through to the ventricles.

- **atrium**
One of two small upper receiving chambers of the heart; plural form is "atria."

- **atrophy**
Shrinkage or near disappearance of tissue or an organ.

- **attached x**
A pair of Drosophila X chromosomes joined at one end and inherited as a single unit.

- **attenuator**
A control region at the promoter end of repressible amino acid operons that exerts transcriptional control based on the translation of a small leader peptide gene. A region adjacent to the structural genes of the trp (tryptophan) operon; in the presence of tryptophan this region acts to reduce the rate of transcription from the structural genes.

- **attenuator stem**
A configuration of the leader transcript that signals transcription termination in attenuator-controlled amino acid operons.

- **atypical hyperplasia**
Cells that are both abnormal (atypical) and increased in number. Benign microscopic breast changes known as atypical hyperplasia moderately increase a woman's risk of developing breast cancer.

- **audiology**
The study of hearing. Often refers to a hearing test (audiogram), which determines hearing loss.

- **audiometric**
An audiometric examination is an examination in which the hearing is measured and evaluated.

- **aura**
Sensation felt before the onset of a convulsion or migraine headache.

- **auricles**
Outside part of the ears.

- **autogamy**
nuclear reorganization in a single Paramecium cell similar to the changes that occur during conjugation.

- **autoimmune disease**
1. Disorder of the body's immune system in which the immune system mistakenly attacks and destroys body tissue that it believes to be foreign. Insulin-dependent diabetes is an autoimmune disease because the immune system attacks and destroys the insulin-producing beta cells. 2. Illnesses which occur when the body tissues are attacked by its own immune system. The immune system is a complex organization within the body that is designed normally to "seek and destroy" invaders of the body, particularly infections.

Patients with these diseases have unusual antibodies in their blood that target their own body tissues.

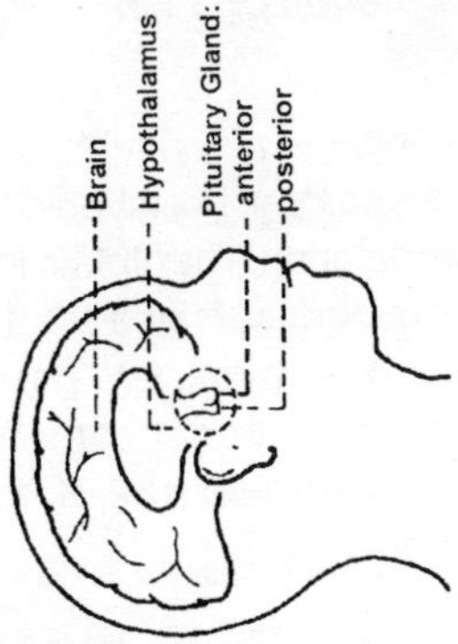


- **autonomic neuropathy**
A disease of the nerves affecting mostly the internal organs such as the bladder muscles, the cardiovascular system, the digestive tract, and the genital organs. These nerves are not under a person's conscious control and function automatically. Also called visceral neuropathy.

- **autonomous replication sequence (ars)**
A segment of a DNA molecule necessary for the initiation of its replication; generally a site recognized and bound by the proteins of the replication system.

- **autophagy**
Digestion of the cell's own organelles.

- **autopolyploid**
A polyploid formed from the doubling of a single genome. Polyploidy in which all the chromosomes come from the same species.

- **autopsy**
Examination of tissues and organs of the body after death.

- **autoradiograph**
A photographic picture showing the position of radioactive substances in tissues; A technique that uses X-ray film to visualize radioactively labeled molecules or fragments of molecules; used in analyzing length and number of DNA fragments after they are separated by gel electrophoresis.

- **autoregulation**
The control of the transcription of a gene by its own gene product.

- **autosomal**
Refers to any of the chromosomes other than the sex-determining chromosomes (i.e., the X and Y) or the genes on these chromosomes; Everyone gets 1 chromosome from their mother and one from their father. The mother's chromosome is always an "X", and the father gives either an "X" (which causes a female child) or a "Y" (which causes a male child). If a disorder is autosomal it is found on both the x and y chromosomes.

- **autosomal disease**
A disease encoded by a gene on one of the 22 pairs of autosomes.

- **autosomal dominant**

A trait that is expressed in an individual who is heterozygous for a particular gene when the mutant allele is on one of the autosomes. Autosomal dominant inheritance An allele which produces an effect regardless of the allele on the homologous chromosome; family histories of patients often show that the condition is present in successive generation (vertical pedigree); parent to child transmission; roughly equally expressed in males and females in the family; severity of the condition/symptoms may vary considerably, even among family members. Male to male transmission is present only in autosomal dominant inheritance.

- **autosomal inheritance**

The pattern of inheritance shown by a disorder or trait determined by a gene on one of the non-sex chromosomes.

- **autosomal modifier**

gene A gene that modifies the action of the autosomes.

- **autosomal recessive**

Describes a trait or disorder requiring the presence of two copies of a gene mutation at a particular locus in order to express observable phenotype; specifically refers to genes on one of the 22 pairs of autosomes (non-sex chromosomes).

- **autosomal set**

The non-sex chromosomes consisting of one from each homologous pair in a diploid species.

- **autosome**

A chromosome not involved in sex determination. The diploid human genome consists of a total of 46 chromosomes: 22 pairs of autosomes, and 1 pair of sex chromosomes (the X and Y chromosomes).

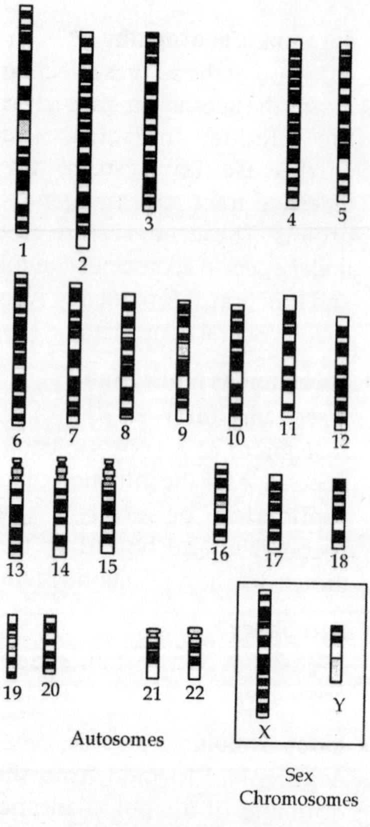

- **autotroph**
  Organism that is able to utilize carbon dioxide as a carbon source.
- **autozygosity**
  Homozygosity in which the two alleles are identical by descent (ie they are copies of an ancestral gene) .
- **auxotroph**
  An organism with specific nutritional requirements.
- **auxotrophic mutant**
  A mutant strain of microorganism that will proliferate only when the medium is supplemented with some specific substance not required by wild-type organisms.
- **avuncular relationship**
  The genetic relationship between nieces and nephews and their aunts and uncles.
- **axoneme**
  A bundle of microtubules and other proteins forming the core of each cilium or flagellum.
- **azoospermia**
  Absence of sperm in semen.
- **b cell**
  A type of lymphocyte that works as part of the immune system by producing antibodies to fight infection.
- **b form dna**
  A right-handed double-helical conformation of DNA normally seen in solution described by Watson and Crick. A second DNA conformation (A form) is seen in unhydrated DNA (fibres or crystals of oligonucleotides).
- **b lymphocytes**
  Antibody-producing lymphocytes involved in humoral immunity.
- **bacillus**
  A rod-shaped bacterium.
- **back mutation**
  The process that causes reversion. A change in a nucleotide pair in a mutant gene that restores the original sequence and hence the original phenotype.
- **backcross**
  A cross between an animal that is heterozygous for alleles obtained from two parental strains and a second animal from one of those parental strains. Also used to describe the breeding protocol of an outcross followed by a backcross.
- **background risk (synonym: population risk)**
  The proportion of individuals in a given population who are affected with a particular disorder or who have mutations in a certain gene; often discussed in the genetic counseling process as a comparison to the patient's personal risk given his/her family history or other circumstances.
- **bacteria**
  Microorganisms that consist of a single cell.Bacteria, like all living things, have their own

genomes. They also have the ability to exchange genes with other bacteria. This "swapping" of DNA may help explain how genes that confer resistance to anti-bacterial drugs have spread among many species.

- **bacterial artificial chromosome (bac)**
  A vector used to clone DNA fragments (100- to 300-kb insert size; average, 150 kb) in Escherichia coli cells. Based on naturally occurring F-factor plasmid found in the bacterium E. coli.

- **bacterial lawn**
  A continuous cover of bacteria on the surface of a growth medium.

- **bacteriophage**
  A virus whose host is a bacterium; commonly called phage.

- **bag of waters**
  A lay person's term for the amniotic sac and amniotic fluid.

- **balanced lethal system**
  An arrangement of recessive lethal alleles that maintains a heterozygous chromosome combination. Homozygotes for any lethal-bearing chromosome perish.

- **balanced polymorphism**
  Two different genetic variants which are stably present in a population, i.e. selective advantages and disadvantages cancel each other out.

- **balanced translocation**
  A rearrangement translocation with no apparent loss or gain of chromosomal material, resulting in a clinically normal but genetically "abnormal" person.

- **balbiani ring**
  A large chromosome puff. The larger polytene chromosomal puffs. See chromosome puff.

- **ballismus**
  Wide flinging or jerking movements of the extremities.

- **band**
  When chromosomes at a particular stage in cell division are stained using one of several types of preparations, a specific pattern of light and dark stripes (bands) appear which can aid in identifying the chromosome and evaluating its structure

- **band level**
  The total number of bands estimated to be present in a haplotype set (23) of chromosomes. When cell division is arrested and staining is performed at an earlier stage of mitosis (prometaphase), chromosomes appear longer, with approximately 700-1200 bands. At a later stage of mitosis (metaphase), chromosomes are more condensed, with approximately 300-600 bands. At higher band levels, the greater resolution increases the ability to

identify more subtle chromosomal abnormalities and their breakpoints.

- **banding**
The differential staining of a chromosome by a variety of techniques that results in a specific pattern of positively and negatively stained bands for each chromosomal pair.

- **banti's syndrome**
An obsolete term used to describe patients with Splenomegaly, hypersplenism and portal hypertension without cirrhosis and without occlusion of the portal venous system.

- **bard button**
A small plastic device with a hole into which a feeding or venting tube is placed.

- **bare lymphocytre syndrome**
A rare autosomal recessive form of severe combined immunodeficiency due to absence of the class II molecules of the major histocompatibility complex.

- **barr body**
The condensed single X-chromosome seen in the nuclei of somatic cells of female mammals; A densely staining mass that represents an inactivated X chromosome. Heterochromatic body found in the nuclei of normal females but absent in the nuclei of normal males.

- **barrett's esophagus**
A change in the cells of the tissue that lines the bottom of the esophagus. The esophagus may become irritated when the contents of the stomach back up (reflux). Reflux that happens often over a period of time can lead to Barrett's esophagus.

- **barth syndrome**
Cardiomyopathy-Neutropenia Syndrome. Marked by elevated levels of 3-methylglutaconic acid in the blood and urine.

- **bart's test**
Prenatal blood test for Down Syndrome.

- **basal body**
A short cylindrical array of microtubules and other proteins, found at the base of a eukaryotic cilium or flagellum, that organises the assembly of the axoneme (the bundle of microtubules and other proteins forming the core of each cilium or flagellum).

- **basal cells**
Small, round cells found in the lower part, or base, of the epidermis.

- **basal ganglia**
A group of structures at the base of the cerebral hemispheres, concerned with involuntary control of movement, among other functions.

- **base**
One of the molecules that form DNA and RNA molecules.

- **base analogue**
A chemical whose molecular structure mimics that of a DNA base; because of the mimicry, the analogue may act as a mutagen.

- **base pair**
The basic units of DNA and RNA, base pairs are chemical structures made up of the chemicals adenine, thymine, guanine and cytosine, which are designated by the letters A, T, G and C, respectively. Adenine always pairs with thymine and guanine always pairs with cytosine, creating the pairs or nucleotides in which genetic information is found. A pair of bases, or molecules (either adenine and thymine or cytosine and guanine), which forms one rung in the DNA ladder. Bases are the letters that spell out genetic code.

- **base sequence**
The order of nucleotide bases in a DNA molecule; determines structure of proteins encoded by that DNA.

- **base sequence analysis**
A method, sometimes automated, for determining the base sequence.

- **batesian mimicry**
Form of mimicry in which an innocuous mimic species gains protection by resembling noxious or dangerous model species.

- **bayes' theorem**
Combining the prior and conditional probabilities of certain events or the results of specific tests to give a joint probability to derive the posterior or relative probability.

- **bayesian analysis**
Mathematical method for calculating probability of the carrier state in mendelian disorders by combining several independent likelihoods.

- **bead theory**
The disproved hypothesis that genes are arranged on the chromosome like beads on a necklace, indivisible into smaller units of mutation and recombination.

- **becker muscular dystrophy**
X-linked condition characterized by progressive muscle weakness and wasting; manifests later in life with progression less severe than Duchenne muscular dystrophy.

- **behavioral genetics**
The study of genes that may influence behavior.

- **bence jones protein**
The antibody of a single species produced in large amounts by a person with multiple myeloma, a tumour of antibody producing plasma cells.

- **benign (bee-nine)**
Not cancerous. Not growing or spreading.

- **benign tumor**
  An abnormal growth that is not cancer and does not spread to other parts of the body.

- **benign variant (synonym: polymorphism)**
  An alteration in a gene distinct from the normal, wild-type allele that does not appear to have a deleterious effect

- **beta (β) thalassaemia**
  Inherited disorder of haemoglobin involving under-production of the β-globin chain occurring most commonly in persons from the Mediterranean region and Indian subcontinent.

- **beta-galactosidase**
  The enzyme that splits lactose into glucose and galactose (coded by a gene (lac z) in the lac operon of Escherichia coli).

- **beta-galactoside acetyltransferase**
  An enzyme that is involved in lactose metabolism and encoded by a gene (lac a) in the lac operon of Escherichia coli.

- **beta-galactoside permease**
  An enzyme involved in concentrating lactose in the cell (coded by a gene (lac y) in the lac operon of Escherichia coli)).

- **beta-oxidation**
  A series of metabolic reactions necessary for burning fatty acids(fats).

- **bias of ascertainment**
  An artefact, which must be taken into account in family studies when looking at segregation ratios, caused by families coming to attention because they have affected individual(s).

- **bicuspid tooth**
  One of four teeth in the adult mouth having two points; located between the canine and molar.

- **bicuspid valve**
  A heart valve having two cusps.

- **bifid uvula**
  The small, cone shaped tissue in the middle of the soft palate is split into two parts.

- **bilateral**
  Appearing on both sides of the body.

- **bile**
  A yellow-green fluid made by the liver. Bile is stored in the gallbladder. It passes through the common bile duct into the duodenum, where it helps digest fat.

- **biliary tract**
  Left, right and common hepatic, cystic, and common bile ducts.

- **bilirubin**
  Orange or yellowish pigment that is the result of breakdown of red blood cells. Excess of bilirubin in the blood produces jaundice.

- **bimodal distribution**
  A statistical distribution having two modes.

- **binary fission**
The process in which a parent cell splits into two daughter cells of approximately equal size. Simple cell division in single-celled organisms.

- **binaural**
Using, pertaining to or involving the function of both ears.

- **binomial expansion**
The terms generated when a binomial expression [eg. (p+q)] is raised to a particular power n [eg. (p+q) ^ n].

- **binomial theorem**
The theorem that gives the terms of the expansion of a binomial expression [eg. (p+q)] raised to a particular power n [eg. (p+q) ^ n].

- **binovular**
Originating from two separate eggs.

- **biochemical disorder**
An inherited disorder involving a metabolic pathway, i.e. an inborn error of metabolism.

- **biochemical genetics**
The study of the relationships between genes and enzymes, specifically the role of genes in controlling the steps in biochemical pathways.

- **bioinformatics**
The science of managing and analyzing biological data using advanced computing techniques. Especially important in analyzing genomic research data; An emerging field of research that applies the tools of advanced computer analysis and molecular biology to organize and understand the vast quantities of data created by genomics research; The discipline of using computers to address information problems in the life sciences; it involves the creation of electronic data bases on genomes, protein sequences, etc.

- **biolistic**
A method (biological ballistics) of transfecting cells by bombarding them with microprojectiles coated with DNA.

- **biological atlas**
Maps describing different aspects of protein function should be compiled into a "biological atlas" By integrating the information contained in the atlas, increasingly meaningful biological hypotheses could be formulated.

- **biological or genetic determinisim**
The premise that our genetic make-up is the only factor determining all aspects of our health and disease.

- **biological species concept**
Organisms are classified in the same species if they are potentially capable of interbreeding and producing fertile offspring.

- **biopsy**
  Removal of a portion (sample) of tissue for pathological examination or diagnostic study.

- **bioremediation**
  The science of using living things, such as plants and micro-organisms, to remove toxins from the environment and restore it to a healthful condition.

- **biosynthesis**
  Use of recombinant DNA techniques to produce molecules of biological and medical importance in the laboratory or commercially.

- **biotechnology**
  A set of biological techniques developed through basic research and now applied to research and product development. In particular, biotechnology refers to the use by industry of recombinant DNA, cell fusion, and new bioprocessing techniques.

- **biparental zygote**
  A Chlamydomonas zygote that contains chloroplast DNA (cpDNA) from both parents, such cells generally are rare since normally cpDNA is inherited uniparentally from the mt+ mating type parent. These rare biparental zygotes allowed mapping of chloroplast genes by recombination.

- **bipolar illness**
  Affective manic-depressive illness.

- **birth defect**
  A physically or mentally disabling condition present in an individual at birth. There are more than 4,000 known birth defects, some of which are fatal. A birth defect may be caused by a faulty gene or by environmental factors during pregnancy, such as radiation exposure.

- **bivalent**
  Structure, formed during prophase of meiosis 1, consisting of synapsed homologous chromosomes.

- **bladder**
  Membranous sac that holds secretions, such as the urinary bladder that collects urine before its elimination.

- **blast**
  BLAST (Basic Local Alignment Search Tool) is a set of tools for comparing sequence information in proteins or DNA by using all available public sequence databases. It is designed to find matches in sequence information by looking for close matches of a small portion of DNA or protein within a larger whole sequence.

- **blastocyst**
  Early embryo consisting of embryoblast and trophoblast; Early stage of an embryo produced by cleavage of an ovum; a liquid-filled sphere whose wall is composed of a single layer of cells; during this stage (about

eight days after fertilization) implantation in the wall of the uterus occurs

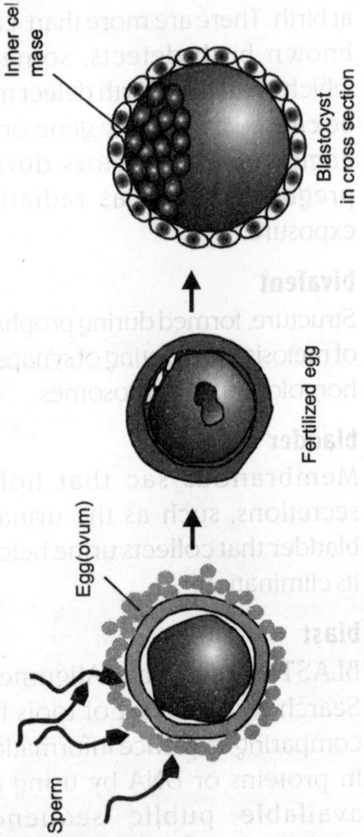


- **blastoderm**
In an insect embryo, the layer of cells that completely surrounds an internal mass of yolk.

- **blastomere**
One of the cells formed by division of the fertilized egg making up the blastula.

- **blastopore**
The embryonic structure present during gastrulation and formed by invagination of the endoderm.

- **blastula**
An early developmental stage of vertebrate embryos formed by cleavage of the fertilized egg, in which the embryo consists of a single layer of cells surrounding a cavity (the blastocoel).

- **blending inheritance**
A discredited model of inheritance suggesting that the characteristics of an individual result from the smooth blending of fluid like influences from its parents.

- **blepharitis**
Inflammation of eyelid.

- **blood chimera**
A mixture of cells of different genetic origin present in twins as a result of an exchange of cells via the placenta between non-identical twins in utero.

- **blood pressure**
The force of the blood on the walls of arteries. Two levels of blood pressure are measured-the higher, or systolic, pressure, which occurs each time the heart pushes blood into the vessels, and the lower, or diastolic, pressure, which occurs when the heart rests. In a blood pressure reading of 120/80, for example, 120 is the systolic pressure and 80 is the diastolic pressure. A reading of 120/80 is said to be the normal range. Blood pressure that is too high can cause health problems such as heart attacks and strokes.

- **blood urea nitrogen (bun)**
  A waste product of the kidneys. Increased levels of BUN in the blood may indicate early kidney damage.
- **blood vessels**
  Tubes that act like a system of roads or canals to carry blood to and from all parts of the body. The three main types of blood vessels are arteries, veins, and capillaries. The heart pumps blood through these vessels so that the blood can carry with it oxygen and nutrients that the cells need or take away waste that the cells do not need.
- **blunt-end ligation**
  The ligating or attaching of blunt-ended pieces of DNA by T4 DNA ligase. Used in creating hybrid vectors.
- **bolus**
  A small rounded mass of food made ready by the tongue and jaw movement for swallowing.
- **bone**
  Bone is the substance that forms the skeleton of the body. It is composed chiefly of calcium phosphate and calcium carbonate. It also serves as a storage area for calcium, playing a large role in calcium balance in the blood.
- **bone density**
  Bone density is the amount of bone tissue in a certain volume of bone. It can be measured using a special x-ray called a quantitative computed tomogram.
- **bone marrow**
  The soft material found in the hollow centre of long bones.

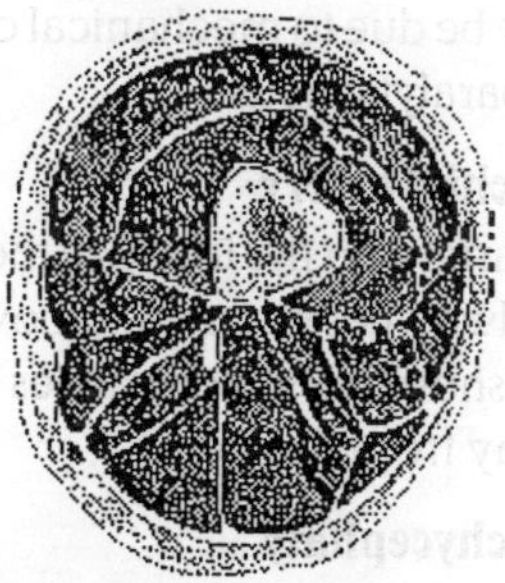

- **bone scan**
  A technique to create images on bones on a computer screen or on film. A small amount of radioactive material is injected and travels through the bloodstream. It collects in the bones, especially in abnormal areas of the bones, and is detected by a scanner.
- **bossing**
  A swelling or protuberance.
- **bottleneck**
  A brief reduction in size of a population which usually leads to random genetic drift.
- **boundary elements**
  Short sequences of DNA, usually 500 bp to 3 kb in size, which block or inhibit the influence of regulatory elements of adjacent genes.

- **bowel**
  Small or large intestine. The small intestine is sometimes called the small bowel. The large intestine is also called the colon.

- **bowel or intestinal obstruction**
  May be due to mechanical causes or paralytic ileus.

- **brachial artery**
  An artery on the inside of the arm, midway between the elbow and the shoulder, which carries blood away from the heart.

- **brachycephaly**
  Shortish head, due to a short anteroposterior (front to back) diameter.

- **brachydactyly**
  A condition in which the fingers or toes are abnormally short, all digits or only one or two.

- **bradycardia**
  A slow heart rate, usually defined as less than 60 beats per minute.

- **brain**
  The brain is that portion of the central nervous system that is located within the skull. It functions as a primary receiver, organizer and distributor of information for the body. It has two (right and left) halves called "hemispheres."

- **brain stem**
  Portion of the brain that connects the hemispheres with the spinal cord. Consists of medulla oblongata, pons and midbrain.

- **branch migration**
  1. The process in which a crossover point between two DNA duplexes slides along the duplexes.
  2. The process by which a single invading DNA strand extends its partial pairing with its complementary strand as it displaces the resident strand from a DNA duplex.

- **brca1**
  A gene that normally helps to restrain cell growth.

- **brca1 breast cancer susceptibility gene**
  A mutated version of BRCA1, which predisposes a person toward developing breast cancer.

- **brca1/brca2**
  Two mutant genes that are responsible for approximately 50 percent of all inherited forms of breast cancer. Normally these genes are tumor suppressors, which limit the growth of tumors. When mutated, these genes fail to do their job correctly, allowing cancers to grow.

- **breakage and reunion**
  The general mode by which recombination occurs. DNA duplexes are broken and reunited in a crosswise fashion according to the Holliday model.

- **breakage-fusion-bridge cycle**
  Damage that happens to a dicentric chromosome during each cell cycle.

- **break-point cluster (bcr)**
  Region of chromosome 22 involved in the translocation seen in the majority of persons with chronic myeloid leukaemia.

- **bridging cross**
  A cross made to transfer alleles between two sexually isolated species by first transferring the alleles to an intermediate species that is sexually compatible with both.

- **broad heritability**
  The proportion of total phenotypic variance at the population level that is contributed by genetic variance.

- **broad ligament**
  The broad ligament is a folded sheet of tissue that drapes over the uterus, fallopian tubes and the ovaries.

- **bronchial tubes**
  1. The main breathing tubes leading from the trachea into the lungs. 2. The large air tubes leading to the lungs. One tube is called a bronchus, both tubes are called bronchi.

- **bronchioles**
  The tiny branches of air tubes in the lungs.

- **bronchoscopy**
  procedure using a lighted scope to examine the airways.

- **bronze diabetes**
  A genetic disease of the liver in which the body takes in too much iron from food. Also called "hemocromatosis.

- **bruise**
  A bruise or "contusion" is an traumatic injury of the soft tissues which results in breakage of the local capillaries and leakage of red blood cells. In the skin it can be seen as a reddish-purple discoloration which does not blanch when pressed upon. When it fades it becomes green and brown as the body metabolizes the blood cells in the skin. It is best treated with local application of a cold pack immediately after injury.

- **brushfield spots**
  A speckled ring about 2/3 of the distance from the pupil to the periphery of the iris with a relative lack of patterning beyond the ring. Found in about 80% of babies with Down syndrome.

- **bruxism**
  Repetitive grinding of the teeth.

- **buccal mucosa**
  The inner lining of the cheeks and lips.

- **bud**
  A daughter cell formed by mitosis in yeast; one daughter cell retains

the cell wall of the parent, and the other (the bud) forms a new cell wall.

- **bulbar**
  Relating to the medulla oblongata which is part of the brain stem.
- **bulbous**
  Spherical or round like a bulb.
- **bullous**
  Characterized by blistering, such as in second-degree burn.
- **bundle-branch block**
  Condition in which portions of the heart's conduction system become defective and unable to conduct the electrical signal normally (can be right or left bundle-branch block).
- **buoyant density**
  A measure of the tendency of a substance to float in some other substance; large molecules are distinguished by their differing buoyant densities in some standard fluid. Measured by density-gradient ultra-centrifugation.
- **buoyant density of dna**
  A measure of the density of DNA determined by the equilibrium point reached by DNA after density gradient centrifugation.
- **bupthalmos**
  Enlargement of the eye ball due to increased pressure and failure of the drainage system.
- **burkitt lymphoma**
  A cancer of the lymphatic system manifested by tumours in the jaw, often associated with a translocation bringing a specific oncogene next to a novel regulatory element.
- **c.a.t. scan**
  Computer Axial Tomographic scan. Radiographic scan of structures within the body: used for diagnostic purposes.
- **c.s.f.**
  The fluid which accumulates round the linings of the brain and the spinal cord
- **ca repeat**
  A short dinucleotide sequence present as tandem repeats at multiple sites in the human genome producing microsatellite polymorphisms.
- **caat box**
  A conserved, non-coding, so-called 'promoter' sequence about 80 bp upstream from the start of transcription.
- **cachexia**
  Malnutrition and wasting due to illness.
- **cag/ctg**
  Abbreviation for cytosine-adenine-guanine triplet nucleotide and cytosine-thymine-guanine triplet nucleotide repeats; they are associated with unstable mutations.

- **calcification**
  Abnormal deposits of calcium and magnesium salts in tissue.

- **calcium**
  A mineral important for strong teeth and bones and for muscle and nerve function. Dairy products are a good source of calcium. Calcium is added to bone by cells called osteoblasts. It is removed from bone by cells called osteoclasts.

- **calculus**
  Accumulation of mineral salts in various parts of the body, such as a kidney stone or on teeth.

- **callus**
  A small area of skin, usually on the foot, that has become thick and hard from rubbing or pressure. Calluses may lead to other problems such as serious infection. Shoes that fit well can keep calluses from forming.

- **calvaric, calvaria**
  Top of the skull or the skull cap.

- **camp (cyclic adenosine monophosphate)**
  A molecule that plays a key role in the regulation of various processes within the cell.

- **campodactyly**
  A permanent and irreducible flexion or flexation (bending) of one or more fingers.

- **canalized character**
  A character whose phenotype is kept within narrow boundaries even in the presence of disturbing environments or mutations.

- **cancer**
  Diseases in which abnormal cells divide and grow unchecked. Cancer can spread from its original site to other parts of the body and can be fatal.

- **cancer family syndrome.**
  A term used to describe the clustering in certain families of particular types of cancers, in which it has been proposed that the different types of malignancy could be due to a single dominant gene, specifically Lynch type II.

- **cancer genetics**
  The study of the genetic causes of cancer.

- **cancer-family syndrome**
  Pedigree in which unusually large numbers of blood relatives develop certain kinds of cancers.

- **candidate gene**
  A gene known to be located in the region of interest whose product has biochemical or other properties suggesting that it may prove to be the disease gene being sought.

- **candidate gene approach**
  Strategy to identify disease-associated genes based on finding candidate genes in a chromosome region in which a disorder is mapped.

- **canine**
One of four teeth found between the molars and incisors; also known as eye teeth.

- **canthi, canthus**
The inside corner of the eye; the angle at either end of the eye.

- **canthic, canthral**
Referring to the inside corner of the eye.

- **cap**
A protein, which binds cyclic AMP, whose presence is necessary for the activation of operons whose activity is repressed by the presence of glucose (catabolite repression) eg. lac (lactose), ara (arabinose), gal (galactose) etc. cAMP-CAP complex binds to a site, the CAP binding site, which is centred at -61 to -62 from the transcription start site in the lac operon promoter.

- **cap site**
The site of initiation of transcription.

- **capillaries**
The smallest of the blood vessels in the body, carrying nourishment to the cells. Capillaries have walls so thin that oxygen and glucose can pass through them and enter the cells, and waste products such as carbon dioxide can pass back into the blood to be carried away and taken out of the body. Sometimes people who have had diabetes for a long time find that their capillaries become weak, especially those in the kidney and the retina of the eye.

- **capillary**
Hair-like blood vessel.

- **capillary array**
Gel-filled silica capillaries used to separate fragments for DNA sequencing. The small diameter of the capillaries permit the application of higher electric fields, providing high speed, high throughput separations that are significantly faster than traditional slab gels.

- **capitate**
One of the largest of the carpal bones in the wrist.

- **capsid**
The protein shell of a virus.

- **capsomere**
Protein clusters making up discrete subunits of a viral protein shell.

- **carbohydrate**
One of the three main classes of foods and a source of energy. Carbohydrates are mainly sugars and starches that the body breaks down into glucose (a simple sugar that the body can use to feed its cells). The body also uses carbohydrates to make a substance called glycogen that is stored in the liver and muscles for future use. If the body does not have enough insulin or cannot use

the insulin it has, then the body will not be able to use carbohydrates for energy the way it should. This condition is called diabetes.

- **carbon source**
  A nutrient (such as sugar) that provides carbon skeletons needed for synthesis of new organic molecules (anabolism).
- **carcinogen**
  Something which causes cancer to occur by causing changes in a cell's DNA.
- **carcinoma**
  Tumour arising from epithelial tissue (eg glands; breast; skin; linings of the urogenital, intestinal and respiratory systems).
- **cardiac**
  Pertaining to the heart.
- **cardiac arrest**
  Sudden stopping of circulation by cessation of the heartbeat.
- **cardiac arrhythmias**
  Abnormal heart rate or rhythm.
- **cardiologist**
  A doctor who sees and takes care of people with heart disease; a heart specialist.
- **cardiomyopathy**
  Any disease that affects the structure or function of the heart.
- **cardiorespiratory**
  Pertaining to the heart and lungs.
- **cardiovascular**
  Relating to the heart and blood vessels (arteries, veins, and capillaries); the circulatory system.
- **cardiovascular system**
  The circulatory system, including the heart, arteries, veins and lymphatics.
- **carotid**
  Referring to the arteries supplying the neck and head.
- **carotid artery**
  Main (right and left) artery of the neck which carries blood to the head and brain.
- **carrier**
  An individual who has a recessive, disease-causing gene mutation at a particular locus on one chromosome of a pair and a normal allele at that locus on the other chromosome; may also refer to an individual with a balanced chromosome rearrangement.
- **carrier rate (synonym carrier freqency)**
  The proportion of individuals in a population who have a single copy of a specific recessive gene mutation
- **carrier testing (synonyms: carrier detection, heterozygote testing)**
  Testing used to identify usually asymptomatic individuals who have a gene mutation for an

autosomal recessive or X-linked recessive disorder

- **cartilage**

Firm, dense, pliable connective tissue (gristle), devoid of blood vessels and not impregnated with calcium (bone), that cushions bones at joints. A more flexible kind of cartilage connects muscles with bones and makes up other parts of the body, such as the larynx and the outside parts of the ears.

- **cascade screening**

Identification within a family of carriers for an autosomal recessive disorder or persons with an autosomal dominant gene following ascertainment of an index case.

- **cassette mechanism**

The mechanism by which homothallic yeast cells alternate mating types, involves two silent transposons (cassettes) and a region where these cassettes can be expressed (cassette player).

- **cassette model**

A model to explain mating-type switching in yeast. Information for both a and alpha mating types is assumed to be present as silent cassettes ; a copy of either type of cassette may be transposed to the mating-type locus, where it is played (transcribed).

- **cat assay**

Reporter gene assay used to measure activity of a promoter under different conditions, such as to define elements of a promoter or to study signals that activate an intact enhancer/promoter. CAT is the abbreviation for the enzyme, chloramphenicol acetyl transferase, the activity of which is measured in the assay.

- **cat scan**

Computerized axial tomography scan. An imaging technique that uses a computer to organize the information from multiple x-ray views and construct a cross-sectional image of areas inside the body. Also called CT scan.

- **catabolite activator protein**

A protein that when bound with cyclic AMP can attach to sites on sugar-metabolizing operons to enhance transcription of these operons.

- **catabolite repression**

Repression (inactivation) of certain sugar-metabolizing operons (eg lac) in favour of glucose utilization when glucose is the predominant carbon source in the environment of the cell.

- **catalase**

An enzyme that catalyses (causes) the decomposition of hydrogen peroxide into water and oxygen.

- **catalyst**

A substance that increases the rate of a chemical reaction without itself being permanently changed.

- **cataplexy**
  Sudden loss of muscle tone.
- **cataract**
  A clouding or loss of transparency of the eye lens that impairs vision. There are many causes of cataracts including aging, diabetes, cortisone medication, trauma, or other diseases.
- **catecholamines**
  Adrenaline by-products found in the urine, where their measurement is used as a test for pheochromocytoma.
- **cavernous hemangiomas**
  Benign tumors consisiting of large blood-filled spaces.
- **ccaat box**
  An invariant DNA sequence at about minus 70 base pairs from the origin of transcription in many eukaryotic promoters.
- **cdna**
  Complimentary DNA produced from an RNA template by the action of an RNA dependent polymerase. A single stranded cDNA is often used as a probe in physical mapping.
- **cdna library**
  A collection of DNA sequences that code for genes. The sequences are generated in the laboratory from mRNA sequences.
- **cdna maps**
  Shows the locations of expressed DNA regions (exons) on the chromosomal map. Because they represent expressed genomic regions, cDNAs are thought to identify the parts of the genome with the most biological and medical significance. A cDNA map can provide the chromosomal location for genes whose functions are currently unknown. For disease- gene hunters, the map can also suggest a set of candidate genes to test when the approximate location of a disease gene has been mapped by genetic linkage techniques.
- **cebocephaly**
  A facial anomaly characterized by a small, flattened nose with a single nostril situated below incomplete or underdeveloped closely set eyes.
- **cecal volvulus**
  blind or closed bowel causing obstruction.
- **cell**
  A microscopic form of life.Cells are complex entities in and of themselves, capable of carrying out the biochemical processes necessary to stay alive and, when the time comes, to die.
- **cell autonomous**
  A genetic trait in multicellular organisms in which only genotypically mutant cells exhibit the mutant phenotype. Conversely, a nonautonomous trait is one in which genotypically

mutant cells cause other cells (regardless of their genotype) to exhibit a mutant phenotype.

• **cell cycle**
The cycle of cell growth, replication of the genetic material and nuclear and cytoplasmic division.

• **cell division**
The process by which two cells are formed from one.

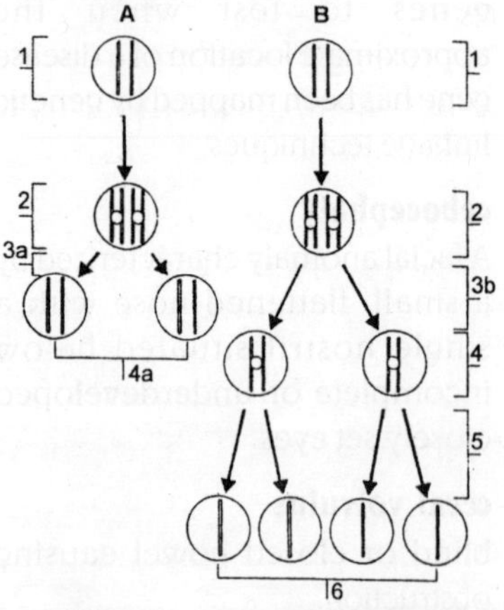


A Mitosis
B Meiosis
1 Diploid parental cell with one pair of homologous chromosomes
2 Chromosomes duplicate to form pairs of chromatids
3 Cell division
3a Mitotic division
3b First meiotic division
4 Daughter cells
4a Diploid, identical to parental cell
4b Haploid, not identical to parental cell
5 Second meiotic division
6 Haploid gametes

• **cell fate**
The ultimate differentiated state to which a cell has become committed.

• **cell line**
A cultured cell type that can be reproduced indefinitely is immortalized.

• **cell lineage**
A pedigree of cells related through asexual division.

• **cell mapping**
The determination of the subcellular location of proteins and of protein- protein interactions by the purification of organelles or protein complexes followed by mass- spectrometric identification of the components. Most proteins are thought to exist in the cell not as free entities but as part of 'cellular machines' which perform cellular functions cooperatively. Systematic identification of protein complexes would permit these machines to be defined and allow 'physical maps' to be created for a variety of cell types and states. Such information is of great value for the assignment of protein function.

• **cell maps**
A cell map specifies the proteins that constitute a given organelle within a given cell type. Cell maps for normal and diseased cells can be constructed which give insight into the role proteins have in disease and can guide the drug development process.

• **cell-free system**
A mixture of cytoplasmic and/or nuclear components from cells and used for in vitro protein synthesis or transcription or DNA replication or other purposes.

- **cell-mediated immunity**

.Immunity which involves the T lymphocytes to fight intracellular infection and is involved in transplantation rejection and delayed hypersensitivity.

- **cellular blastoderm**

The stage of the blastoderm, initially a syncytium, in insects after the nuclei have each been separately packaged into a cell membrane.

- **centimorgan**

The unit of linkage that refers to the distance between two gene loci determined by the frequency with which recombination occurs between them. Two loci are said to be one centimorgan apart if recombination is observed between them in 1% of meioses.

- **central dogma**

The original postulate that genetic information can be transferred only from nucleic acid to nucleic acid and from nucleic acid to protein, that is from DNA to DNA from DNA to RNA and from RNA to protein (although information transfer from RNA to DNA was not excluded and is now known to occur [reverse transcription]). Transfer of genetic information from protein to nucleic acid never occurs.

- **central nervous system**

Consists of the brain and spinal cord.

- **centric fragment**

A piece of chromosome containing a centromere.

- **centric fusion**

The fusion of the centromeres of two acrocentric chromosomes to form a Robertsonian translocation.

- **centriole**

A short cylindrical organelle, found in pairs arranged at right angles to each other at the centre of a microtubule organizing centre (MTOC) or centrosome, found in eukaryotes (except in higher plants). A centriole is similar in structure to the basal body found at the base of eukaryotic cilia and flagella and organises the axoneme, the bundle of microtubules and other proteins forming the core of each cilium or flagellum. The centrosome organizes formation of a spindle during mitosis or meiosis.

- **centromere**

The middle portion of a chromosome where two sister chromatids (chromosome strands) join together.

- **centromere marker**

Locus located close to a centromere.

- **centromeric fission**

Creation of two chromosomes from one by splitting the centromere.

- **centrosome**
  The primary microtubule organising center (MTOC) of animal cells, that divides prior to cell division each daughter MTOC acts as one pole of the spindle apparatus. The centrosome usually contains a pair of centrioles.

- **cephalocaudal**
  From head to tail. Refers to neurological development that proceeds from the head downward.

- **cephalohematoma**
  A bruised area beneath the outer layer of the skull of a newborn.

- **cephalometric analysis**
  Comprehensive dental evaluation to determine dental defects such as high palate, clefts, micrognathia, and ankyloglossia.

- **cerebellar ataxia**
  Lesions of the cerebellum.

- **cerebellum**
  A large portion of the base of the brain which serves to coordinate voluntary movements, posture, and balance, located in the back of the skull behind the brainstem.

- **cerebral**
  Related to the two major hemispherical components of the brain, which serve the "higher" mental functions.

- **cerebral embolism**
  A clot that travels through blood vessels from the site where it formed and blocks blood flow in the brain.

- **cerebral hemispheres**
  The two halves of the cerebrum, the largest part of the brain.

- **cerebral palsy**
  A disorder of movement and posture due to a defect of the immature brain.

- **cerebrospinal fluid**
  The watery fluid that fills the spaces in and around the brain and spinal cord. Also called CSF.

- **cerebrovascular**
  Pertaining to the blood vessels of the brain.

- **cerebrovascular disease**
  Damáge to the blood vessels in the brain, resulting in a stroke. The blood vessels become blocked because of fat deposits or they become thick and hard, blocking the flow of blood to the brain. Sometimes, the blood vessels may burst, resulting in a hemorrhagic stroke. People with diabetes are at higher risk of cerebrovascular disease.

- **cerebrum**
  Largest portion of the brain, consisting of two hemispheres; responsible for thinking, feelings and voluntary movement.

- **cervical**
  Relating to the bones of the neck or the neck of the womb.

- **cg island**
  Unmethylated cytosine-guanine sequences that are often found near the 5' ends of some genes.

- **chain termination mutation**
  A mutation that generates a stop codon, thus preventing further synthesis of the polypeptide chain.

- **character**
  An attribute of individuals within a species for which heritable differences can be defined.

- **character difference**
  Alternative forms of the same attribute within a species.

- **charcot foot**
  A foot complication associated with diabetic neuropathy that results in destruction of joints and soft tissue. Also called "Charcot's joint" and "neuropathic arthropathy.

- **charcot-marie tooth disease**
  A condition characterized by degeneration of the motor and sensory nerves that control movement and feeling in the arm below the elbow and the leg below the knee; transmitted in autosomal dominant, autosomal recessive and X-linked forms.

- **chargaff's rule**
  Chargaff's observation that in the base composition of DNA the quantity of adenine equaled the quantity of thymine and the quantity of guanine equaled the quantity of cytosine.

- **charon phage**
  Phage lambda derivative used as vector in DNA cloning.

- **chemical base**
  An essential building block. DNA contains four complementary bases adenine, which pairs with thymine, and cytosine, which pairs with guanine. In RNA, thymine is replaced by uracil.

- **chemical cleavage mismatch**
  A DNA mutation detection system which involves the addition of the chemicals hydroxylamine and osmium tetroxide which react with free cytosine and thymine nucleotides respectively. By denaturing the double stranded DNA being screened and allowing it to hybridize with a single stranded radiolabelled DNA probe, any mismatched cytosine or thymine nucleotides will be exposed and therefore be susceptible to reaction with the hydroxylamine and osmium tetroxide. The addition of piperidine results in cleavage of the DNA being screened at any such sites allowing identification of mutations.

- **chemotaxis**
  The attraction of phagocytes to the site of infection by components of complement.

- **chi site**
  Sequence of DNA at which the RecBCD protein cleaves one of the strands during recombination.
- **chiasma (plural chiasmata)**
  A cross-shaped structure commonly observed between nonsister chromatids during meiosis; the site of crossing-over. X-shaped configuration seen in tetrads during the latter stages of prophase 1 of meiosis. They represent physical crossovers between DNA molecules.
- **chiasmata**
  Cross-overs between chromosomes in meiosis.
- **chimera (pl. chimaera)**
  An organism that contains cells or tissues with a different genotype. These can be mutated cells of the host organism or cells from a different organism or species.
- **chimera**
  An individual composed of two populations of cells with different genotypes.
- **chimeraplasty**
  An experimental targeted repair process in which a desirable sequence of DNA is combined with RNA to form a chimeraplast. These molecules bind selectively to the target DNA. Once bound, the chimeraplast activates a naturally occurring gene-correcting mechanism. Does not use viral or other conventional gene-delivery vectors.
- **chimeric plasmid**
  Hybrid or genetically mixed plasmid used in DNA cloning.
- **chi-square distribution**
  The sampling distribution of the chi-square statistic. A family of curves whose shapes depend on degrees of freedom.
- **chi-square test**
  A statistical test used to determine the probability of obtaining the observed results by chance, under a specific hypothesis.

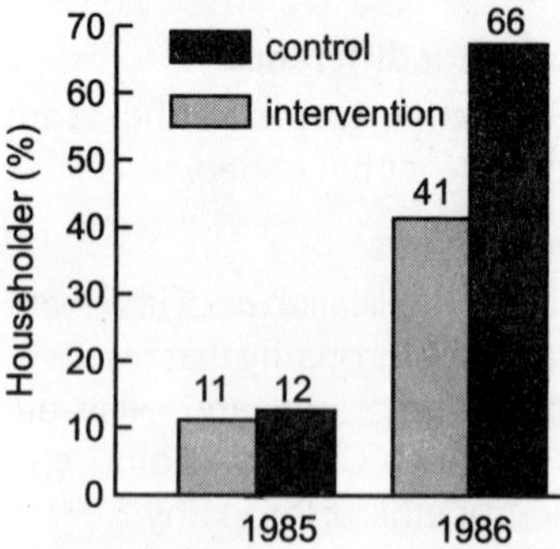


- **chloroplast**
  The organelle that carries out photosynthesis and starch grain formation. A chlorophyll-containing organelle in plants that is the site of photosynthesis.
- **chloroplast chromosome**
  Circular DNA found in the photosynthesizing organelle (chloroplast) of plants instead of the cell nucleus where most genetic material is located.

- **choana**
  The opening into the nasopharynx of the nasal cavity on either side.
- **choanal**
  Petaining to the choana - the opening into the nasopharynx of the nasal cavity on either side. Obstruction or interruption of bile flow from the liver.
- **cholesterol**
  A fat-like substance found in blood, muscle, liver, brain, and other tissues in people and animals. The body makes and needs some cholesterol. Too much cholesterol, however, may cause fat to build up in the artery walls and cause a disease that slows or stops the flow of blood. Butter and egg yolks are foods that have a lot of cholesterol.
- **chordee**
  fibrous band of tissue along the base of the penis causing a downward curve
- **chorea**
  Disorder characterized by irregular, spasmodic, involuntary movements of individual muscles or small muscle groups of the face, fingers and toes.
- **choreoathetosis**
  Sudden, involuntary movements of limbs and facial muscles.
- **chorion**
  Layer of cells covering a fertilized ovum some of which, the chorion frondosum, will later form the placenta.
- **chorionic villus sampling**
  A procedure performed vaginally via the cervix or abdominally between the 8th and 12th week of pregnancy to detect genetic defects in the fetus. A few milligrams of Cells are aspirated (sucked out) from the chorion - a layer of embryonic tissue surrounding the fetus (fetal placenta) - and are analyzed for chromosomal abnormalities.
- **choroid**
  Thin membrane covering the retina that contains major blood vessels.
- **chromatid**
  One of the two side by side replicas produced by chromosome replication in mitosis or meiosis. Subunit of a chromosome after replication and prior to anaphase of meiosis II or mitosis. At anaphase of meiosis II or mitosis when the centromeres divide and the sister chromatids separate each chromatid becomes a chromosome.
- **chromatid conversion**
  Gene conversion that is inferred from the existence of identical sister-spore pairs in a fungal octad that shows a non-Mendelian allele ratio.
- **chromatid interference**
  A situation in which the occurrence of a crossover

between any two nonsister chromatids can be shown to affect the probability of those chromatids being involved in other crossovers in the same meiosis.

- **chromatin**

The substance of chromosomes; now known to include DNA, chromosomal proteins, and chromosomal RNA. The nucleoprotein material of the eukaryotic chromosome.

- **chromatin fibre fish.**

Use of extended chromatin or DNA fibres with fluorescent in situ hybridization to physically order DNA clones or sequences.

- **chromocenter**

The point at which polytene chromosomes appear to be attached together.

- **chromomere**

A small beadlike structure visible on a chromosome during prophase of meiosis and mitosis. Dark regions of chromatin condensation in eukaryotic chromosomes at meiosis or mitosis.

- **chromosomal analysis**

The process of counting and analysing the banding pattern of the chromosomes of an individual.

- **chromosomal deletion**

The loss of part of a chromosome's DNA.

- **chromosomal fragments**

Acentric chromosomes which can arise as a result of segregation of a paracentric inversion and which are usually incapable of replication.

- **chromosomal inversion**

Chromosome segments that have been turned 180 degrees. The gene sequence for the segment is reversed with respect to the rest of the chromosome.

- **chromosomal maps**

Genes or other identifiable DNA fragments are assigned to their respective chromosomes, with distances measured in base pairs. These markers can be physically associated with particular bands (identified by cytogenetic staining) primarily by in situ hybridization, a technique that involves tagging the DNA marker with an observable label (e.g., one that fluoresces or is radioactive). The location of the labeled probe can be detected after it binds to its complementary DNA [cDNA] strand in an intact chromosome.

- **chromosome**

The self-replicating genetic structure of cells containing the cellular DNA that bears in its nucleotide sequence the linear array of genes. In prokaryotes, chromosomal DNA is circular, and the entire genome is carried on one chromosome. Eukaryotic genomes consist of a number of chromosomes whose DNA is associated with different kinds of proteins.

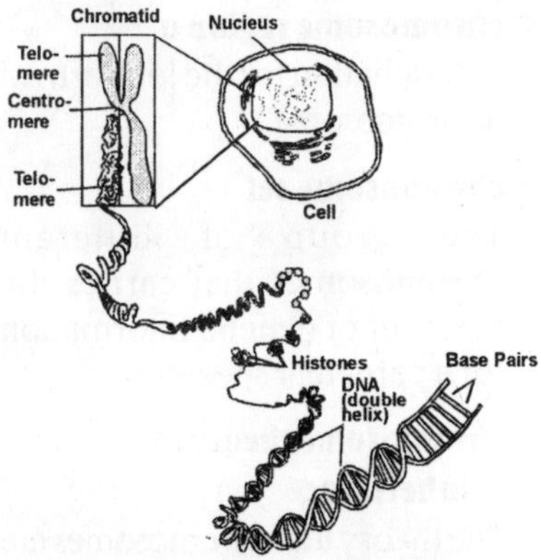


A linear end-to-end arrangement of genes and other DNA, sometimes with associated protein and RNA. The form of the genetic material in viruses and cells. A circle of DNA in prokaryotes; a DNA or an RNA molecule in viruses; a linear nucleoprotein complex in eukaryotes.

- **chromosome aberration**
Any type of change in the chromosome structure or number.

- **chromosome abnormalities**
These can be either structural or numerical. Structural abnormalities include translocations, deletions or insertions, duplications and amplifications. Numerical abnormalities are either a gain or loss of chromosomes.

- **chromosome banding**
A technique for staining chromosomes so that bands appear in a unique pattern particular to the chromosome.

- **chromosome breakage studies**
Cytogenetic testing to detect an increased rate of chromosomal breakage or rearrangement in metaphase cells by exposing cell cultures to clastogenic agents such as diepoxybutane (DEB) or mitomycin C (MMC); cell cultures not exposed to the DNA clastogenic agent are used as controls to measure the spontaneous rate of chromosomal breakage or rearrangement.

- **chromosome instability**
The presence of breaks and gaps in the chromosomes from persons with a number of disorders associated with an increased risk of neoplasia.

- **chromosome jumping**
A technique of isolating clones from a genomic library that are not contiguous by skipping a region between known points on the chromosome. Done usually to bypass regions that are difficult or impossible to walk through or regions known not to be of interest.

- **chromosome loss**
Failure of a chromosome to become incorporated into a daughter nucleus at cell division.

- **chromosome mapping**
  Any method used for determining the location of and relative distances between genes on a chromosome.
- **chromosome marker**
  Any distinct and heritable feature of chromosome structure that can be used to follow (usually by microscopy) that chromosome or chromosome region in breeding experiments.
- **chromosome mutation**
  Any type of change in the chromosome structure or number.
- **chromosome painting**
  Attachment of certain fluorescent dyes to targeted parts of the chromosome. Used as a diagnositic for particular diseases, e.g. types of leukemia; The use of fluorescent-tagged chromosome-specific dispersed repeat DNA sequences to visualize specific chromosomes or chromosome segments by in situ DNA hybridization and fluorescence microscopy.
- **chromosome puff**
  A swelling at a site along the length of a polytene chromosome; the site of active transcription. A diffuse uncoiled region in a polytene chromosome where transcription is actively taking place.
- **chromosome rearrangement**
  A chromosome mutation involving new juxtapositions of chromosome parts.
- **chromosome region p**
  A designation for the short arm of a chromosome.
- **chromosome region q**
  A designation for the long arm of a chromosome.
- **chromosome set**
  The group of different chromosomes that carries the basic set of genetic information for a particular species.
- **chromosome theory of inheritance**
  The theory that chromosomes are linear sequences of genes. The unifying theory stating that inheritance patterns may be generally explained by assuming that genes are located in specific sites on chromosomes.
- **chromosome walking**
  A technique which produces sets of overlapping DNA clones for studying segments of DNA larger than can be cloned individually. A method for the analysis of large regions of DNA, in which a each end of a large single cloned DNA fragment is used separately to screen recombinant DNA genome library for other clones containing neighbouring sequences.
- **chromosome-mediated gene transfer**
  The technique of transferring chromosomes or parts of

chromosomes to somatic cell hybrids to enable more detailed chromosome mapping.

- **chronic**
  A disease, disorder, or condition that has been, or will be, around for a relatively long time. Present over a long period of time. Diabetes is an example of chronic disease.

- **cilia**
  Eyelashes; or, microscopic hair-like projections lining the nose and bronchi.

- **circle of willis**
  A ring of arteries deep in the brain interconnecting the pairs of internal carotid arteries and vertebral arteries to supply the brain with oxygen-rich blood.

- **circulation**
  The flow of blood through the heart and blood vessels of the body.

- **circulatory system**
  The circulatory system is a composed of the heart, arteries, capillaries and veins. It serves to transport blood low in oxygen from the body to the lungs and heart (veins) and oxygenated blood from the lungs and heart throughout the body (arteries).

- **cirrhosis**
  Progressive fibrous tissue growth in an organ such as the liver.

- **cirrhosis**
  A Chronic degenerative disease of the liver.

- **cis**
  Meaning on the near side of; refers to geometric configurations of atoms or mutations on the same molecule or chromosome.

- **cis configuration (synonym cis, coupling)**
  Term which indicates that an individual who is heterozygous at two neighboring loci has the two mutations in question on the same chromosome

- **cis conformation**
  In a heterozygote involving two mutant sites (a,b) within a gene or within a gene cluster, the arrangement ab/AB.

- **cis dominance**
  The ability of a gene to affect genes next to it on the same chromosome.

- **cis-dominant**
  mutations (eg of an operator) that alter the functioning of genes on that same piece of DNA.

- **cis-trans complementation test**
  A mating test to determine whether two different recessive mutations (a1;a2) on opposite chromosomes (trans, a1+/+a2) of a diploid or partial diploid will not complement (i.e., have a mutant phenotype) each other; but the same two recessive mutations on

the same chromosome (cis, a1a2/++) in a diploid or partial diploid show a wild-type phenotype. A test for allelism. A test to determine whether two mutant sites are in the same functional unit or gene.

- **cistron**

Term coined by Benzer for the smallest genetic unit that does not show genetic complementation when two different mutations are in trans during a cis-trans complementation test; but shows wild-type phenotype when the same mutations are in cis. Synonymous with gene. Originally defined as a functional genetic unit within which two mutations cannot complement. Now equated with the term gene, as the region of DNA that encodes a single polypeptide (or functional RNA molecule such as tRNA or rRNA).

- **cladogenesis**

The evolutionary process whereby one species splits into two or more species.

- **class switching**

Term used for the normal change in antibody class from IgM to IgG in the immune response.

- **classical gene families.**

Multigene families which show a high degree of sequence homology.

- **classical pathway**

One of the two ways of activation of complement, in this instance, involving antigen-antibody complexes.

- **clb method**

A technique devised by Muller to rapidly screen fruit flies for recessive X chromosome lethal mutations. The ClB chromosome carries a recessive lethal (l) a dominant marker (B) and an inversion (crossover suppressor C).

- **cleft lip**

An abnormal fissure of the lip which failed to close during development

- **cleft lip and/or palate**

A gap in the soft palate and roof of the mouth, sometimes extending through the upper lip. Results when the various parts of a lip or palate don't grow together to make a single lip or hard palate and is usually correctable. Affects eating, speech production, hearing and tooth formation. Clefting occurs during the sixth through thirteenth week of pregnancy.

- **cleft lip/palate**

Congenital condition with cleft lip alone, or with cleft palate; cause is thought to be multifactorial.

- **cleft palate**

An abnormal fissure of the back of the mouth which failed to close during development.

- **cleft uvula**

An abnormal fissure in the roof of the mouth which failed to close during development.

- **clinal selection**
  Selection that changes gradually along a geographic gradient.
- **clinical**
  Pertaining to information gathered from direct observation of patients, as distinct from laboratory findings.
- **clinical genetics**
  That part of medical genetics concerned with health and illness in individuals and families.
- **clinical heterogeneity**
  Refers here to the production of clinically different phenotypes from mutation in the same gene.
- **clinical trial**
  A scientifically controlled study carried out in people with a particular disease or class of diseases, usually to test the effectiveness of a new treatment. In cancer research, a clinical trial generally refers to the evaluation of treatment methods such as surgery, drugs or radiation techniques, although methods of prevention, detection or diagnosis may also be the subject of such studies.
- **clinodactyly**
  Fingers or toes permanently fixed in a bent position; an abnormal bending of the toes or fingers most common in the fifth digit.
- **clitoral enlargement**
  Structure of the female genatalia located behind the labia majora.
- **cloacal**
  Describes the common uro-genital and rectal chamber in the human embryo.
- **clone**
  An exact copy made of biological material such as a DNA segment (e.g., a gene or other region), a whole cell, or a complete organism; An identical copy of a DNA sequence or entire gene; one or more cells derived from and identical to a single ancestor cell; to isolate a gene or specific sequence of DNA
- **clone contigs**
  Assembly of clones which have been mapped and ordered to produce an overlapping array.
- **clone-based physical maps**
  The physical map of the human genome published by Nature is a clone- based physical map of 3.2 gigabases (25 times larger than any previously mapped genome). This approach involved generating an overlapping series of clones for the whole genome. With a fingerprinted BAC map clones could be selected for sequencing ensuring comprehensive coverage of the genome.
- **cloned dna**
  Any DNA fragment that passively replicates in the host organism after it has been joined to a cloning vector.

- **clonic**
  Referring to clonus, rapid contractions and relaxations of a muscle.

- **cloning**
  Using specialized DNA technology to produce multiple, exact copies of a single gene or other segment of DNA to obtain enough material for further study. This process, used by researchers in the Human Genome Project, is referred to as cloning DNA. The resulting cloned (copied) collections of DNA molecules are called clone libraries. A second type of cloning exploits the natural process of cell division to make many copies of an entire cell. The genetic makeup of these cloned cells, called a cell line, is identical to the original cell. A third type of cloning produces complete, genetically identical animals such as the famous Scottish sheep, Dolly.

- **cloning in silico**
  The use of a number of computer programs which can search genomic DNA sequence databases for sequence homology to known genes, as well as DNA sequences specific to all genes such as the conserved intron/exon splice junctions, promoter sequences, polyadenylation sites and stretches of open-reading frames (ORFs) to identify novel genes.

- **cloning vector**
  DNA molecule originating from a virus, a plasmid, or the cell of a higher organism into which another DNA fragment of appropriate size can be integrated without loss of the vector's capacity for self-replication; vectors introduce foreign DNA into host cells, where the DNA can be reproduced in large quantities. Examples are plasmids, cosmids, and yeast artificial chromosomes; vectors are often recombinant molecules containing DNA sequences from several sources.

- **clonus**
  Involuntary, rapid contractions and relaxations of a muscle.

- **clubbing**
  Enlargement of the end of toes or fingers.

- **coagulation**
  Clotting of the blood.

- **coarctation**
  Condition of narrowing or stricture.

- **coccyx**
  Fused bone at the base of the spine; tailbone.

- **cochlea**
  A structure in the inner ear that converts sound coming from the middle ear into electrical signals that are transmitted to the brain.

• **code dictionary**
A listing of the 64 possible codons and their translational meanings (the corresponding amino acids).

• **coding region**
(synonym open reading frame) All exons of a gene that contribute to the protein product(s) of the gene

• **coding strand**
The DNA strand with the same sequence as the transcribed mRNA (given U in RNA and T in DNA) and containing the linear array of codons which interact with anticodons of tRNA during translation to give the primary sequence of a protein. Compare with anticoding strand.

• **codominance**
Situation in which two different alleles for a genetic trait are both expressed; The situation in which a heterozygote shows the phenotypic effects of both alleles equally. (eg blood group antigens).

• **codominant**
Alleles are codominant if each is expressed independent of the presence of the other. Example: AB blood type.

• **codon**
In DNA or RNA, a sequence of three nucleotides that codes for a certain amino acid or signals the termination of translation (stop or termination codon). A sequence of three bases in DNA or RNA that specifies an amino acid or a stop signal in protein synthesis.

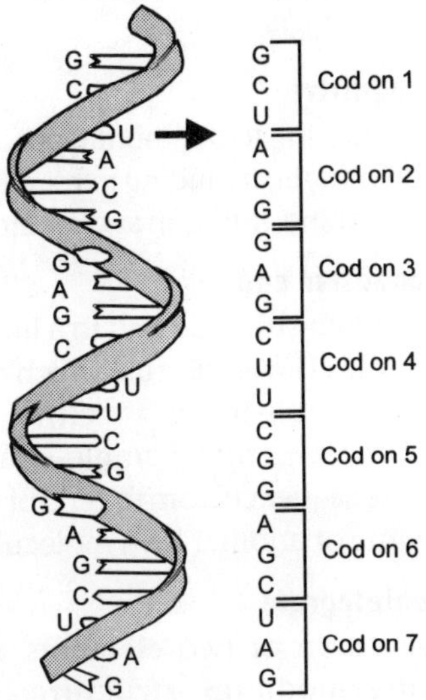


**RNA**
Ribonucleic acid

• **codon preference**
The idea that for amino acids with several codons one or a few are preferred and are used disproportionately. They would correspond with tRNAs that are abundant.

• **coefficient of coincidence**
In a three point cross the number of observed double crossovers divided by the number expected based on the observed occurrence of single crossovers. The ratio of the observed number of double recombinants to the expected number.

- **coefficient of relationship (r)**
The proportion of alleles held in common by two related individuals.

- **cognitive**
Pertaining to the mental process of thought, including perception, reasoning, intuition and memory.

- **cohesive end**
A single-stranded end to a linear duplex DNA molecule which can hydrogen-bond with a complementary single-strand base sequence from the end of the same or another DNA molecule.

- **cointegrate**
A fusion of two elements. An intermediate structure in replicative transposition. The product of the fusion of two circular elements to form a single, larger circle.

- **coisogenic or congenic**
Nearly identical strains of an organism; they vary at only a single locus.

- **col plasmid**
Plasmid that produces an antibiotic (colicin) used by the host to kill other strains of bacteria.

- **colinearity**
The one to one linear correspondence between the order of codons in a coding sequence and the order of amino acids in the protein encoded. A linear map of mutation sites within a gene corresponds to the linear location of amino acid substitutions within the polypeptide encoded by that gene.

- **collateral vessels**
Small branches of arteries and veins that develop to bypass narrowed or blocked segments.

- **coloboma**
A defect or misshaping of the iris, present at birth. The absence of a portion of ocular tissue resulting in a notch or cleft-like defect in the structure, usually resulting from the failure to close part of a fetal fissure (e.g., coloboma of iris, coloboma of retina).

- **colon**
The long, coiled, tube like organ that removes water from digested food. The remaining material, solid waste called stool, moves through the colon to the rectum and leaves the body through the anus. The colon is sometimes called the large bowel or the large intestine.

- **colonoscopy**
Examination of the colon through a flexible, lighted instrument called a colonoscope.

- **colony**
A visible clone of cells.

- **colorectal**
Pertaining to the colon and rectum.

- **colostomy**
Artificial opening in the abdomen connecting the large intestine to the outside of the body.

- **coma**
A sleep-like state; not conscious.

- **common ancestry**
The state of two individuals when they are blood relatives. When two parents have a common ancestor their offspring will be inbred.

- **common cancers**
The cancers which occur commonly in humans, such as bowel and breast cancer.

- **common diseases**
The diseases which occur commonly in humans, e.g. cancer, coronary artery disease, diabetes, etc.

- **community genetics**
The branch of medical genetics concerned with screening and the prevention of genetic diseases on a population basis.

- **community genomics (also called environmental genomics)**
The study of communities of organisms in nature using the tools of genomics.Sequencing the DNA of microorganisms found in a liter of ocean water is an example of community genomics.

- **comparative genome mapping**
Comparative genome mapping in the sequence-based era:early experience with human chromosome 7.

- **comparative genomic hybridization (synonym CGH)**
A molecular cytogenetic method for detecting loss and gain of chromosomal material; a map is produced showing DNA sequence copy number as a function of chromosomal location.

- **comparative genomics**
The science of comparing the genome sequences of humans and other species in order to discover similarities and differences in biology.For instance, scientists who study evolution might compare the genomes of humans and chimpanzees, while scientists who study the bacterium E.coli might compare strains that harm humans and those that do not.

- **compartment**
The existence of boundaries within the organism beyond which a specific clone of cells will never extend during development.

- **competence factor**
A surface protein that binds extracellular DNA and enables the cell to be transformed.

- **competent**
Able to take up exogenous DNA and thereby be transformed;

Making bacterial cell membrane permeable to DNA by a variety of different methods including exposure to certain salts or high voltage; A series of at least 10 serum proteins in humans (and other vertebrates) that can be activated by either the 'classical' or the 'alternative' pathways and which interact in sequence to bring about the destruction of cellular antigens.

- **complementarity**
  The correspondence of DNA bases in the double helix such that adenine in one strand is opposite thymine in the other strand and cytosine in one strand is opposite guanine in the other. This relationship explains Chargaff's rule.

- **complementary dna (cdna)**
  Synthetic DNA reverse transcribed from a specific RNA through the action of the enzyme reverse transcriptase. DNA synthesized by reverse transcriptase using RNA as a template.

- **complementary rna (crna)**
  Synthetic RNA produced by transcription from a specific DNA single stranded template.

- **complementary sequence**
  Nucleic acid base sequence that can form a double-stranded structure with another DNA fragment by following base-pairing rules (A pairs with T and C with G). The complementary sequence to GTAC for example, is CATG; The complementary sequence to G-T-A-C, for instance, is C-A-T-G. Cytosine (C): A base; one of the molecular components of DNA and RNA. Always bonds with guanine (C-G). A sequence of bases that can form a double-stranded structure by matching base pairs.

- **complementary strands**
  The specific pairing of the bases in the DNA of the purines adenine and guanine with thymine and cytosine.

- **complementation**
  The production of a wild-type phenotype when two different mutations are combined in a diploid or a heterokaryon. The production of the wild-type phenotype by a cell or an organism that contains two mutant genes. If complementation occurs the mutations are almost certainly non-allelic (ie in different genes).

- **complementation analysis**
  A genetic test for determining whether two mutations producing a similar phenotype are allelic.

- **complementation group**
  A group of mutant genes which do not complement each other. A cistron (determined by the cis-trans complementation test).

- **complementation test**
  A mating test to determine whether two different recessive mutations (a1;a2) on opposite chromosomes (trans, a1+/+a2) of a diploid or partial diploid will not complement (i.e., have a mutant phenotype) each other; but the same two recessive mutations on the same chromosome (cis, a1a2/++) in a diploid or partial diploid show a wild-type phenotype; a test for allelism. A test to determine whether two mutant sites are in the same functional unit or gene.

- **complete ascertainment**
  A term used in segregation analysis for a type of study which identifies all affected individuals in a population.

- **complete linkage**
  The state in which two loci are so close together that alleles of these loci are virtually never separated by crossing over.

- **complete medium**
  A culture medium that is enriched to contain all of the growth requirements of a strain of organisms.

- **complex disorder**
  A disease that involves multiple genetic and environmental factors.Obesity, heart disease, and schizophrenia are examples of diseases that have multiple causes.

- **complex trait**
  Trait that has a genetic component that does not follow strict Mendelian inheritance. May involve the interaction of two or more genes or gene-environment interactions.

- **component of fitness**
  A particular aspect in the life cycle of an organism upon which natural selection acts.

- **composite transposon**
  A transposon constructed of two IS (insertion sequence) elements flanking a control region that frequently contains host genes.

- **compound heterozygote**
  An individual who has two different abnormal alleles at a particular locus, one on each chromosome of a pair; usually refers to individuals affected with an autosomal recessive disorder.

- **conception**
  The union of an egg and a sperm that forms a cell capable of surviving and maturing, which results in pregnancy.

- **concordance**
  The amount of similarity in phenotype between individuals; When both members of a pair of twins exhibit the same trait they are said to be concordant. If only one twin has the trait they are said to be discordant.

- **conditional knockout**
  A mutation that is only expressed under certain conditions, e.g. raised temperature.
- **conditional mutation**
  A mutation that has the wild-type phenotype under certain (permissive) environmental conditions and a mutant phenotype under other (restrictive) conditions.
- **conditional probability**
  Observations or tests which can be used to modify prior probabilities using Bayesian calculation in risk estimations.
- **conditional-lethal mutation**
  A mutation that is lethal under one condition but not lethal under another condition.
- **conditionally toxic or suicide gene**
  Genes that are introduced in gene therapy and which, under certain conditions or after the introduction of a certain substance, will kill the cell.
- **confidence limits**
  A statistical term for a pair of numbers that predict the range of values within which a particular parameter lies for a given level of confidence (probability).
- **confidentiality**
  In genetics, the expectation that genetic material and the information gained from testing that material will not be available without the donor's consent.
- **confined placental mosaicism**
  The occurrence of a chromosomal abnormality in chorionic villus samples obtained for first trimester prenatal diagnosis in which the fetus has a normal chromosomal complement.
- **confined placental mosaicism**
  Mosaicism that is seen only in the placenta but not in the fetus.
- **conformation-sensitive gel electrophoresis (synonym: CSGE)**
  A type of mutation scanning in which a segment of DNA is screened for mismatch pairing between normal and mutated base pairs.
- **congenic mouse strain**
  A strain that differs from another in the region containing one genetic locus.
- **congenital**
  Any trait present at birth, whether the result of a genetic or nongenetic factor.
- **congenital defects**
  Problems or conditions that are present at birth.
- **congenital heart defect**
  The baby is born with a structural problem of the heart so that the blood does not flow normally.

- **congenital hypertrophy of the retinal pigment epithelium (chrpe)**
  Abnormal retinal pigmentation which, when present in persons at risk for familial adenomatous polyposis, is evidence of the heterozygous state.
- **congenital lipoid hyperplasia**
  Overgrowth of fatty-like cells in the adrenal glands (Male Psuedohermaphroditism; 20-22 Demolase Deficiency.
- **congestion**
  The presence of excessive blood or fluid, such as mucus, in an organ or tissue.
- **congestive heart failure**
  Heart failure caused by loss of pumping power by the heart, resulting in fluids collecting in the body. Congestive heart failure often develops gradually over several years, although it also can happen suddenly. It can be treated by drugs and in some cases, by surgery. Congestive heart failure (CHF), also called congestive cardiac failure (CCF) or just heart failure, is a condition that can result from any structural or functional cardiac disorder that impairs the ability of the heart to fill with or pump a sufficient amount of blood throughout the body. It is not to be confused with "cessation of heartbeat", which is known as asystole, or with cardiac arrest, which is the cessation of normal cardiac function in the face of heart disease. Because not all patients have volume overload at the time of initial or subsequent evaluation, the term "heart failure" is preferred over the older term "congestive heart failure".
- **conjunction**
  The mucous membrane lining the eyelids and the front of the eye.
- **connective tissue**
  General term for all tissues of the body which support and connect various organs and other structures.
- **consanguineous**
  Having at least one common ancestor in the preceding few generations
- **consanguineous marriage**
  A marriage between 'blood relatives', that is between persons who have one or more ancestors in common, most frequently between first cousins.
- **consanguinity**
  Genetic relatedness between individuals descended from at least one common ancestor
- **consensus sequence**
  A sequence of nucleotides or amino acids in common between regions of homology in different but related DNA or RNA or protein sequences; A GGGCGGG sequence promoter element to the 5' side of genes in eukaryotes

involved in the control of gene expression.

- **conservative change**
An amino acid change that does not affect significantly the function of the protein.

- **conservative replication**
A postulated mode of DNA replication in which an intact double helix acts as a template for a new double helix; known to be incorrect. A disproved model of DNA synthesis suggesting that one-half of the daughter DNA molecules should have both strands composed of newly polymerized nucleotides.

- **conservative substitution**
Single base pair substitution which, although resulting in the replacement by a different amino acid, if chemically similar, has no functional effect.

- **conserved sequence**
A base sequence in a DNA molecule (or an amino acid sequence in a protein) that has remained essentially unchanged throughout evolution.

- **constant region**
A region of an antibody molecule that is nearly identical with the corresponding regions of antibodies of different specificities.

- **constipation**
The inability to pass bowel movements easily.

- **constitutional**
Present in the fertilized gamete.

- **constitutional heterozygosity**
The presence in an individual at the time of conception of obligate heterozygosity at a locus when the parents are homozygous at that locus for different alleles.

- **constitutive**
Always expressed in an unregulated fashion (when referring to gene control).

- **constitutive ablation**
Gene expression that results in cell death.

- **constitutive heterochromatin**
Heterochromatin that surrounds the centromere. Specific regions of heterochromatin always present and in both homologs of a chromosome.

- **constitutive mutation**
A mutation which causes transcription to be no longer under regulatory control.

- **constricted**
Smaller than normal.

- **constrictions**
Abnormal closing or reduction in size of an opening or passageway.

- **construction of a human genomic library**
A genomic library comprises a set of bacteria, each carrying a different small fragment of human DNA. For simplicity, cloning of just

a few representative fragments (colored) is shown. In reality, all the gray DNA fragments will also be cloned.

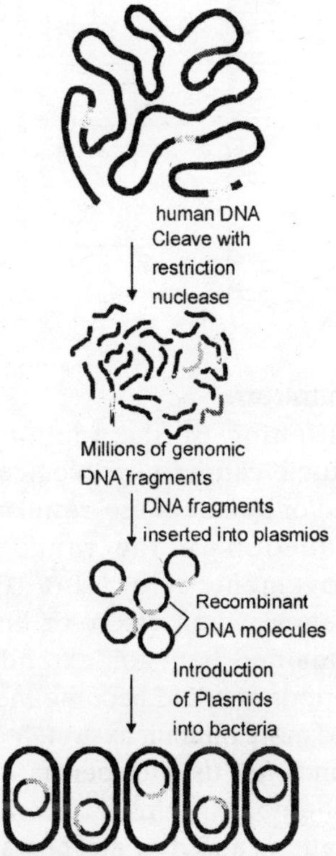


- **consultand**

The individual (not necessarily affected) who presents for genetic counseling and through whom a family with an inherited disorder comes to medical attention

- **contig**

Group of cloned (copied) pieces of DNA representing overlapping regions of a particular chromosome.

- **contig map**

A map depicting the relative order of a linked library of overlapping clones representing a complete chromosomal segment; A virtual map showing the relative order of a library of small, overlapping linked clones representing the complete segment from a single chromosome or sequence of DNA; Overlapping of cloned or sequenced DNA to construct a continuous region of a gene, chromosome or genome; Contig maps are important because they provide the ability to study a complete, and often large segment of the genome by examining a series of overlapping clones which then provide an unbroken succession of information about that region. The bottom- up approach involves cutting the chromosome into small pieces, each of which is cloned and ordered. The ordered fragments form contiguous DNA blocks (contigs). Currently, the resulting library of clones varies in size from 10,000 bp to 1 Mb. An advantage of this approach is the accessibility of these stable clones to other researchers Contig construction can be verified by FISH [fluorescence in situ hybridization], which localizes cosmids to specific regions within chromosomal bands. Consist of a linked library of small overlapping clones representing a complete chromosomal segment. While useful for finding genes localized to a small area (under 2 Mb), contig maps are difficult to extend over large stretches of a chromosome because all regions are not clonable. DNA probe techniques can be used to fill in the gaps, but they are time consuming.

- **contiguous gene syndrome**
  A constellation of findings caused by a small chromosome deletion or duplication that spans two or more adjacent genes

- **continuous replication**
  The uninterrupted replication of DNA in the 5' to 3' direction using a 3' to 5' template.

- **continuous trait**
  A trait, such as height, for which there is a range of observations or findings, in contrast to traits which are all or none, cf. discontinuous, such as cleft lip and palate.

- **continuous variation**
  Variation measured on a continuum rather than in discrete units or categories (e.g. height in human beings). Variation where individuals cannot be classified as belonging to one of a set of discrete classes. Characters showing continuous variation are referred to as quantitative.

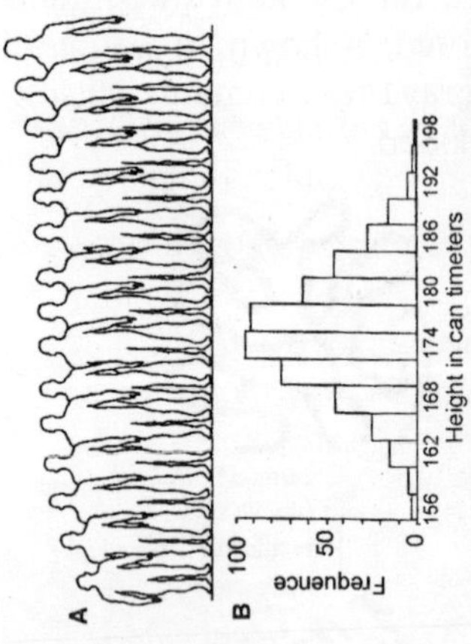


A Height in human males as an example of continuous variation  B Histogram showing variation in height in a group of human males

- **contracture**
  Stiffening or shortening of muscle caused physiologically and/or by lack of use; result in a reduction of the range of movement of a joint. For example, if an elbow or knee remained bent for extended periods, it could become more and more difficult to straighten; Abnormal usually permanent condition of joint flexion and fixation caused by atrophy and shortening of muscle fibers or loss of normal elasticity of skin; muscle contractions.

- **contraindication**
  A condition that makes a treatment not helpful or even harmful.

- **control gene**
  A gene which can turn other genes on or off, i.e. regulate.

- **controlling element**
  A term used by maize geneticists to indicate a mobile genetic element capable of producing an unstable mutant target gene; two types exist, the regulator and the receptor elements.

- **convulstion**
  A sudden attack usually characterized by loss of consciousness and sustained or rhythmic contractions of some or all voluntary muscles. Convulsions are most often a manifestation of a seizure disorder (epilepsy).

- **copper fist**
  Configuration of a DNA-binding protein that resembles a fist closed around a penny. In this case the penny is copper ions; the knuckles of the fist of the yeast ACE1 protein interact with the promoter of the metallothionein gene, enhancing its transcription.

- **copy number**
  The number of copies of a transgene integrated into a host genome; used to describe transgenic animals.

- **copy-choice hypothesis**
  An incorrect hypothesis that stated that recombination resulted from the switching of the DNA-replicating enzyme from one DNA homologue to the other.

- **copy-choice model**
  A model of the mechanism for crossing over, suggesting that crossing over occurs during chromosome division and can occur only between two supposedly new nonsister chromatids; the experimental evidence does not support this model.

- **cor pulmonale**
  Right-sided heart failure which can occur after serious lung disease, such as in persons with cystic fibrosis.

- **cordocentesis**
  The procedure of obtaining fetal blood samples for prenatal diagnosis.

- **corepressor**
  The metabolite that when bound to the repressor (of a repressible operon) forms a functional unit that can bind to its operator and block transcription.

- **cornea**
  Transparent part of the eye in front of the iris and pupil.

- **corneal**
  Related to the cornea of the eye, the transparent coating over the front of the eye.

- **cornelia de lange syndrome**
  condition involving growth deficiency, significant developmental delay, anoxmalies of the extremities and a characteristic facial appearance.

- **corona radiata**
  Cellular layer surrounding the mature oocyte.

- **coronary arteries**
  Arteries supplying blood to the heart muscle itself.

- **coronary disease**
  Damage to the heart. Not enough blood flows through the vessels because they are blocked with fat or have become thick and hard; this harms the muscles of the heart.

- **corpus callosum**
  Part of the brain which joins one cerebral hemisphere to the other.

- **corpus luteum**
  The zona granulosa and theca cells remaining in the ovary after ovulation and some surrounding capillaries and connective tissue evolve into the corpus luteum. The corpus luteum produces progesterone and, in the event of fertilization, provides the required progesterone until the placenta is formed. The corpus luteum also produces some estrogen. In the absence of fertilization, the life span of the corpus luteum is 14 days.

- **correction**
  The production (possibly by excision and repair) of a properly paired nucleotide pair from a sequence of hybrid DNA that contains a mismatched base pair.

- **correlation**
  Statistical measure of the degree of association or resemblance between two parameters.

- **correlation coefficient**
  A statistic that gives a measure of how closely two variables are related. A statistical measure of the extent to which variations in one variable are related to variations in another.

- **cortex**
  The outer portion of an organ, as distinguished from the inner or medullary portion.

- **cortical**
  Referring to the outer layer.

- **cortical blindness**
  Blindness caused by malformation or damage to the cortex of the brain.

- **cosegregation**
  The inclusion of two or more linked genes on a chromosome in the same gamete leading to their transmission together

- **cosmid**
  Artificially constructed cloning vector containing the cos gene of phage lambda. Cosmids can be packaged in lambda phage particles for infection into E. coli; this permits cloning of larger DNA fragments (up to 45kb) than can be introduced into bacterial hosts in plasmid vectors; A hybrid plasmid that contains cos sites at each end. Cos sites are recognized during head filling of lambda phages. Cosmids are useful for cloning large segments of foreign DNA (up to 50 kb).

- **cosmid maps**
"Constructing chromosome- and region-specific cosmid maps of the human genome".

- **cot value**
The product of Co (the original concentration of denatured DNA) and t (time in seconds), giving a useful index of DNA renaturation. Cot1/2 is the value when 50% renaturation has occurred which can be used to estimate the length of unique DNA in a sample.

- **cotransduction**
The simultaneous transduction of two or more genes. The simultaneous transduction of two bacterial marker genes.

- **cotransformation**
The simultaneous transformation of two bacterial marker genes.

- **co-twins**
Both members of a twin pair, whether dizygotic or monozygotic.

- **counsellee**
Person receiving genetic counselling.

- **coupling**
Arrangement of wild-type and mutant alleles at two linked loci in which both mutants are on the same chromosome and both wild-type alleles on the homologue (ab/AB); When a certain allele at a particular locus is on the same chromosome with a specific allele at a closely-linked locus.

- **coupling conformation**
Linked heterozygous gene pairs in the arrangement, AB/ab.

- **covariance**
A statistical measure used in computing the correlation coefficient between two variables; the covariance is the mean of (x- x(bar))(y-y(bar)) over all pairs of values for the variables x and y, where x(bar) is the mean of the x values and y(bar) is the mean of the y values. A statistical value measuring the simultaneous deviations of x and y variables from their means.

- **cpdna**
Chloroplast DNA.

- **cpeo**
Chronic Progressive External Ophthalmoplegia Syndrome. The combination of ptosis and restricted eye movements is referred to as opthalmoplegia.

- **cpg dinucleotides**
The occurrence of the nucleotides cytosine and guanine together in genomic DNA which is frequently methylated and which is associated with spontaneous deamination of cytosine converting it to thymine as a mechanism of mutation.

- **cpg islands**
Areas of a multiple CG repeats in DNA.

- **cranial nerves**
  Twelve nerves that connect the brain with the muscles and sense organs of the face, neck, eyes, ears, nose, and mouth.

- **craniofacial**
  Referring to the skull and face.

- **craniofacial dysmorphism**
  Abnormalities of the head and face.

- **craniolacunae**
  Incomplete formation of the bones of the vault of the fetal skull so there are nonossified areas in the calvaria.

- **craniosynostosis**
  Premature closing sutures (joints of the bones) of the skull.

- **creatinine**
  A chemical found in the blood and passed in the urine. A test of the amount of creatinine in blood or in blood and urine shows if the kidney is working right or if it is diseased. This is called the creatinine clearance test.

- **cri-du-chat syndrome**
  A chromosomal condition (monosomy 5p). Name comes from the distinctive mewing cry of affected infants; characterized by significant mental deficiency, low birthweight, failure to thrive and short stature; deletion of a small section of the short arm of chromosome 5.

- **crisscross inheritance**
  Transmission of a gene from male parent to female child to male grandchild for example, X-linked inheritance.

- **critical region**
  The specific portion of a chromosome or a gene that, when altered in some way (deleted, duplicated, or otherwise mutated), produces the characteristic set of phenotypic abnormalities associated with a particular syndrome or disorder.

- **cross**
  The deliberate mating of two parental types of organisms in genetic analysis.

- **crossbreed**
  Fertilization between separate individuals.

- **crossing over**
  The breaking during meiosis of one maternal and one paternal chromosome, the exchange of corresponding sections of DNA, and the rejoining of the chromosomes. This process can result in an exchange of alleles between chromosomes; The exchange of a segment of DNA between two homologous chromosomes during meiosis leading to a novel combination of genetic material in the gamete; A phenomenon, also known as recombination, that sometimes occurs during the formation of

sperm and egg cells (meiosis); a pair of chromosomes (one from the mother and the other from the father) break and trade segments with one another.

- **crossover suppression**
  Reduction of crossing over within an inversion loop in inversion heterozygotes due to physical constraints during synapsis. Crossing over within an inversion loop, when it does occur, leads to defective (deleted and duplicated) crossover chromosomes and mortality of zygotes carrying them.

- **crossovers**
  The exchange of genetic material between two paired chromosome during meiosis.

- **cross-reacting material (crm)**
  Immunologically detected protein or enzyme which is functionally inactive.

- **cruciform configuration**
  A region of DNA having a sequence at one end repeated but inverted at the other end, so that each strand may pair with itself to form a helix extending sideways from the main helix.

- **cryotherapy**
  A method of stunting the growth of tissues by freezing them. Used most commonly on retinal angiomas.

- **cryptic chromosome translocation**
  A chromosome translocation or rearrangement detected by special techniques (e.g., fluorescent in situ hybridization [FISH], telomeric detection) because it is too small to be seen with conventional cytogenetic techniques.

- **cryptic coloration**
  Coloration that allows an organism to match its background and hence become less vulnerable to predation or recognition by prey.

- **cryptic splice site**
  A mutation in a gene leading to the creation of the sequence of a splice site which results in abnormal splicing of the mRNA.

- **cryptorchism, cryptorchidism**
  Failure of one or both of the testicles to descend into the scrotum.

- **csge (synonym conformation-sensitive gel electrophoresis)**
  A type of mutation scanning in which a segment of DNA is screened for mismatch pairing between normal and mutated base pairs.

- **ct scan**
  A computerized tomography technique which uses X-ray slices for images.

- **cubitus valgus**
  Abnormal outward bending (valgus) of the elbow (cubitus).

- **culture**
  Tissue or cells multiplying by a sexual division, grown for experimentation.

- **cusp**
  A segment of a heart valve.

- **cuspid**
  Tooth with one point, sometimes called the canine tooth.

- **custom mutation analysis**
  Molecular genetic testing for a given specific mutation developed on an as-needed basis in a clinical laboratory for diseases for which testing is not otherwise clinically available. Situations in which custom mutation analysis may be used include: a) testing for at-risk family members when a disease-causing mutation has been identified in an affected family member in a research laboratory; b) prenatal testing for families in which a disease-causing mutation has been identified in an affected family member by a laboratory not offering prenatal testing.

- **custom prenatal testing**
  Prenatal testing offered to families in which disease-causing mutations have been identified in an affected family member in either a research or clinical laboratory; testing is not otherwise clinically available for prenatal diagnosis.

- **cutaneous**
  Referring to the skin.

- **cutis hyperelastica**
  A congenital condition characterized by excessive elasticity of the skin, loose jointedness, easy bruisability, and the development of false tumors at the joints.

- **cyanosis**
  A condition in which a lack of oxygen in the blood causes the blood to be darker and the skin to look bluish.

- **cyanotic heart disease**
  Birth defects of the heart which permit oxygen-depleted (blue) blood to circulate to the body without passing through the lungs.

- **cyanotic, cyanosis**
  Bluish discoloration of the skin or mucus membranes due to lack of oxygen.

- **cyclic amp (camp)**
  A form of AMP (adenosine monophosphate) used frequently as a second messenger in eukaryotics and in catabolite repression in prokaryotes.

- **cyclopia**
  An abnormality characterized by the development of a single eye, located in the area normally occupied by the root of the nose, and a missing nose or a nose in

the form of a proboscis (a tubular appendage) located above the eye.

- **cys**
  Cysteine (an amino acid).

- **cyst**
  A hollow tumour in the form of a membranous sac filled with fluid or soft tissue; May occur normally in tissues from time to time, or which may grow up around irritations in tissues.

- **cystic**
  Referring to a fluid filled sac, as the gall bladder or urinary bladder.

- **cystic fibrosis**
  A hereditary disease in which the primary symptoms are breathing difficulties and respiratory infections due to an accumulation of mucus in the lungs. The symptoms of this disease usually develop in infancy; A potentially lethal human disease of secretory cells, showing excess lung mucus secretion, and inherited as an autosomal recessive on chromosome 7. CF is caused by mutations in a gene encoding the cystic fibrosis membrane conductance regulator, a transmembrane protein involved in ion transport; an inherited disease in which a thick mucus clogs the lungs and blocks the ducts of the pancreas.

- **cystic fibrosis transmembrane conductance regulator (cftr)**
  The gene product of the cystic fibrosis gene responsible for chloride transport and mucin secretion.

- **cytidine**
  The nucleoside containing cytosine as its base.

- **cytochrome**
  A type of protein whose function is to carry electrons or protons (hydrogen ions) by virtue of the reversible charging/discharging of an iron atom or iron/sulfur atoms in the center of the protein. Cytrochromes are central molecules of electron transport in the process known as oxidative phosphorylation. The "chrome" means color, and these cytochromes are divided into four groups. (a, b, c, d) according to their ability to absorb or transmit certain colors of light; A class of protein, found in mitochondrial membranes, whose main function is oxidative phosphorylation of ADP to form ATP.

- **cytogenetic maps**
  The visual appearance of a chromosome when stained and examined under a microscope. Particularly important are visually distinct regions, called light and dark bands, which give each of the chromosomes a unique appearance. This feature allows a person's chromosomes to be

studied in a clinical test known as a karyotype, which allows scientists to look for chromosomal alterations.

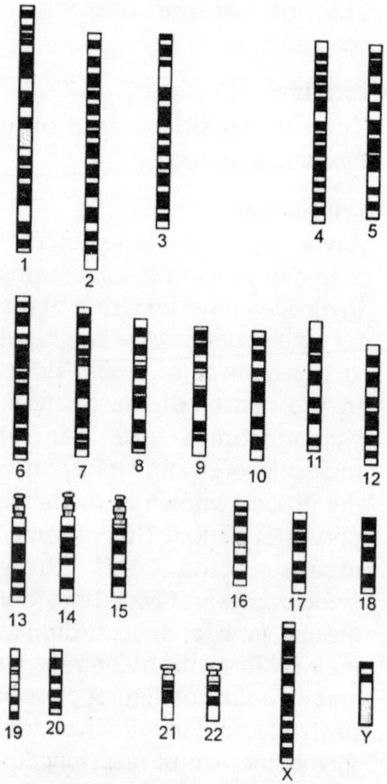


- **cytogeneticist**

One who studies human chromosomes and their abnormalities.

- **cytogenetics**

The study of the physical appearance of chromosomes; The study of the structure, function, and abnormalities of human chromosomes; The microscopic study of chromosomes; The cytological approach to genetics, mainly involving microscopic studies of chromosomes.

- **cytohet**

A cell containing two genetically distinct types of a specific organelle.

- **cytokinesis**

The division of the cytoplasm of a cell into two daughter cells; Division of the cytoplasm to form two daughter cells in meiosis and mitosis.

- **cytological band**

An area of the chromosome that stains differently from areas around it.

- **cytological map**

A type of chromosome map whereby genes are located on the basis of cytological findings obtained with the aid of chromosome mutations.

- **cytomegaly**

Characterized by enlarged cells.

- **cytopathies**

A pathologic process or disease of the cell or components of the cell.

- **cytoplasm**

The cellular substance outside the nucleus in which the cell's organelles are suspended; The material between the nuclear and cell membranes; includes fluid (cytosol) organelles, and various membranes.

- **cytoplasmic inheritance**
  Inheritance via genes found in cytoplasmic organelles. Extra-chromosomal inheritance controlled by non-nuclear genomes.

- **cytoplasmic trait**
  A genetic characteristic in which the genes are found outside the nucleus, in chloroplasts or mitochondria. Results in offspring inheriting genetic material from only one parent.

- **cytosine**
  One of the four bases that make up the letters ATGC in DNA. Cytosine ("C") always pairs with guanine ("G").

- **cytosol**
  The fluid portion of the cytoplasm, outside the organelles.

- **cytotoxic t cells**
  A subclass of T lymphocytes sensitized to destroy cells bearing certain antigens.

- **cytotoxic t lymphocyte (tc)**
  T lymphocyte responsible for attacking cancerous host cells or cells infected with an invading bacterium or virus.

- **darwinian fitness**
  The relative probability of survival and reproduction for a genotype.

- **data warehouse**
  A collection of databases, data tables, and mechanisms to access the data on a single subject.

- **dauermodification**
  The persistence for several generations of an environmentally induced trait.

- **de novo**
  New, for the first time; Spontaneous.

- **de novo mutation (synonym de novo gene mutation, new gene mutation, new mutation)**
  An alteration in a gene that is present for the first time in one family member as a result of a mutation in a germ cell (egg or sperm) of one of the parents or in the fertilized egg itself

- **deafness**
  Partial or complete loss of hearing.

- **deafness, conductive**
  Due to impairment in conduction of sound waves through the bones and structures in the middle and outer ear.

- **deafness, sensorineural**
  A type of hearing impairment that is caused by damage in the inner ear or nerve pathways to the brain (cochlear hair cells or auditory nerve damage). Certain sounds are heard less distinctly than others, causing distortion and reduced understanding of speech. The aging process, heredity, birth defects, certain drugs, head injury, tumors, and exposure to loud noise can all lead to this type

of hearing loss. While this kind of hearing loss is usually not medically correctable, people with sensorineural hearing loss can often be helped by using a hearing aid or other amplification device.

- **debridement**
  The removal of infected, hurt, or dead tissue.
- **deep vein thrombosis**
  A blood clot in the deep veins of the leg.
- **deeply furrowed palate**
  Grooved roof of the mouth.
- **deficiency**
  Lack or shortage of something; The absence of part of the normal genome or chromosome set. See deletion.
- **degenerate code**
  A code in which several code words have the same meaning. The genetic code is degenerate because there are many instances in which different codons specify the same amino acid. A genetic code in which some amino acids may each be encoded by more than one codon.
- **degenerate codon**
  A codon that specifies the same amino acid as another codon.
- **degrees of freedom**
  An estimate of the number of independent categories in a particular statistical test or experiment.
- **deletion**
  A loss of part of the DNA from a chromosome; can lead to a disease or abnormality; Absence of a segment of DNA; may be as small as a single base or as large as one or more genes; A kind of genetic mutation that results when a chromosome loses a piece of DNA, leading to disease or other abnormalities.
- **deletion chromosome**
  A chromosome containing a deletion.
- **deletion map**
  A description of a specific chromosome that uses defined mutations —specific deleted areas in the genome— as 'biochemical signposts,' or markers for specific areas.
- **deletion mutation**
  A mutation in which one or more (sequential) nucleotides is lost by the genome. If the number lost is not divisible by 3 and is in a coding region, the result is a frame shift mutation.
- **deme**
  A locally interbreeding population.
- **dementia**
  Lossor severe impairment of cognition and mental functions

due to a disease or disease process.

- **denaturation**

1)The separation of the two strands of a DNA double helix, or 2) the severe disruption of the hydrogen bonded structure of any complex molecule without breaking the covalent bonds of its chains.

- **denaturation map**

A map of a stretch of DNA showing the locations of local denaturation loops, which correspond to regions of high AT content.

- **denatured**

Loss of natural configuration (of a molecule) through heat or other treatment. Fully denatured DNA is single-stranded.

- **denaturing gradient gel electrophoresis**

Identification of mutations by electrophoresis of double-stranded DNA samples through a denaturing gradient, such as urea. Certain mutations affect the migration pattern by changing the point in the gel at which the DNA denatures; mutant sequences can be distinguished from wild-type sequences by comparing the electrophoretic pattern.

- **denominator element**

Gene on an autosome of Drosophila that helps regulate the sex switch (sxl) to the off condition (maleness). Refers to the denominator of the X/A (number of X chromosomes/autosomes) genic balance equation that determines sex in insects.

- **densitometry**

Method of identifying gene dosage or expression by measurement of light absorption on an autoradiogram (film) of a band (or spot) representing a DNA, RNA, or protein sample; useful in detecting duplication mutations and heterozygous deletion mutations

- **density**

A quality of a tissue to be soft or solid. Muscle is less dense than bone; a sac filled with fluid is less dense than a hard tumor.

- **density-gradient centrifugation**

A method of separating macromolecules by their:

(1) differential rate of sedimentation in a centrifugal gradient

(2) differential bouyancy in a density gradient.

- **deoxyribonucleic acid (dna)**

The chemical found in the nucleus of the cell that holds the genetic instructions for making all living organisms.

- **deoxyribose**

A type of sugar that is one component of DNA (deoxyribo-nucleic acid).

- **depauperate fauna**
  A fauna, especially common on islands, lacking many species found in similar habitats elsewhere.

- **derepressed**
  The condition of an operon that is transcribing because repressor control has been lifted. May apply more generally to any gene being transcribed.

- **derivative chromosome**
  Term used to denote an abnormal chromosome consisting of segments from two or more chromosomes joined together as the result of a translocation, insertion, or other rearrangement

- **dermatitis**
  An inflammatory condition of the skin.

- **dermatologist**
  A doctor who specializes in the diagnosis and treatment of skin problems.

- **dermis**
  The lower or inner layer of the two main layers that make up the skin.

- **determinant**
  A spatially localized molecule that causes cells to adopt a particular fate or set of related fates; The process of commitment of cells to particular fates.

- **deterministic**
  Referring to events that have no random or probabilistic aspects but proceed in a fixed predictable fashion.

- **development**
  The process whereby a single cell becomes a differentiated organism. The process of orderly change that an individual goes through in the formation of structure.

- **developmental delay**
  Slowed down process of moving from simple abilities to more advanced abilities.

- **dgge (synonym denaturing gradient gel electrophoresis)**
  Identification of mutations by electrophoresis of double-stranded DNA samples through a denaturing gradient, such as urea. Certain mutations affect the migration pattern by changing the point in the gel at which the DNA denatures; mutant sequences can be distinguished from wild-type sequences by comparing the electrophoretic pattern.

- **diabetes insipidus**
  A disease of the pituitary gland or kidney, not diabetes mellitus. Diabetes insipidus is often called "water diabetes" to set it apart from "sugar diabetes." The cause and treatment are not the same as for diabetes mellitus. "Water diabetes" has diabetes in its name

because most people who have it show most of the same signs as someone with diabetes mellitus- they have to urinate often, get very thirsty and hungry, and feel weak. However, they do not have glucose (sugar) in their urine. It is a metabolic disorder due to injury of the neurohypophyseal system, which results in a deficient quantity of antidiuretic hormone being released or produces, and thus in failure of tubular reabsorption of water in the kidney. As a consequence, there is a passage of a large amount of urine of low specific gravity, and great thirst; it is often attended by voracious appetite, loss of strength, and emaciation. It may be inherited, acquired, or idiopathic.

- **diabetes mellitus**

A disease that occurs when the body is not able to use sugar as it should. The body needs sugar for growth and energy for daily activities. It gets sugar when it changes food into glucose (a form of sugar). A hormone called insulin is needed for the glucose to be taken up and used by the body. Diabetes occurs when the body cannot make use of the glucose in the blood for energy because either the pancreas is not able to make enough insulin or the insulin that is available is not effective. The beta cells in areas of the pancreas called the islets of Langerhans usually make insulin. In insulin-dependent diabetes (IDDM), the pancreas makes little or no insulin because the insulin-producing beta cells have been destroyed. This type usually appears suddenly and most commonly in younger people under age 30. Treatment consists of daily insulin injections or use of an insulin pump, a planned diet and regular exercise, and daily self-monitoring of blood glucose. In insulin-dependent diabetes, if the level of insulin is too low for a long period of time, the body begins to break down its stores of fat for energy. This causes the body to release acids (ketones) into the blood. The result is called ketoacidosis, a severe condition that may put a person into a coma if not treated right away. The causes of diabetes are not known. Scientists think that insulin-dependent diabetes may be more than one disease and may have many causes. They are looking at hereditary (whether or not the person has parents or other family members with the disease) and at factors both inside and outside the body, including viruses. In noninsulin-dependent diabetes (NIDDM), the pancreas makes some insulin, sometimes too much. The insulin, however, is not effective (see Insulin Resistance). NIDDM is controlled by diet and exercise and daily monitoring of glucose levels. Sometimes oral drugs that lower blood glucose levels or insulin injections are needed. This type of diabetes usually gradually, most often in people over 40 years of age. NIDDM accounts for 90 to 95 percent of diabetes.Noninsulin-dependent diabetes appears to be closely associated with obesity and with the body resisting the action of insulin.

- **diabetic amyotrophy**

  A disease of the nerves leading to the muscles. This condition affects only one side of the body and occurs most often in older men with mild diabetes. See also: Neuropathy.

- **diabetic coma**

  A severe emergency in which a person is not conscious because the blood glucose (sugar) is too low or too high. If the glucose level is too low, the person has hypoglycemia; if the level is too high, the person has hyperglycemia and may develop ketoacidosis.

- **diabetic ketoacidosis (dka)**

  Severe, out-of-control diabetes (high blood sugar) that needs emergency treatment. DKA happens when blood sugar levels get too high. This may happen because of illness, taking too little insulin, or getting too little exercise. The body starts using stored fat for energy, and ketone bodies (acids) build up in the blood. Ketoacidosis starts slowly and builds up. The signs include nausea and vomiting, which can lead to loss of water from the body, stomach pain, and deep and rapid breathing. Other signs are a flushed face, dry skin and mouth, a fruity breath odor, a rapid and weak pulse, and low blood pressure. If the person is not given fluids and insulin right away, ketoacidosis can lead to coma and even death.

- **diabetic myelopathy**

  Spinal cord damage found in some people with diabetes.

- **diabetic retinopathy**

  A disease of the small blood vessels of the retina of the eye. When retinopathy first starts, the tiny blood vessels in the retina become swollen, and they leak a little fluid into the center of the retina. The person's sight may be blurred. This condition is called background retinopathy. About 80 percent of people with background retinopathy never have serious vision problems, and the disease never goes beyond this first stage. However, if retinopathy progresses, the harm to sight can be more serious. Many new, tiny blood vessels grow out and across the eye. This is called neovascularization. The vessels may break and bleed into the clear gel that fills the center of the eye, blocking vision. Scar tissue may also form near the retina, pulling it away from the back of the eye. This stage is called proliferative retinopathy, and it can lead to impaired vision and even blindness. See also: Photocoagulation or vitrectomy for treatments.

- **diabetogenic**

Causing diabetes; some drugs cause blood glucose (sugar) to rise, resulting in diabetes.

- **diabetologist**

A doctor who sees and treats people with diabetes mellitus.

- **diagnosis**

Identification of a disease or disorder; The process to find if a person has a certain medical problem or disease and how it will affect the person's health and abilities; or the decision reached by this process.

- **diagnostic testing**

Testing designed to confirm or exclude a known or suspected genetic disorder in a symptomatic individual or, prenatally, in a fetus at risk for a certain genetic condition.

- **diakinesis**

The final stage of prophase 1 of meiosis when chiasmata terminalize.

- **dialysis**

Technique of removing waste and toxins from the blood, used primarily when the kidneys malfunction or in cases of overdose of a drug. The two types of dialysis are: hemodialysis and peritoneal dialysis. In hemodialysis, the patient's blood is passed through a tube into a machine that filters out waste products. The cleansed blood is then returned to the body. In peritoneal dialysis, a special solution is run through a tube into the peritoneum, a thin tissue that lines the cavity of the abdomen. The body's waste products are removed through the tube. There are three types of peritoneal dialysis. Continuous ambulatory peritoneal dialysis (CAPD), the most common type, needs no machine and can be done at home. Continuous cyclic peritoneal dialysis (CCPD) uses a machine and is usually performed at night when the person is sleeping. Intermittent peritoneal dialysis (IPD) uses the same type of machine as CCPD, but is usually done in the hospital because treatment takes longer; A method for removing waste such as urea from the blood when the kidneys can no longer do the job. The two types of dialysis are: hemodialysis and peritoneal dialysis. In hemodialysis, the patient's blood is passed through a tube into a machine that filters out waste products. The cleansed blood is then returned to the body. In peritoneal dialysis, a special solution is run through a tube into the peritoneum, a thin tissue that lines the cavity of the abdomen. The body's waste products are removed through the tube. There are three types of peritoneal dialysis. Continuous ambulatory peritoneal dialysis (CAPD), the most common type, needs no machine and can be done at home. Continuous cyclic peritoneal dialysis (CCPD) uses a machine and is usually performed at night when the person is sleeping. Intermittent peritoneal dialysis (IPD) uses the same type of machine as CCPD, but is usually done in the hospital because treatment takes longer. Hemodialysis and peritoneal dialysis may be used to treat people with diabetes who have kidney failure.

- **diaphragm**
  The thin muscular partition below the lungs and heart that separates the chest cavity from the abdominal cavity.
- **diaphyses**
  Shafts of the long bones.
- **diarrhea**
  A condition in which fecal matter is discharged from the bowel more often than usual and in a more or less liquid state.
- **diastasis recti**
  Gap between midline abdominal muscles.
- **diastrophic**
  Bent or curved condition of bones or distortion of other structures.
- **dicentric**
  Refers to an aberrant chromosome that contains two centromeres.
- **dicentric chromosome**
  A chromosome with two centromeres.
- **dictyotene**
  A prolonged diplonema of primary oocytes that can last many years.
- **dideoxy method**
  A method of DNA sequencing that uses chain-terminating (dideoxy) nucleotides.
- **differentiation**
  The changes in cell shape and physiology associated with the production of the final cell types of a particular organ or tissue.
- **diffuse**
  Spread about and not limited to a specific area.
- **digital**
  Referring to the digits (fingers and toes).
- **dihybrid**
  An organism heterozygous at two loci.
- **dihybrid cross**
  A cross between two individuals identically heterozygous at two loci for example, AaBb/AaBb.

- **dilated**
  Larger than normal.
- **dimerization**
  The chemical union of two identical molecules.
- **dimorphism**
  A polymorphism involving only two forms.
- **dioecious plant**
  A plant species in which male and female organs appear on separate individuals.
- **diplepia**
  Paralysis that affects both sides of the body, due to injury of both hemispheres of the brain. More commonly affects the legs more than the arms.
- **diploid**
  A full set of genetic material consisting of paired chromosomes, one from each parental set. Most animal cells except the gametes have a diploid set of chromosomes. The diploid human genome has 46 chromosomes.
- **diplonema (diplotene stage)**
  The stage of prophase of meiosis I in which chromatids appear to repel each other.
- **direct dna analysis (synonym direct DNA)**
  The use of any test method, such as sequence analysis, mutation scanning, or mutation analysis to detect a mutation in a gene.
- **directed evolution**
  A laboratory process used on isolated molecules or microbes to cause mutations and identify subsequent adaptations to novel environments.
- **directed mutagenesis**
  Alteration of DNA at a specific site and its reinsertion into an organism to study any effects of the change.
- **directed mutagenesis**
  Altering some specific part of a cloned gene and reintroducing the modified gene back into the organism.
- **directed sequencing**
  Successively sequencing DNA from adjacent stretches of chromosome.
- **directional selection**
  A type of selection that removes individuals from one end of a phenotypic distribution and thus causes a shift in the distribution. Selection that changes the frequency of an allele in a constant direction, either toward or away from fixation for that allele.
- **disassortative mating**
  The mating of two individuals with dissimilar phenotypes.
- **discontinuous replication**
  Replication of DNA in short 5' to 3' segments using the 5' to 3' strand as a template while going

backward away from the replication fork.

- **discontinuous variation**

Variation that falls into discrete categories (e.g., the colour of garden peas).

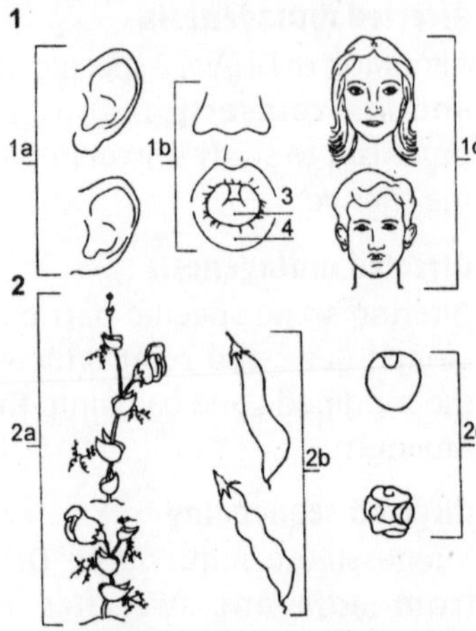


1 Discontinuous variation in humans
1a Free earlobes and attached ear lobes
1b Tongue rolling
1c Female and male
2 Discontinuous variation in peas
2a Long and short stems
2b Smooth and constricted pods
2c Round and wrinkled seeds

- **discordant**

A twin pair (or set of individuals) in which one member exhibits a certain trait and the other does not.

- **discrete generations**

Generations that have no overlapping reproduction. All reproduction takes place between individuals in the same generation.

- **disease**

An interruption, cessation or disorder of body functions, systems, or organs; Any deviation from the normal structure or function of any part, organ, or system of the body that is manifested by a characteristic set of symptoms and signs whose pathology and prognosis may be known or unknown.

- **disease-associated genes**

Alleles carrying particular DNA sequences associated with the presence of disease.

- **disease-causing mutation**

A gene alteration that causes or predisposes an individual to a specific disease

- **dispersive replication**

Disproved model of DNA synthesis suggesting more-or-less random interspersion of parental and new segments in daughter DNA molecules. A postulated mode of DNA replication combining aspects of conservative and semi-conservative replication; known to be incorrect.

- **disruptive selection**

A type of selection that removes individuals from the centre of a phenotypic distribution and thus causes the distribution to become bimodal. Disruptive selection favors two extremes of a phenotypic distribution, with selection occurring against the mean phenotype or intermediate form (1 and 2). Eventually this gives rise to a bimodal distribution

(3) in which two distinct forms predominate.

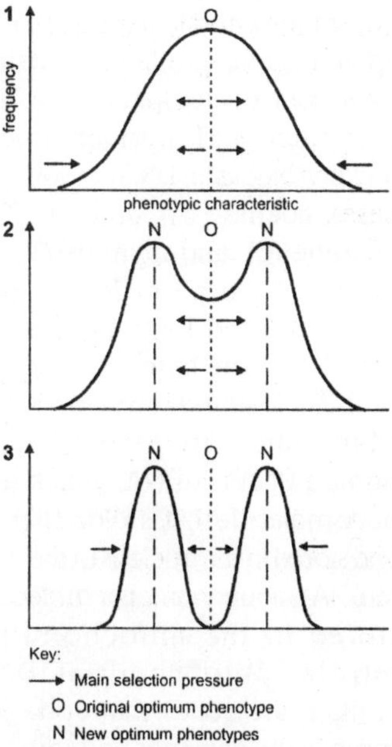


- **distal**

  Farthest from one point of reference/the midline of the body;

- **distribution function**

  A graph of some precise quantitative measure of a character against its frequency of occurrence.

- **diuretic**

  A drug that increases the flow of urine to rid the body of extra fluid.

- **diverticulum**

  A pouch-like herniation through the muscular wall of a tubular organ.

- **dizygotic**

  The product of fertilization of 2 separate eggs by 2 separate sperm; nonidentical twin pair.

- **d-loop**

  Configuration found during DNA replication of chloroplast and mitochondrial chromosomes wherein the origin of replication is different on the two strands. The first structure formed is a displacement loop or D-loop.

- **dna**

  The molecule that encodes genetic information. DNA is a double-stranded molecule held together by weak bonds between base pairs of nucleotides.

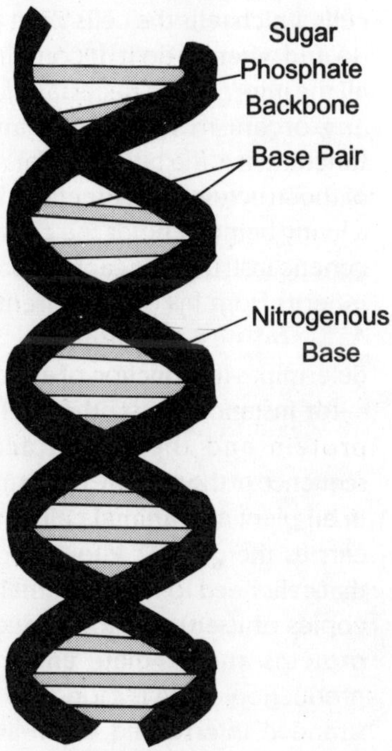

The four nucleotides in DNA contain the bases adenine (A), guanine (G), cytosine (C), and thymine (T). In nature, base pairs form only between A and T and between G and C; thus the base sequence of each single strand can be deduced from that of its partner; The molecule which encodes the genes responsible for the structure and function of an organism and allows for transmission of genetic information from one generation to the next; The substance of heredity; It is the biochemical molecule of which chromosomes and genes are composed. It is the primary genetic material of all cells which tells the cells what to do and when to do it. It contains all the information necessary for any organism to develop and function. It is the blueprint for all of the structures and functions of a living being. It holds the coded genetic instructions each person inherits from his or her parents. As coding sequences, it determines the function of a gene —for instance the synthesis of a protein and the amino acid sequence of the protein. It is found in all plant and animal cells and carries the genetic information that cells need to replicate (make copies of itself) and to produce proteins and regulate enzyme production . DNA is a long, two-stranded, intertwined, chain-like molecule held together by weak bonds between base pairs of nucleotides (polysugar and phosphate chemical groups). The chain resembles a ladder twisted into a double helix, spiral shape. The four nucleotides, or chemical building blocks, in DNA contain the bases: adenine (A), guanine (G), cytosine (C), and thymine (T). In nature, base pairs form only between A and T and between G and C; thus the base sequence of each single strand can be deduced from that of its partner. Most human DNA is nDNA, which is a huge molecule that is folded tightly and stored in the nucleus of the cell. MtDNA is a much smaller molecule stored in the mitochondria. mtDNA: Mitochondrial DNA contain the genes that code for some of the enzymes and some of the necessary molecules needed to make those enzymes of the respiratory chain. Mitochondria are the only part of the body cell with their own separate and unique DNA. Regardless, most of the mitochondria and the respiratory chain are coded by nDNA. MtDNA is inherited only from the mother. nDNA: Nuclear DNA; located in the nucleus of the cell, this DNA contains the blueprints for cells which make up the body.

- **dna bank**

A service that stores DNA extracted from blood samples or other human tissue; The process through which DNA is extracted from any of a number of possible cell sources and stored indefinitely by freezing or refrigerating for future testing; done when a specific test is not presently available or when the decision to have testing has not been made.

- **dna chip**

  A part of the microarray technology scientists use in gene sequencing to understand how the thousands of genes in a genome interact simultaneously.

- **dna clone**

  A section of DNA that has been inserted into a vector molecule, such as a plasmid or a phage chromosome, and then replicated to form many identical copies.

- **dna construct**

  A DNA sequence that has been modified to yield a recombinant DNA molecule.

- **dna fingerprint**

  The largely individual-specific autoradiographic banding pattern produced when DNA is digested with a restriction endonuclease that cuts outside a family of VNTRs, and a Southern blot of the electrophoretic gel is probed with a VNTR-specific probe.

- **dna fingerprint technique**

  A method employed to determine differences in amino acid sequences between related proteins; relies upon the presence of a simple tandem-repetitive sequences that are scattered throughout the human genome.

- **dna fingerprinting**

  A technique for identifying a person or an organism. A "DNA fingerprint" is a composite of short, repetitive segments of DNA that vary from person to person. DNA (deoxyribonucleic acid) fingerprinting (or genetic fingerprinting) is an example of the use of sophisticated biochemical techniques in the analysis of genetic material.

  1. VNTRs (a) can be amplified (copied many times) (b) from a very small tissue or body-fluid sample by PCR (the polymerase chain reaction).
  2. Using gel electrophoresis, the copied VNTRs are separated, according to their length, into invisible bands in an agar gel (c).
  3. The bands containing the VTNRs are transferred to a nitrocellulose membrane (d).
  4. A radioactive DNA probe solution (e) is then added. The probe will bind to VNTRs with complementary base sequences. Unbound probes are washed off.
  5. X-ray film is placed against the membrane. On the developed film (f) appears the unique pattern of bands known as the DNA fingerprint.

These bands have been made visible by the DNA probe. The position of the bands show the lengths of all the VNTRs that the probe has bound to. Even though two individuals are quite likely to have the same number of repeats in a particular VNTR, they are very unlikely to have the same number of repeats in all their VNTRs and so will have different DNA fingerprints.

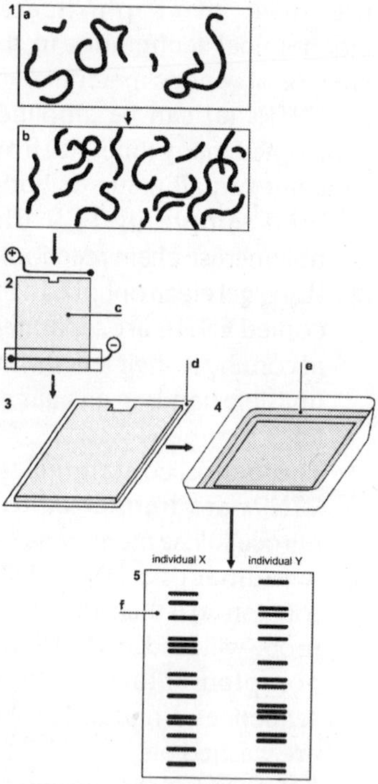


- **dna glycosylase**
endonuclease initiating excision repair at various damaged or improper bases in DNA.

- **dna gyrase**
A topoisomerase that relieves supercoiling in DNA by creating a transient break in the double helix.

- **dna hybridization**
A molecular technique for binding specific segments of single stranded DNA or RNA through base pairing with complementary sequences of single stranded DNA molecules attached or trapped on a nitrocellulose filter.

- **dna ligase**
An enzyme that closes nicks or discontinuities in one strand of double-stranded DNA by creating an ester bond between adjacent 3' OH and 5' PO4 ends on the same strand; Enzyme that catalyzes religation (reconnection) of 2 fragments of DNA.

- **dna marker**
Any unique DNA sequence which can be used in hybridization, PCR or restriction mapping experiments to identify that sequence. See expressed sequence tag and sequence tagged site.

- **dna microarray**
A wafer similar to a computer chip that can be used to swiftly screen for the presence of particular genetic sequences.

- **dna microarray (also called gene chip)**

A device for monitoring the activity of genes.Most DNA microarrays are glass slides or microchips "embedded" with thousands of genes.DNA microarrays have many applications in research and have been used, for instance, to identify genes involved in cancer and to develop drugs.

- **dna polymerase**

An enzyme that can synthesize new DNA strands using a DNA template; several such enzymes exist. One of several classes of enzymes that polymerize DNA nucleotides using single or double-stranded DNA as a template; Enzymes that accurately copy a DNA template by polymerizing nucleotides to form a DNA that is complementary to the template. Different DNA polymerases are responsible for replication and repair of DNA. Polymerases extend the chain by adding nucleotides to the 3' end of the growing DNA.

- **dna probe**

A segment of DNA specifically designed to be complementary to a target sequence of chromosomes, genes or gene sequences. The synthetic piece of DNA is coupled with a fluorescent indicator, or tag, so that the chromosomes or genes it binds (or hybridizes) to can be directly visualized.

- **dna rearrangements**

Recombination of DNA segments, eg, in cells of the immune system, the variable (V), diversity (D), and joining (J) regions somatically rearrange to generate functional antibody genes.

- **dna repair genes**

Genes encoding proteins that correct errors in DNA sequencing; Certain genes that are part of a DNA repair pathway; when altered, they permit mutations to pile up throughout the DNA.

- **dna replication**

The use of existing DNA as a template for the synthesis of new DNA strands. In humans and other eukaryotes, replication occurs in the cell nucleus. The process by which the DNA molecule unwinds and makes an exact copy of itself.

- **dna sequence**

The relative order of base pairs, whether in a DNA fragment, gene, chromosome, or an entire genome; The sequence of genetic "letters," or nucleotides, in a piece of DNA.For instance: ACGTACGTACGT; "Plus and minus" or "primed synthesis" method, developed by Sanger, DNA is synthesized in vitro in such a way that it is radioactively labeled and the reaction terminates specifically at the position corresponding to a given base; the "chemical" method. ssDNA is subjected to several chemical cleavage protocols that selectively make breaks on one side of a particular base; Deoxyribonucleic acid (DNA) carries genetic material (inherited information), which needs to be passed on to new cells. In preparation for cell division, the DNA replicates (copies) itself so that each new cell can have its own exact copy of the DNA.

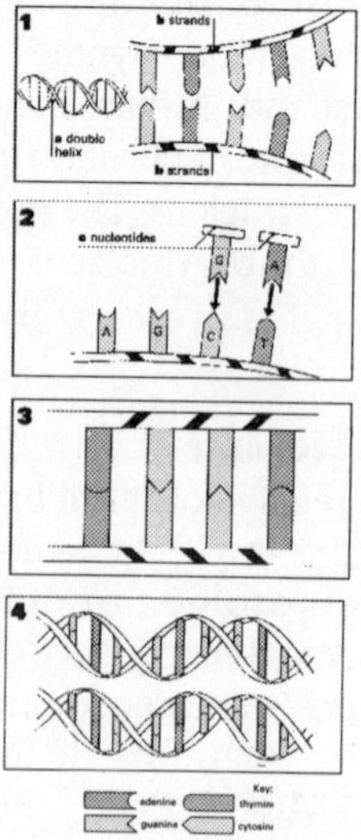


1. The DNA double helix (**a**) uncoils and separates into two strands (**b**). These act as "molds" for new strands.
2. Free nucleotides (individual base-sugar-phosphate units) (**c**) attach to exposed complementary bases on the original strands: adenine (A) attaches to thymine (T), and guanine (G) attaches to cytosine (C).
3. The free nucleotides bond to form new strands, attached by the bases to the old ones.
4. The end result is two DNA molecules identical to the original. Each one consists of one new and one old strand or series of nucleotides.

- **dna/rna**

(Deoxy)ribonucleic acid. First discovered in nuclei of cells (thus, they are also called "nucleic acid"). DNA together with RNA are molecules that carry genetic information. DNA consists of double chains of nucleotides. RNA usually consists of a single chain. DNA/RNA are polymerized chains of nucleotides. The polymerization of the nucleotide chain occurs by joining the hydroxyl group on the 3' carbon of the sugar to the phosphate of an adjacent nucleotide. Thus, at one end of the chain, there is an unjoined hydroxyl or phosphate group at the 5' carbon (5' end of the chain); at the other end, there is an unjoined hydroxyl group at the 3' carbon (3' end of the chain).

- **dna-based testing**
(synonym DNA testing, molecular genetic testing) Testing that involves the analysis of DNA, either through linkage analysis, sequencing, or one of several methods of mutation detection

- **dna-dna hybridization**
When DNA is heated to denaturation temperatures to form single strands and then cooled double helices will re-form (renaturation) at regions of sequence complementarity. This technique is useful for determining sequence similarity among DNAs of different origin and the amount of sequence repetition within one DNA.

- **dna-rna hybridization**
When a mixture of DNA and RNA is heated to denaturation temperatures to form single strands and then cooled RNA can hybridize (form a double helix) with DNA that has a complementary nucleotide sequence. Useful for determining relationships between DNAs and RNAs.

- **dnase(deoxyribonuclease)**
An enzyme that degrades DNA to nucleotides.

- **docking protein**
Responsible for attaching (docking) a ribosome to a membrane by interacting with a signal particle attached to a ribosome destined to be membrane bound.

- **domain**
A discrete portion of a protein with its own function. The combination of domains in a single protein determines its overall function; A specific region or amino acid sequence in a protein associated with a particular function or corresponding segment of DNA

- **dominance variance**
Genetic variance at a single locus attributable to dominance of one allele over another.

- **dominant**
A gene that almost always results in the expression of a certain characteristic in an individual, even though an individual's genome only possesses one copy of the gene. This gene always has a 50-50 chance of being passed on to a child; A mode of inheritance in which only a gene from one parent is required for a trait to appear in an offspring; A gene (allele) which is expressed clinically in a heterozygous state. In a dominant disorder only one mutant allele need be present as it covers up, or masks, the normal allele; An allele that determines phenotype even when heterozygous. Also the trait controlled by that allele.

- **dominant allele**
  A gene that is expressed, regardless of whether its counterpart allele on the other chromosome is dominant or recessive. Autosomal dominant disorders are produced by a single mutated dominant allele, even though its corresponding allele is normal.

- **dominant gene**
  A gene (allele) that almost always results in a specific characteristic, for example, a disease, even though the parent's genome possesses only one copy. In a dominant disorder only one mutant allele need be present as it covers up, or masks, the normal allele. Whith a dominant gene, the chance of passing on the gene (and therefore the disease) to children is 50-50 in each pregnancy. A gene that is expressed, regardless of whether its counterpart allele on the other chromosome is dominant or recessive. Autosomal dominant disorders are produced by a single mutated dominant allele, even though its corresponding allele is normal.

- **dominant negative mutation**
  A mutation whose gene product adversely affects the normal, wild-type gene product within the same cell, usually by dimerizing (combining) with it. In cases of polymeric molecules, such as collagen, dominant negative mutations are often more deleterious than mutations causing the production of no gene product (null mutations or null alleles).

- **dominant phenotype**
  The phenotype of a genotype containing the dominant allele; the parental phenotype that is expressed in a heterozygote.

- **donor site**
  Guanine-thymidine sequence that defines the splice site at the 5' end of an intron.

- **dorsal**
  The back of a body part, with reference to the standard anatomical convention.

- **dosage analysis**
  Method of measuring the quantity of a variety of analytes, including DNA, RNA, and protein, by comparison with a known standard; can be used to determine the number of copies of a sequence of DNA (i.e:, to test for duplication and deletion mutations) either by visual comparison of band intensity or numerical quantification by densitometry. If extra copies of a gene are present, intensity is greater than 100% on a gel or film; whereas, if one copy of the

gene is missing, the intensity is approximately 50%.

- **dosage compensation**

A mechanism by which species with sex chromosomes ensure that the homogametic sex does not have too much or the heterogametic sex too little activity of loci on the homogametic sex chromosome. The process, in organisms using a chromosomal sex determination mechanism (such as XX versus XY), that allows standard structural genes on the homogametic sex chromosome to be expressed at the same levels in females and males, regardless of the number of homogametic sex chromosomes. In mammals, dosage compensation operates by maintaining only a single active X chromosome in each cell, while in Drosophila it operates by hyperactivating the single male X chromosome.

- **dot blotting**

A technique of blotting cloned DNA without prior restriction digestion and electrophoresis. Autoradiography reveals dots indicating probe hybridization.

- **double crossover**

Two crossovers occurring in a chromosomal region under study.

- **double digest**

The product formed when two different restriction endonucleases act on the same sample of DNA.

- **double helix**

The twisted-ladder shape that two linear strands of DNA assume when complementary nucleotides on opposing strands bond together; The spiraling lattice of double-stranded DNA that contains the genetic information pertinent to the organism. The sides of the lattice — its spine — are composed of sugar and phosphate molecules. The crosspieces, or rungs, are made up of base pairs, also known as nucleotides.

- **double hemiplegia**

Paralysis that involves both sides of the body, with one side being more greatly affected.

- **double heterozygote**

An individual who is heterozygous for a mutation at each of two separate genetic loci

- **double infection**

Infection of a bacterium with two genetically different phages.

- **double reduction**

The condition in polyploids in which a heterozygous individual produces homozygous gametes.

- **doublesex**

Locus (dsx) in Drosophila in which some mutations convert both males and females into intersexes. Encodes male and female specific proteins produced by differential splicing of the primary transcript in each sex.

- **down syndrome**

A congenital disease caused by an extra copy of chromosome 21 (trisomy 21).

- **downstream**

A convention used to describe features of a DNA sequence, gene or mRNA related to the position and direction (5' to 3') of transcription by RNA polymerase or translation by the ribosome. Downstream (or 3' to) is in the direction of transcription (or translation) whereas upstream (5' to) is in the direction from which the polymerase (or ribosome) has come. Conventionally DNA sequences, gene maps and RNA sequences are drawn with transcription (or translation) from left to right and so downstream is towards the right.

- **draft sequence**

The sequence generated by the HGP as of June 2000 that, while incomplete, offers a virtual road map to an estimated 95% of all human genes. Draft sequence data are mostly in the form of 10,000 base pair-sized fragments whose approximate chromosomal locations are known.

- **duchenne muscular dystrophy**

A lethal muscle disease in humans caused by mutation in a huge gene coding for the muscle protein dystrophin; inherited as an X-linked recessive phenotype.

- **duchenne muscular dystrophy (dmd)**

An x-linked hereditary disease characterized by the absence of a protein known as dystrophin which causes degeneration and necrosis of skeletal muscle fibres. The incidence of this disorder is about 1 in 3500 male births and of these a third are estimated to be new mutational events.

- **duchenne/becker muscular dystrophy**

The most common and severe form of muscular dystrophy; transmitted as an X-linked trait. X-linked recessive. Symptoms include onset at 2-5 years with difficulty with gait and stairs, enlarged calf muscles, progression to wheelchair by adolescence, shortened life span.

- **duct**

A channel that carries body fluids. Breast ducts transport milk from the breast's lobules out to the nipple.

- **ductus arteriosis**

An artery that allows blood in the fetus to bypass the lungs until the lungs expand at birth. It normally closes soon after birth.

- **due date**

The estimated calendar date when your baby will be born. It is also called the estimated date of confinement (EDC).

- **duodenal stricture**
  Part of the intestine (duodenum) narrows abnormally.

- **duodenum**
  The beginning portion of the small intestine, starting at the lower end of the stomach and extending to the jejunum.

- **duplication**
  The presence of an extra segment of DNA, resulting in redundant copies of a portion of a gene, an entire gene, or a series of genes, usually caused by unequal crossing-over during gene replication when gametes are formed in meiosis;

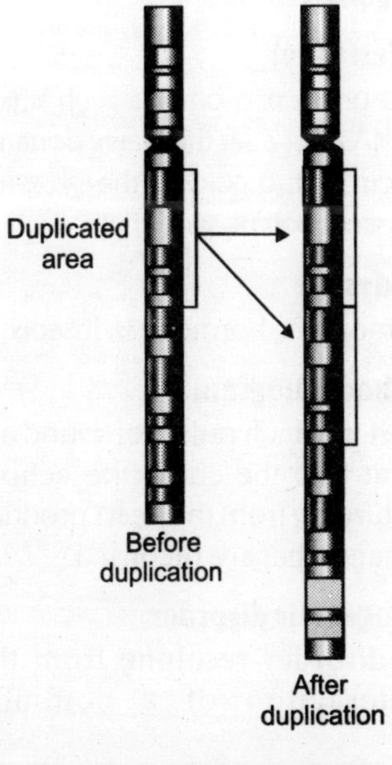


A particular kind of mutation: production of one or more copies of any piece of DNA, including a gene or even an entire chromosome.

- **dupuytren's contracture**
  A condition that causes the fingers to curve inward and may also affect the palm. The condition is more common in people with diabetes and may precede diabetes.

- **dura mater**
  The tough outer membrane covering the brain and spinal cord.

- **dwarf**
  An abnormally short undersized person whose body is not normally proportioned; Conditions of short stature with adult height under 4'10" as adult, usually with normal intelligence and lifespan. Ehlers Danlos Syndrome connective tissue condition including problems with tendons, ligaments, skin, bones, cartilage, and membranes surrounding blood vessels and nerves. Symptoms include joint laxity, elastic skin, dislocations. Many forms: autosomal dominant, autosomal recessive, X-linked forms.

- **dyad**
  Two sister chromatids attached to the same centromere. A pair of sister chromatids joined at the centromere, as in mitosis and meiosis.

- **dysarthia**
  The inability to form words and speak clearly.

- **dysethesia**
  Unpleasant sensation that is produced in response to normal stimuli.

- **dysfunction**
  A system or organ doesn't work or function as it should.

- **dysgenesis**
  Defective or abnormal formation of an organ mainly during embryonic development.

- **dyskeratosis**
  Abnormal or premature keratinization of epithelial cells.

- **dyskinesia**
  A physical condition caused by partial impairment of the coordination of voluntary muscles, which results in obvious clumsy movements and poor physical control.

- **dysmorphology**
  The clinical study of malformation syndromes

- **dysostosis**
  Defective formation of bone.

- **dysphagia**
  Difficult or painful swallowing.

- **dysphasia**
  Lack of coordination in speech, and failure to arrange words in an understandable way; due to brain lesion. Aphasia is the complete or near complete absence of speech, and is used to describe a more severe situation than dysphasia.

- **dyspraxia**
  Inability to perform coordinated movements, especially speech, with no apparent problem in the muscles or nerves.

- **dystomia**
  Abnormally small mouth.

- **dystonia**
  Acute tonic muscular spasms, often of the tongue, jaw, eyes, and neck, but sometimes of the whole body. Sometimes occurs during the first few days of antipsychotic drug administration.

- **dystrophy**
  A disorder, usually congenital, of the structure or functions of an organ or tissue.

- **e (exit site)**
  Site on the ribosome through which tRNAs pass after they have donated their amino acid to the growing nascent polypeptide chain.

- **ecdysone**
  A moulting hormone in insects.

- **echocardiogram**
  Test in which pulses of sound are sent into the chest; the echoes returning from the heart produce images that are recorded.

- **ecogenetic disorder**
  A disorder resulting from the interaction of a common

environmental factor with a specific genetic predisposition, e.g., cigarette smoking causing emphysema in alpha- antitrypsin deficiency.

- **ectodermal**
  Referring to the outermost layer of cells of an organism.
- **ectopia**
  Congenital displacement or malposition of any organ or body part; an organ situated in an unusual place.
- **ectopia cordis**
  Congenital condition in which the heart is exposed on the chest wall due to maldevelopment of the sternum and pericardium.
- **ectopia lentis**
  Displacement of the lens of the eye.
- **ectopic**
  Abnormal placement, such as of a fertilized egg in a fallopian tube.
- **ectopic expression**
  The occurrence of gene expression in a tissue in which it is normally not expressed. Such ectopic expression can be caused by the juxtaposition of novel enhancer elements to a gene during genetic manipulation of transgenic organisms.
- **ectopic integration**
  In a transgenic organism, the insertion of an introduced gene (transgene) at a site other than its usual locus.
- **eczema**
  Non-contagious disease of the skin characterized by redness, itching, scaling and lesions with discharge. Frequently becomes encrusted. Eczema primarily affects young children. The underlying cause is usually an allergy to many things, including foods, wool, skin lotions. The disorder may begin in month-old babies. It usually subisdes by age 3 but may flare again at age 10 to 12 and last through puberty.
- **edema**
  A swelling or puffiness of some part of the body such as the ankles. Water or other body fluids collect in the cells and cause the swelling.
- **electrocardiogram (e.c.g. or e.k.g.)**
  A graphic record of electrical activity within the heart; typically used to diagnose various heart conditions or to confirm a diagnosis of heart attack.
- **electroencephalogram (e.e.g.)**
  A record of the activity and types of brain waves illustrated as a graph.
- **electrolytes**
  An element which uses ions to conduct normal electrical current in the body.

- **electromyogram (e.m.g.)**
An electrical test of muscle contraction.

- **electron transport chain (etc)**
Also known as the respiratory chain: The mitochondrial enzymes (also known as complexes I, II, III and IV) that are needed to generate the electron and proton "gradient" that is utilized by complex V to generate ATP.

- **electronic fetal monitor**
A machine that continuously records fetal heartbeat or maternal uterine contractions. It may be attached externally to a woman's abdomen by two belts or through the vagina with an electrode on the baby's scalp.

- **electrophoresis**
A method of separating large molecules (such as DNA fragments or proteins) from a mixture of similar molecules. An electric current is passed through a medium containing the mixture, and each kind of molecule travels through the medium at a different rate, depending on its electrical charge and size. Agarose and acrylamide gels are the media commonly used for electrophoresis of proteins and nucleic acids.

- **electroporation**
A process using high-voltage current to make cell membranes permeable to allow the introduction of new DNA; commonly used in recombinant DNA technology.

- **elongation factors (ef-ts, ef-tu, ef-g)**
Proteins necessary for the proper elongation and translocation processes during translation at the ribosome in prokaryotes. Replaced by eEF1 and eEF2 in eukaryotes.

- **elsi**
Acronym for the ethical, legal and social implications of the Human Genome Project.

- **embolectomy**
The surgical removal of blood clot from arteries or veins.

- **emboli**
Small clots of the blood.

- **embolism**
Obstruction of a blood vessel by a blood clot, air bubble, fat deposit, or other foreign substance.

- **embryo**
Term used for the baby during the first 8 weeks of life in the uterus.

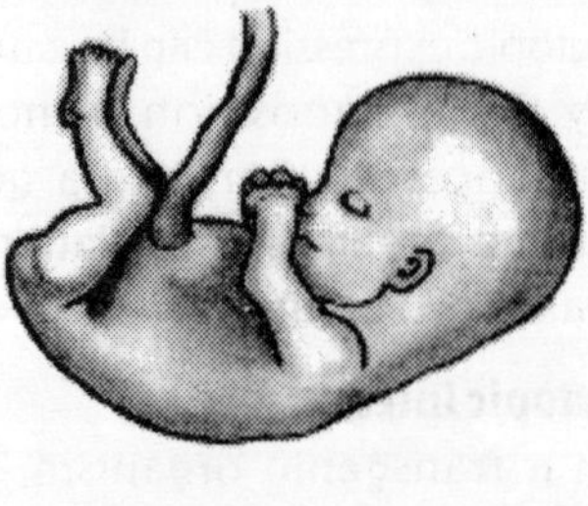

- **embryo biopsy**
Potential method for preimplantation diagnosis of genetic disorders used in conjunction with in vitro fertilization in which cells are removed and analyzed at a very early stage in embryonic development.

- **embryonic (or tissue) polarity**
The production of axes of asymmetry in a developing embryo or tissue primordium.

- **embryonic stem cells**
Cells derived from early embryos that can replicate indefinitely and differentiate into many cell types. Stem cells serve as a continuous source of new cells; they may become incorporated into many tissues to produce chimeric animals when introduced into early embryos, i.e., blastocysts.

- **embryotoxon**
A congenital eye condition in which the margin of the cornea is opaque.

- **emphysema**
A condition where the lungs are unable to perform properly, causing shortness of breath.

- **empiric risk**
Risk of recurrence for multifactorial or polygenic disorders based on family studies (observed risk).

- **en-, endo-**
Prefixes meaning inside or within.

- **enamel**
Hard outer covering of the teeth.

- **enamel dystrophy**
Lack of tooth enamel.

- **encephalocele**
Protrusion of the brain or part of the brain through a fissure in the bones of the skull.

- **encephalopathy**
Any disease of the brain; Progressive degeneration of tissue of the brain.

- **endocarditis**
Inflammation of the lining of the heart.

- **endocrine glands**
Glands that release regulatory substances such as hormones directly into the bloodstream. They affect how the body uses food (metabolism). They also influence other body functions. One endocrine gland is the pancreas. It releases insulin so the body can use sugar for energy.

- **endocrinologist**
A physician specializing in the treatment of the endocrine system, its hormones, and glands, which includes the adrenal glands, pancreas and a number of other organs and glands. Diabetes is an endocrine disorder.

• **endogenous**
Grown or made inside the body. Insulin made by a person's own pancreas is endogenous insulin. Insulin that is made from beef or pork pancreas or derived from bacteria is exogenous because it comes from outside the body and must be injected.

• **endolymphatic sac**
The large bulb-like end of the endolymphatic duct which connects to the semicircular canals of the ear.

• **endometrium**
The inner layer of the uterus.

• **endomitosis**
Chromosomal replication without nuclear or cellular division that results in cells with many copies of the same chromosome.

• **endonuclease**
An enzyme that breaks the internal phosphodiester bonds in a DNA molecule.

• **endonuclease**
Enzyme that cleaves bonds between nucleotides of single- or double-stranded DNA or of RNA at specific sequences of nucleotides.

• **endopolyploidy**
An increase in the number of chromosome sets caused by replication without cell division.

• **endoscopy**
The visualization of the interior of the organs and cavities of the body with a lighted optical instrument.

• **endosperm**
Triploid tissue in a seed, formed from fusion of two haploid female and one haploid male nucleus.

• **end-stage renal disease (esrd)**
The final phase of kidney disease; treated by dialysis or kidney transplantation.

• **enforced outbreeding**
Deliberate avoidance of mating between relatives.

• **enhancer**
A cis-regulatory sequence that can elevate levels of transcription from an adjacent promoter. Many tissue specific enhancers can determine spatial patterns of gene expression in higher eukaryotes. Enhancers can act on promoters over many tens of kilobases of DNA and can be 5' or 3' to the promoter they regulate. A eukaryotic DNA sequence that increases transcription of a region even if the enhancer is distant from the region being transcribed.

• **enhancer trap**
A transgenic construction inserted in a chromosome which is used to identify tissue-specific enhancers in the genome. In such a construct, a promoter sensitive to enhancer regulation is fused to a reporter gene, such that expression patterns of the reporter gene

identify the spatial regulation conferred by nearby enhancers.

- **enteral**
  Through the digestive tract.

- **enucleate cell**
  A cell having no nucleus.

- **enucleation**
  Referring to kidney or pancreas, removal of a tumor with only a small margin of healthy tissue to ensure that all the unhealthy tissue is out. This is sometimes referred to as a lumpectomy, or removal of the tumor (lump) only. In ophthalmology, enucleation means removal of the eye. If the retina has detached, the blood supply to the eye is reduced and the eye may deteriorate, causing discomfort. If this occurs, enucleation of the eye may be recommended. A good prosthesis (artificial eyeball), can bemade to look like a healthy eye.

- **env gene**
  Encodes capsule or envelope protein of a retrovirus.

- **environment**
  The combination of all the conditions external to the genome that potentially affect its expression and its structure.

- **environmental genomics (also called community genomics)**
  The study of communities of organisms in nature using the tools of genomics.Sequencing the DNA of microorganisms found in a liter of ocean water is an example of environmental genomics.

- **environmental variance**
  The variance due to environmental variation.

- **enzyme**
  A protein that acts as a catalyst, speeding the rate at which a biochemical reaction proceeds but not altering the direction or nature of the reaction.

**Mechanism of enzyme activity**

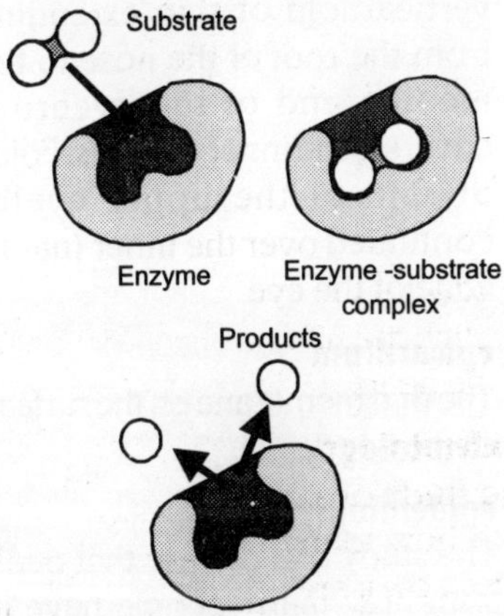


- **enzyme assay**
  Measurement of enzyme activity with a particular substrate; can be assessed in a variety of ways including quantification of the end product or colorimetric analysis ,

- **eosinophilic granuloma**
  A type of xanthomatosis characterized by the presence of rarefactions of cysts in one or

more bones and sometimes associated with eosinophilia.

- **epephora**
  An overflow of tears from obstruction of the lacrimal ducts of the eye.
- **epibulbar**
  Located on the eyeball; Upon a bulb or any kind, specifically, upon the eyeball.
- **epicanthic folds**
  The fold of skin extending from the upper eyelid to or over the inner corner of the eye nearest the nose (the inner canthus); vertical fold of skin extending from the root of the nose to the median end of the eyebrow, covering the inner canthus; Folds of skin of the upper eyelid continued over the inner (nasal) edge of the eye.
- **epicardium**
  The thin membrane on the surface of the heart.
- **epidemiology**
  The study of a disease that deals with how many people have it, where they are, how many new cases develop, and how to control the disease.
- **epidermis**
  The outer surface layer of the skin that contains both squamous and basal cells.
- **epididymis**
  A gland which lies behind the testicle, in the scrotum, on the path to the vas deferens, the vessel which carries the sperm from the testicle to the prostate gland, and is important for sperm maturation, mobility and storage.
- **epigenetic**
  A factor that changes the phenotype without changing the genotype; The study of "environmental," or non-genetic, factors inside cells that influence the ways genes produce proteins.
- **epiglottis**
  The small flap of cartilage that covers the trachea during swallowing so that food does not enter the lungs.
- **epinephrine**
  One of the secretions of the adrenal glands. It helps the liver release glucose (sugar) and limit the release of insulin. It also makes the heart beat faster and can raise blood pressure; also called adrenalin.
- **epineural**
  On the outside of a nerve trunk.
- **epiphyses**
  Growing ends of bones.
- **epiphysis**
  A secondary bone forming centre attached to a bone and separated from it by cartilage.

- **episome**

A genetic element in bacteria that can replicate free in the cytoplasm or can be inserted into the main bacterial chromosome and replicate with the chromosome. Term used by Jacob and Wollman for genetic elements that can either exist independently in a cell or become integrated into the host chromosome.

- **epispadias**

A congenital deformity in which the urethra opens on the upper surface of the penis.

- **epistasis**

Two or more genes acting together to produce a particular characteristic (such as purple flowers) is called epistasis. In this example, the trait being studied is flower color in sweet peas.

**Flower color**

In sweet peas, flower color is determined by two genes, *C* and *P*. These genes both have two alleles (forms): *C* (colored) and *c* (colorless); *P* (purple) and *p* (white). *C* and *P* are dominant – expressed in preference to the recessive ("weaker") forms of *c* and *p* respectively.

**Purple flowers** The plants need a dominant allele of both genes to be able to have purple flowers – that is those with the genotype (genetic constitution): *CC PP*; *Cc PP*; *CC Pp*; or *Cc Pp* will have purple flowers.

**White flowers** Plants that lack a *C* or a *P* allele will have white flowers.

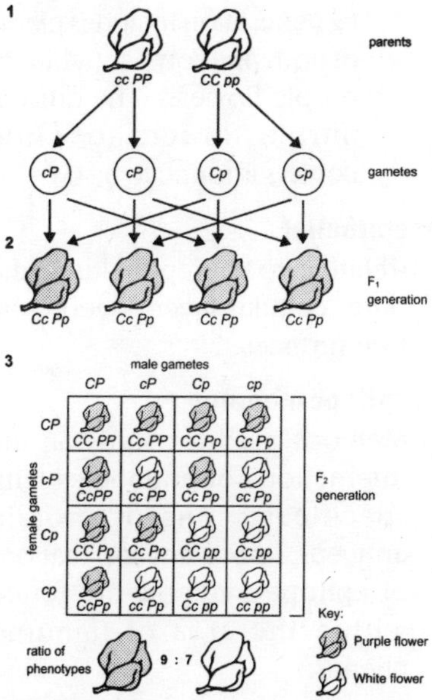


**How flower color is inherited**

1. Parental (P) generation A pure-breeding, white flowered plant lacking a *C* allele is crossed with a pure-breeding, whiteflowered plant that lacks a *P* allele.
2. First (F1) generation The F1 offspring all have purple flowers because they each have a copy of both the *C* allele and the *P* allele. These are called dihybirds.
3. Second (F2) generation The F1 offspring are crossfertilized to produce the F2 offspring. This is called a dihybrid cross. A Punnet square is used to

calculate how the F1 gametes (pollen grains) combine to produce the F2 offspring. The F2 generation includes plants of both phenotypes (white or purple flowers). The ratio of purple flowers to white flowers is found to be 9:7.

- **epithelial**
  Relating to the epithelium, the outer cellular layer covering all free surfaces.

- **epitope mapping**
  Methods used for studying the interactions of antibodies with specific regions of protein antigens. Important applications of epitope mapping are found within the area of immuno chemistry.

- **equational division**
  The second meiotic division is an equational division because it does not reduce chromosome numbers. A nuclear division that maintains the same ploidy level of the cell.

- **equivalence group**
  A set of immature cells that all have the same developmental potential. In many cases cells of an equivalence group end up adopting different fates from one another.

- **erythema**
  Area of reddened skin due to small blood vessels dilating in the skin.

- **erythrocytes**
  The hemoglobin-containing cell found in the blood of vertebrates.

- **escherichia coli**
  Common bacterium that has been studied intensively by geneticists because of its small genome size, normal lack of pathogenicity, and ease of growth in the laboratory.

- **esophageal**
  Referring to the esophagus, the tube from the mouth to the stomach, or more precisely, from the pharynx to the stomach.

- **esophageal sphincter**
  A circular band of muscle where the esophagus is attached to the stomach.

- **esophagitis**
  Inflammation of the esophagus.

- **esophagostomy**
  procedure of draining the esophagus to the outside.

- **esophagus**
  The "Tube" which carries food from the mouth to the stomach.

- **ethics**
  The study of fundamental principles which defines values and determines moral duty and obligation.

- **ethidium**
  A molecule that can intercalate into DNA double helices when the helix is under torsional stress.

- **ethmocephaly**
The least common facial anomaly. It consists of a proboscis separating narrow-set eyes with an absent nose and microphthalmia (abnormal smallness of one or both eyes).

- **ethmoid sinuses**
Air cells or space inside the bone opening to the Nasal cavity.

- **etiology**
The study of what causes a disease; also the cause or causes of a certain disease.

- **euchromatin**
The chromatin that shows the staining behavior characteristic of the majority of the chromosomal complement; A chromosome region that stains poorly or not at all; thought to contain the normally functioning genes. Region of eukaryotic chromosome that is diffuse during interphase. Presumably the actively transcribing DNA of the chromosomes.

- **eugenics**
The study of improving a species by artificial selection; usually refers to the selective breeding of humans; The science of improving humanity by encouraging breeding of those presumed to have the most desirable genes, thereby altering the genetic composition of that society.

- **eukaryote**
Cell or organism with membrane-bound, structurally discrete nucleus and other well-developed subcellular compartments. Eukaryotes include all organisms except viruses, bacteria, and bluegreen algae.

- **eukaryotic cell**
A cell containing a nucleus.

- **euploid**
Any chromosome number that is a multiple of the haploid number

- **euploidy**
The condition of a cell or organism that has one or more complete sets of chromosomes.

- **eustachian tube**
A structure that extends from the throat to the middle-ear cavity and controls air flow between the two.

- **eventraction**
Abnormal protrusion of the intestines from the abdomen.

- **evolution**
In Darwinian terms a gradual change in phenotypic frequencies in a population that results in individuals with improved reproductive success.

- **evolutionary genetics**
Evolutionary study of genes has been purely theoretical, but it can provide useful information for guiding gene mapping. People are

now finding, for example, that a lot of things are not true associations; instead, they are an artifact of association. You can make such mistakes when you are looking at two individuals who share a common ancestry. Understanding the phylogeny helps us, for example, understand horizontal gene transfer between microorganisms. For humans or other sexually reproducing organisms, the use of phylogenetic information improves resolution for making associations by helping to avoid type I errors - that is, finding an association that is actually merely due to sharing a recent common ancestor, or, in other words, being closely related.

- **evolutionary rate**

The rate of divergence between taxonomic groups measurable as amino acid substitutions per million years.

- **ex determination**

The mechanism in a given species by which sex is determined; in many species sex is determined at fertilization by the nature of the sperm that fertilizes the egg.

- **excision**

Surgical removal for diagnostic and/or therapeutic purposes.

- **excision repair**

A process whereby cells remove part of a damaged DNA strand and replace it through DNA synthesis using the undamaged strand as a template. The repair of a DNA lesion by removal of the faulty DNA segment and its replacement with a new segment.

- **exconjugant**

Each of the two cells that separates after conjugation has taken place. A female bacterial cell that has just been in conjugation with a male and that contains a fragment of male DNA.

- **exogenote**

DNA that a bacterial cell has taken up through one of its sexual processes.

- **exogenous dna**

DNA originating outside an organism that has been introduced into the organism.

- **exon**

The part of a gene that contains the code for producing the gene's protein. In humans, exons are often separated by long regions of DNA called introns, or "junk DNA," that have no apparent function. The protein coding DNA sequence of a gene. A region of a gene that is present in the final functional transcript (mRNA) from that gene. Any non-intron section of the coding sequence of a gene; together the exons constitute the mRNA and are translated into protein.

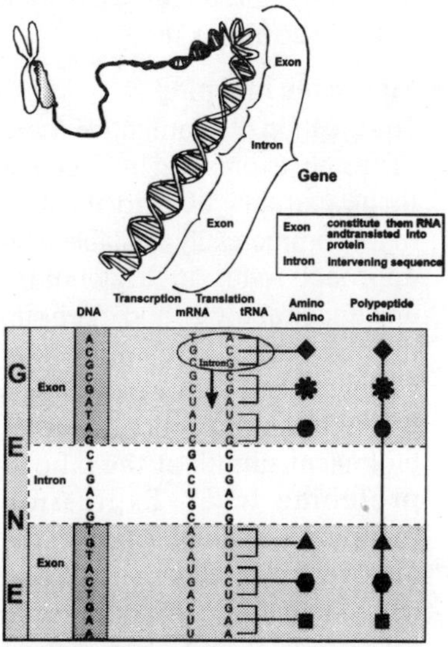


- **exon scanning**

The process by which certain exons (coding regions within a gene), under highest suspicion to contain a specific mutation, are subjected to testing via conformation sensitive gel electrophoresis (CSGE), single-stranded conformational-polymorphism (SSCP), denaturing gradient gel electrophoresis (DGGE), or other means deemed most appropriate, to confirm the presence of a mutation before use of further testing, such as sequencing, to delineate the exact nature of the mutation; used to expedite analysis when the disorder in question can be caused by numerous possible mutations within a gene.

- **exon shuffling**

The hypothesis put forward by Walter Gilbert that exons code for functional units of a protein and that evolution of new genes has proceeded by recombination or exclusion of exons.

- **exonuclease**

An enzyme that cleaves nucleotides one at a time from an end of a polynucleotide chain. An enzyme that hydrolyzes phosphodiester bonds from either the 3' or 5' terminus of a polynucleotide molecules.

- **exophthalmos**

Protrusion of the eyeballs (Bug-eyed).

- **exostoses**

Bony outgrowths or tumors.

- **exostosis**

A bony growth that grows on a bone.

- **experimental design**

A branch of statistics that attempts to outline the way in which experiments should be carried out so the data gathered will have statistical value.

- **expiration**

Letting a breath out; exhalation.

- **exploitation competition**

A form of competition that revolves around the superior ability to gather resources rather than an active interaction among organisms for these resources.

- **expressed sequence tag**

A unique DNA sequence derived from a cDNA library (therefore from a sequence which has been transcribed in some tissue or at some stage of development). The EST can be mapped, by a combination of genetic mapping procedures, to a unique locus in the genome and serves to identify that gene locus.

- **expression**

The observable effects of an active gene.

- **expression imbalance map eim**

A new visualization method, for detecting mRNA expression imbalance regions, reflecting genomic losses and gains at a much higher resolution than conventional technologies such as comparative genomic hybridization (CGH). Simple spatial mapping of the micro-array expression profiles on chromosomal location provides little information about genomic structure, because mRNA expression levels do not completely reflect genomic copy number and some microarray probes would be of low quality. The EIM, which does not employ arbitrary selection of thresholds in conjunction with hyper-geometric distribution- based algorithm, has a high tolerance of these complex factors.

- **expression mapping**

The creation of quantitative maps of protein expression from cell or tissue extracts, akin to the EST maps commercially available. This approach relies on 2D gel maps and image analysis, and opens up the possibility of studying cellular pathways and their perturbation by disease, drug action or other biological stimuli at the whole-proteome level. Expression mapping is a valuable tool in the discovery of disease markers and its use in gaining information in toxicological and drug- action studies seems assured. It is unclear at present how successful this approach will be in elucidating cellular pathways and their importance in disease processes, and how much the precise measurement of protein levels matters when compared with the rough guide provided by the measurement of mRNA levels the ability to measure protein- level changes directly would seem to carry inherent advantages and it seems likely that expression proteomics will be a useful tool in drug target discovery and in studying the effects of various biological stimuli on the cell.

- **expression vector**

A vector that has been designed to express cloned genes in a particular cell type.

- **expressivity**
  The extent to which a gene is clinically evident (expressed) in an individual. Variable expressivity refers to the variation in severity of symptoms produced by the same gene in different individuals.

- **extensor**
  A muscle which causes extension (as distinct from flexion) of a joint, generally meaning alignment of the components, or movement of the distal component towards the back of the body.

- **extraneous movement**
  Any irrelevant movement, such as unnecessary tapping of feet or fingers.

- **extremities**
  The arms and hands (upper extremitites) and the legs and feet (lower extremities).

- **extremophile**
  An organism that lives in an extreme environment such as ice in Antarctica, Chilean deserts, and thermal vents deep in the ocean.Most extremophiles are microorganisms, but a few species of plants and animals, including certain worms and snails, endure extremely harsh conditions.

- **extrophy**
  Congenital condition in which an internal organ is malformed.

- **extrusion**
  Outward displacement of the contents of an organ.

- **f-(minus) cell**
  In Escherichia coli, a cell having no fertility factor; a female cell.

- **f'(prime) factor**
  A fertility factor into which a portion of the bacterial chromosome has been incorporated.

- **f+(plus) cell**
  In Escherichia coli, a cell having a free fertility factor; a male cell.

- **f1 generation**
  The first filial generation, produced by crossing two parental lines.

- **f1 hybrids**
  The first generation of animals generated from two different inbred strains. These animals are genetically identical to one another but different from either inbred parent.

- **f2 generation**
  The second filial generation, produced by selfing or intercrossing the F1.

- **f2 hybrids**
  The progeny produced from matings between F1 animals. These animals are different from one another and will contain different mixtures of the genetic variations that were present in the original inbred progenitors.

- **facet, medial**
  A bony prominence on the vertebral arch which forms a joint with similar projection on the upper or lower aspect of an adjacent vertebra.

- **facetectomy**
  Surgical removal of a facet.

- **facial**
  Referring to the face, the front portion of the head.

- **facial palsy**
  Loss of sensation or the ability to control movement in the facial muscles.

- **facioscapulohumeral**
  Affecting the face, shoulder and upper arm.

- **factorial**
  The product of all integers from the specified number down to one (unity).

- **facultative heterochromatin**
  Heterochromatin located in positions that are composed of euchromatin in other individuals of the same species, or even in the other homologue of a chromosome pair.

- **failure to thrive**
  A group of symptoms when infants or children are not gaining weight properly; A chronic disorder of infancy and childhood characterized by growth failure, malnutrition and variable degrees of the delay in motor and social development. Possible causes of FTT are varied; illness, oral-motor feeding and swallowing disorders, inadequate food resources and problems with parent-child interaction.

- **fallopian tube**
  The channel carrying eggs from the ovary to the uterus; Structures between the ovaries and the uterus through which the egg travels to the uterus.

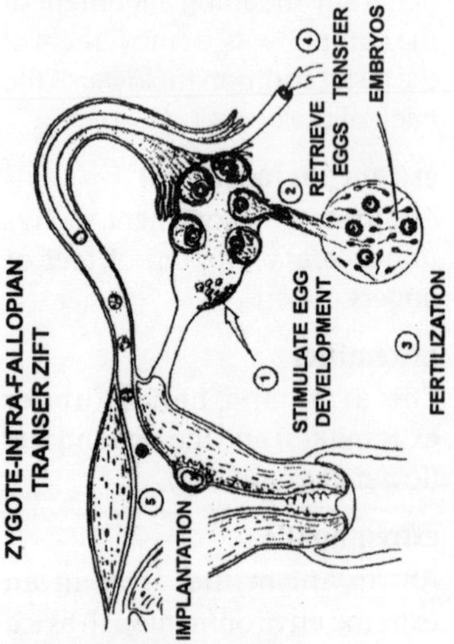


- **false negative result**
  A test result which indicates that an individual is unaffected and/or does not have a particular gene mutation when he or she is actually affected and/or does have a gene mutation; i.e., a negative test result in an affected individual.

- **false positive result**
  A test result which indicates that an individual is affected and/or

has a certain gene mutation when he or she is actually unaffected and/or does not have the mutation; i.e., a positive test result in a truly unaffected individual

- **familial**
  A phenotype that occurs in more than one family member; may have genetic or non-genetic etiology; It occurs in families, whether or not transmitted genetically. It occurs more often in the relatives of an affected person than in the general population; traits that tend to "run in families" (e.g., diabetes, neural tube defects).Chicken pox is considered familial, but is not genetic

- **familial adenomatous polyposis**
  An inherited condition in which hundreds of potentially cancerous polyps develop in the colon and rectum.

- **familial cancer**
  Cancer, or a predisposition toward cancer, that runs in families.

- **familial trait**
  A trait shared by members of a family.

- **family history**
  The genetic relationships and medical history of a family; when represented in diagram form using standardized symbols and terminology, usually referred to as a pedigree; Information about an individual's family concerning its medical background and usually concentrating on the history of disease, birth defects and reproduction.

- **family selection**
  A breeding technique of selecting a pair on the basis of the average performance of their progeny.

- **family-specific mutation**
  In a family, the sequence alteration observed that causes or predisposes to a particular disease; the mutation may be rare or common

- **fanconi's anemia**
  An heritable disease in human beings with a syndrome of congenital malformations (decreased blood cells, short stature, patchy dark skin pimentation, predisposition to cancer especially leukaemia) inherited as an autosomal recessive.

- **fascia**
  Sheet of thick-fiber tissue which surrounds the body beneath the skin. Fascia also encloses muscles. Inflammation of the fascia is referred to as facilities.

- **fate map**
  A map of an embryo showing areas that are destined to develop into specific adult tissues and organs. A map of the developmental fate of a zygote or early embryo showing the adult

organs that will develop from material at a given position on the zygote or early embryo.

- **fats**

One of the three main classes of foods and a source of energy in the body. Fats help the body use some vitamins and keep the skin healthy. They also serve as energy stores for the body. In food, there are two types of fats: saturated and unsaturated. Saturated fats are solid at room temperature and come chiefly from animal food products. Some examples are butter, lard, meat fat, solid shortening, palm oil, and coconut oil. These fats tend to raise the level of cholesterol, a fat-like substance in the blood. Unsaturated fats, which include monounsaturated fats and polyunsaturated fats, are liquid at room temperature and come from plant oils such as olive, peanut, corn, cottonseed, sunflower, safflower, and soybean. These fats tend to lower the level of cholesterol in the blood. See also: Carbohydrate; protein.

- **fatty acids**

A basic unit of fats. When insulin levels are too low or there is not enough glucose (sugar) to use for energy, the body burns fatty acids for energy. The body then makes ketone bodies, waste products that cause the acid level in the blood to become too high. This in turn may lead to ketoacidosis, a serious problem.

- **fecal occult blood test**

A test to check for hidden blood in stool. (Fecal refers to stool. Occult means hidden.).

- **fecundity selection**

The forces acting to cause one genotype to be more fertile than another genotype.

- **feedback inhibition**

A post-translational control mechanism in which the end product of a biochemical pathway inhibits the activity of the first enzyme of this pathway.

- **femor**

The thigh bone, in the upper leg between the hip and knee.

- **femoral**

Referring to the thigh bone.

- **fenestration**

Refers to the surgical creation of a new opening in the labyrinth of the ear to restore hearing.

- **fertility**

The ability to have children.

- **fertility factor (f factor)**

The plasmid that allows a prokaryote to conjugate with and pass DNA into an F- cell. A bacterial episome whose presence confers donor ability (maleness).

- **fetal**

Referring to a fetus, or unborn baby.

- **fetal alcohol syndrome**
  A link between excessive alcohol consumption during pregnancy and birth defects; characteristics include small head and eyes, folds of the skin that obscure the inner juncture of the eyelids, short, upturned nose, and thin lips.

- **fetal distress**
  Change in fetal activity or heartbeat, or meconium-stained amniotic fluid, indicating the fetus is in potential jeopardy.

- **fetal hydrops**
  Fluid retention of the fetus or newborn infant.

- **fetal movement**
  Movement of the fetus in the womb.

- **fetoscopy**
  A procedure for examining the unborn baby using a needlelike camera, which is inserted into the womb to video scan the fetus for visible abnormalities.

- **fetus**
  Term for an unborn baby from the end of the 8th week after conception until birth.

- **fever**
  A fever is a body temperature above the normal of 98.6 degrees F. (37 degrees C.). It is usually measured with a thermometer.

- **fibroma**
  A benign (non-cancerous) neoplasm of fibrous or connective tissue.

- **fibrosis**
  Development of fibrous tissue in an organ.

- **fibrous ankylosis**
  Overgrowth of fibrous tissue in the joints.

- **fibrovascular**
  Degeneration of the fibrous content of the vascular system.

- **fibula**
  The smaller of the two bones in the lower leg between the knee and ankle.

- **fibular**
  Relating to the fubula, the smaller of the two bones in the lower leg between the knee and ankle.

- **fibular head**
  Upper end of the outer bone of the lower leg, felt as a prominence of the outer part of the knee, just below the kneecap.

- **filial generation**
  Offspring generation. F1 is the first offspring or filial generation; F2 is the second; and so on. Successive generations of progeny in a controlled series of crosses, starting with two specific parents (the P generation) and selfing or intercrossing the progeny of each new (F1; F2; . . . ) generation; Each generation of offspring in a breeding program, designated F1, F2, etc.

- **filter enrichment**
A technique for recovering auxotrophic mutants in filamentous fungi (in which non-auxotrophic organisms are filtered off leaving a residue of non-growing auxotrophs).

- **fingerprint**
1. The characteristic spot pattern produced by electrophoresis of the polypeptide fragments obtained through denaturation of a particular protein with a proteolytic enzyme. 2. See DNA fingerprint; In genetics, the identification of multiple specific alleles on a person's DNA to produce a unique identifier for that person.

- **finished dna sequence**
High-quality, low error, gap-free DNA sequence of the human genome. Achieving this ultimate 2003 HGP goal requires additional sequencing to close gaps, reduce ambiguities, and allow for only a single error every 10,000 bases, the agreed-upon standard for HGP finished sequence.

- **first division segregation (fds)**
The allele arrangement (4+4) of spores within an ordered ascus that indicates the lack of recombination between a locus and its centromere. A linear pattern (4+4) of spore phenotypes within an ordered ascus for a particular allele pair, produced when the alleles go into separate nuclei at the first meiotic division, showing that no crossover has occurred between that allele pair and the centromere.

- **first-degree relative**
Any relative who is one meiosis away from a particular individual in a family (i.e., parent, sibling, offspring)

- **fish (synonym fluorescent in situ hybridization)**
A technique used to identify the presence of specific chromosomes or chromosomal regions through hybridization (attachment) of fluorescently-labeled DNA probes to denatured chromosomal DNA. Examination under fluorescent lighting detects the presence of the hybridized fluorescent signal (and hence presence of the chromosome material) or absence of the hybridized fluorescent signal (and hence absence of the chromosome material); A mapping technique that uses fluorescent tags to identify specific locations of chromosomes.

- **fish-interphase**
A technique used to identify the presence of specific chromosomes or chromosomal regions through hybridization (attachment) of fluorescently-labeled DNA probes to denatured chromosomal DNA. Examination under fluorescent lighting detects the presence of

the hybridized fluorescent signal (and hence presence of the chromosome material) or absence of the hybridized fluorescent signal (and hence absence of the chromosome material). With interphase FISH, probes are introduced directly to the interphase cell. Interphase FISH is often used for rapid detection of specific types of aneuploidy in fetal cells and for the detection of certain deletions, duplications and other abnormalities in tumor cells. In contract to metaphase FISH, interphase FISH does not permit visualization of the actual chromosomes; therefore, certain structural rearrangements or aneuploidy will not be detected.

- **fish-metaphase**

  There are over 20,000 living species of fish. They range in size from the .31-in. (7.9-mm) Paedocypris that lives in tropical swamps in Sumatra to the 45-ft (14-m) whale shark. Many are brightly colored, and many have shapes and patterns that serve as camouflage. They are found in all marine, fresh, and brackish waters throughout the world and at all depths. Members of different species of fish tolerate water temperatures ranging from freezing to over 100°F (38°C). With metaphase FISH, cells progress through the division process until metaphase, when chromosomes are condensed and can be individually distinguished. In contrast to interphase FISH, metaphase FISH permits visualization of the actual chromosomes as well as the general location of the abnormality on the chromosome. A number of fishes that are born in freshwater spend their adult lives in the ocean, returning to their birthplace to spawn; the reverse of this migration occurs in some fishes born in the ocean.

- **fissure**

  A split where there is usually no opening.

- **fistula**

  Abnormal passageway that forms between body structures or from a normal body structure to the body surface.

- **fitness (w)**

  The relative reproductive success of a genotype as measured by survival; fecundity or other life history parameters.

- **fixed allele**

  An allele for which all members of the population under study are homozygous, so that no other alleles for this locus exist in the population.

- **fixed breakage point**

  According to the heteroduplex DNA recombination model, the point from which unwinding of the DNA double helices begins, as a prelude to formation of heteroduplex DNA.

- **flanking marker**

  An identifiable, polymorphic region of DNA (i.e., marker) located to the side of a gene (i.e., flanking), as opposed to an intragenic marker which is located within the gene itself. Flanking markers are used in linkage analysis to track the coinheritance of the gene in question.

- **flanking microsatellite analysis**

  The use of highly variable repetitive sequences found in microsatellite regions adjacent to genes or other areas of interest as markers for linkage analysis, DNA fingerprinting, or other diagnostic application

- **flanking sequence**

  A region of a gene preceding or following the transcribed region.

- **flexion**

  Movement decreasing the angle between two bones such as bending the elbow.

- **flexion contracture**

  A bent joint that doesn't extend.

- **flow cytometry**

  Analysis of biological material by detection of the light-absorbing or fluorescing properties of cells or subcellular fractions (i.e., chromosomes) passing in a narrow stream through a laser beam. An absorbance or fluorescence profile of the sample is produced. Automated sorting devices, used to fractionate samples, sort successive droplets of the analyzed stream into different fractions depending on the fluorescence emitted by each droplet.

- **flow karyotyping**

  Use of flow cytometry to analyze and separate chromosomes according to their DNA content.

- **fluctuation test**

  A test used in microbial genetics to establish the random nature of mutation, or to measure mutation rates. An experiment by Luria and Delbruck that compared the variance in number of mutations among small cultures with subsamples of a large culture to determine the mechanism of inherited change in bacteria.

- **fluorescein angiography**

  A method of taking a picture of the flow of blood in the vessels of the eye by tracing the progress of an injected dye, named for the fluorescent contrast dye which is used. This procedure produces an image of the blood vessels of the retina, sometimes in full motion video so that the ophthalmologist can see the health of the blood vessels and how the blood moves through them.

- **focus map**

  A fate map of areas of the Drosophila blastoderm destined to become specific adult structures.

based on the frequencies of specific kinds of mosaics.

- **fokker-planck equation**
  An equation that describes diffusion processes. It is used by population geneticists to describe random genetic drift.

- **follicle**
  Shaft through which hair grows.

- **fontanelle**
  Soft spots in the newborn's head.

- **footprinting**
  A technique to determine the length of nucleic acid in contact with a protein. While in contact the free DNA is digested. The remaining DNA is then isolated and characterized.

- **foramen magnum**
  Passage in the bottom of the back of the skull through the occipital bone through which the spinal cord enters the spinal column.

- **forcepts**
  Surgical instrument used for grasping or compressing tissue.

- **forensics**
  The use of DNA for identification. Some examples of DNA use are to establish paternity in child support cases; establish the presence of a suspect at a crime scene, and identify accident victims.

- **foreskin**
  The fold of skin which covers the head of a penis.

- **formylmethionine(fmet)**
  A specialized amino acid that is the very first one incorporated into the polypeptide chain in the synthesis of proteins in Prokaryotes.

- **forward mutation**
  A mutation that converts a wild-type allele to a mutant allele.

- **founder**
  Refers to animals generated from genetically altered eggs or embryos, is, eggs microinjected with a transgene.

- **founder effect**
  A gene mutation observed in high frequency in a specific population due to the presence of that gene mutation in a single ancestor or small number of ancestors; Genetic drift observed in a population founded by a small non representative sample of a larger population; The high frequency of a mutant gene in a rapidly expanding population founded by a small ancestral group when one or more of the founders were, by chance, carriers of the mutant gene.

- **f-pili**
  Sex pili. Hair-like projections on an F+, an F' or Hfr bacterium involved in anchorage during conjugation and presumably through which DNA passes.

- **fracture**

A fracture is a break in the bone or cartilage. It usually is a result of trauma. It can, however, be a result of disease of the bone, such as osteoporosis, or an abnormal formation of the bone in rare congenital (from time of birth) diseases, such as osteogenesis imperfecta. Fractures are classified by their character and location. Examples of classification include "spiral fracture of the femur", "greenstick fracture of the radius", "impacted fracture of the humerus", "linear fracture of the ulna", "oblique fracture of the metatarsal", "compression fracture of the vertebrae", and "depressed fracture of the skull". Fractures are also named by the trauma event that caused the bone breakage. Examples include "boxer's fracture" of the metacarpal bone of the hand, "blowout fracture" of the bones behind the eye, and "stress fracture" of the bones of tibia. Some fractures are also named by conditions associated with the bone breakage.

- **fracture, compound**

A fracture in which there is an associated open wound of the skin which leads directly to the broken bone.

- **fragile site**

A chromosomal region that has a tendency to break; A non-staining gap of variable width that usually involves both chromatids and is always at exactly the same point on a specific chromosome derived from an individual or kindred.

- **fragile x syndrome**

A frequent genetic cause of mental retardation.

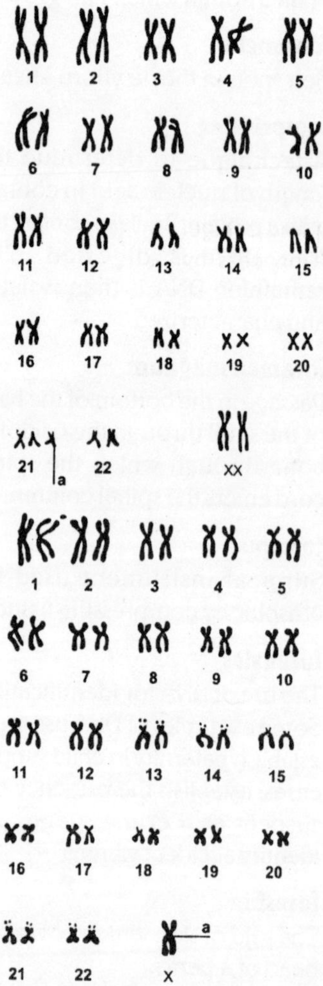

A mutation causes a repetition of the letters CGG in a gene on the X chromosome. The more repeats of this code on a person's X chromosome, the more impaired he or she is likely to be.

- **frameshift**

A mutation in which there is an addition or deletion of one, two or a small number (not a multiple of three) of nucleotides that causes the codon reading frame to shift to one of two others from the point of the mutation during translation. Consequently the amino acid sequence of the protein is altered from the point of the mutation to the carboxy terminus.

- **frameshift mutation**

An insertion or deletion involving a number of base pairs that is not a multiple of three and consequently disrupts the triplet reading frame, usually leading to the creation of a premature termination (stop) codon and resulting in a truncated protein product; The insertion or deletion of a nucleotide pair or pairs, causing a disruption of the translational reading frame.

- **fraternal twin**

Siblings born at the same time as the result of fertilization of two ova by two sperm. They share the same genetic relationship to each other as any other siblings.

- **fraternal twins**

Twins that develop from two fertilized eggs and develop in two placentas. Many times such twins do not resemble one another closely.

- **free-floating cecum**

A blind pouch at the beginning of the large intestine.

- **frenectomy**

Surgical removal of excess tissue in the mouth, under the upper lip between the two front teeth.

- **frenula**

Restraining portion or structure.

- **frenulae**

Fold of skin that attaches the lip to the gums.

- **frenulum**

A shorter than average connection between the floor of the mouth and the underside of the tongue.

- **frequency histogram**

A step curve in which the frequencies of various arbitrarily bounded classes are graphed.

- **frequency-dependent fitness**

Fitness differences whose intensity changes with changes in the relative frequency of genotypes in the population.

- **frequency-dependent selection**

Selection that involves frequency-dependent fitness. Selection of a genotype depending on its frequency in the population.

- **frequency-independent selection**
  Selection in which the fitnesses of genotypes are independent of their relative frequency in the population.

- **frequency-interdependent fitness**
  Fitness that is not dependent upon interactions with other individuals of the same species.

- **frontal bossing**
  A prominent forehead.

- **frontal lobe**
  The largest area of the brain that lies in the front of the cranial cavity and is important for control of voluntary movement or activity, and cognition and feelings.

- **fructose**
  A type of sugar found in many fruits and vegetables and in honey. Fructose is used to sweeten some diet foods. It is considered a nutritive sweetener because it has calories.

- **fruiting body**
  In fungi, the organ in which meiosis occurs and sexual spores are produced.

- **full gene sequence**
  The complete order of bases in a gene. This order determines which protein a gene will produce.

- **full penetrance allele**
  In autosomal dominant, autosomal recessive, and X-linked disorders caused by nucleotide repeat expansion, an abnormally large allele that is associated with disease manifestations

- **fulminant**
  Rapid, intense and severe.

- **functional alleles**
  Mutants that fail to complement each other in a cis-trans complementation test.

- **functional gene tests**
  Biochemical assays for a specific protein, which indicates that a specific gene is not merely present but active.

- **functional genomics**
  The study of genes, their resulting proteins, and the role played by the proteins the body's biochemical processes.

- **functional maps**
  In addition to the raw data, it will be important to design the proper visualization tools to graphically represent the functional relationships contained in different maps. Finally, it will be important to consider the possibility that functional maps need to be related back to particular tissues or even cell types.

- **fundal height**
  The distance from the top of the pregnant uterus to the pubic bone;

measured to help estimate fetal age.

- **fundamental number**
The number of chromosome arms in a somatic cell of a particular species.

- **fundoplication**
Surgical procedure which ties the top of the stomach around the esophagus to prevent reflux.

- **fundus**
The top part of the uterus.

- **fundus of the eye**
The back or deep part of the eye, including the retina

- **funduscopy**
A test to look at the back area of the eye to see if there is any damage to the vessels that bring blood to the retina. The doctor uses a device called an ophthalmoscope to check the eye.

- **fusion**
The joining of two parts to become a single unit.

- **gain-of-function dominant**
A mutation in which dominance is caused by changing the specificity or expression pattern of a gene or gene product, rather than simply by reducing or eliminating the normal activity of that gene or gene product.

- **gait**
A particular pattern or style in which a person walks.

- **galactose**
A type of sugar found in milk products and sugar beets. It is also made by the body. It is considered a nutritive sweetener because it has calories.

- **gallbladder**
A pear-shaped organ located under the liver that stores bile and then releases it into the small intestine.

- **gamete**
Mature male or female reproductive cell (sperm or ovum) with a haploid set of chromosomes (23 for humans); An haploid cell.gel electrophoresis the process by which nucleic acids (DNA or RNA) or proteins are separated by size according to movement of the charged molecules in an electrical field; A germ cell having a haploid chromosome complement. Gametes from parents of opposite sexes fuse to form zygotes. A specialized haploid cell that fuses with a gamete from the opposite sex or mating type to form a diploid zygote; in mammals, an egg or a sperm.

- **gametic selection**
The forces acting to cause differential reproductive success of one allele over another in a heterozygote.

- **gametogenesis**
The meiotic process by which mature gametes (ova and sperm)

are formed. Oogenesis refers specifically to the production of ova and spermatogenesis to the production of sperm.

- **gametophyte**

  The haploid stage of a plant life cycle that produces gametes (by mitosis). It alternates with a diploid sporophyte generation. The haploid gamete-producing stage in the life cycle of plants; prominent and independent in some species but reduced or parasitic in others.

- **gamette**

  An ovum (egg) or sperm.

- **gamma globulin**

  A protein found in the blood that helps fight infection.

- **gangrene**

  The death of body tissue. It is most often caused by a loss of blood flow, especially in the legs and feet.

- **gastric**

  Pertaining to the stomach.

- **gastric atrophy**

  A condition in which the stomach muscles shrink and become weak. It results in a lack of digestive juices.

- **gastroesophageal reflux**

  Backward flow of food through the esophagus after it has been in the stomach.

- **gastrointestinal**

  Pertaining to stomach, small intestine, large intestine, colon, rectum and sometimes the liver, pancreas and gallbladder.

- **gastrointestinal tract**

  The digestive tract, where the body processes and uses food.

- **gastroparesis**

  A form of nerve damage that affects the stomach. Food is not digested properly and does not move through the stomach in a normal way, resulting in vomiting, nausea, or bloating and interfering with diabetes management.

- **gastroschisis**

  A defect in the abdominal wall ususlly accompanied by protrusion of the viscera (internal organs).

- **gastroscopy**

  Visual inspection of the stomach by means of a lighted scope inserted through the esophagus.

- **gastrostomy**

  Surgical opening into the stomach from the outside to enable a feeding tube to be passed.

- **gastrulation**

  The process of movements and infoldings of embryonic cells destined to become endoderm in early animal embryos, immediately following blastula (or blastoderm) stage, generating the blastopore.

- **gavage**
  feeding with a tube through the nose, pharynx and esophagus into the stomach.

- **g-banding**
  Technique for producing banding patterns in eukaryotic chromosomes. Bands are produced by staining with Giemsa stain after pretreating chromosomes with trypsin. Each homologous chromosome pair has a unique pattern of g-bands, enabling recognition of particular chromosomes.

- **gc-rich area**
  Many DNA sequences carry long stretches of repeated G and C which often indicate a gene-rich region.

- **gel**
  A dense net work of fine particles dispersed with water (Jell-O is a gel). Used to separate different-sized strands of DNA.

- **gel-shift**
  An assay used to detect specific protein binding to DNA. Such binding creates complexes that migrate more slowly during gel electrophoresis than free DNA. Also known as mobility-shift assay.

- **gene**
  The fundamental physical and functional unit of heredity. A gene is an ordered sequence of nucleotides located in a particular position on a particular chromosome that encodes a specific functional product (i.e., a protein or RNA molecule); A piece of DNA used by cells to manufacture proteins, which carry out the business of cells.Each human gene is a template for one or more proteins; The definition of a gene is a tricky one. Often, it is defined as a segment of DNA that codes for a functional product, the functional product being either a polypeptide chain or an RNA molecule. But more broadly, a gene can be defined as the fundamental unit of heredity which carries information from one generation to the next. In that sense, it can also include segments of DNA such as those that do not code for any product but rather have specific sequences for binding other regulatory molecules.

- **gene amplification**
  Repeated copying of a piece of DNA; a characteristic of tumor cells; Any process by which specific DNA sequences are replicated disproportionately greater than their representation in the parent molecules; during development, some genes become amplified in specific tissues; A process by which the cell increases the number of a particular gene within the genome. The process by which the number of copies of a

chromosomal segment is increased in a cell.

- **gene chip technology**
  Development of cDNA microarrays from a large number of genes. Used to monitor and measure changes in gene expression for each gene represented on the chip.

- **gene cloning**
  The production of a lineage of cells all of which contain one kind of DNA fragment of interest derived from a population of many kinds of DNA fragments. Operationally by: inserting (recombining) a population of DNA molecules, known to contain the DNA of interest, into a population of vector DNA molecules in such a way that each vector molecule contains only a single DNA molecule from the original population; transforming a population of host cells with the vector DNA recombinants such that each host cell takes up only one vector; growing single host cells separately (cloning) by plating at low density to form a collection of separate colonies; screening the colonies (clones) formed for the presence of the DNA of interest.

- **gene conversion**
  The transfer of DNA sequences between two very similar genes, most often by unequal crossing over during meiosis; can be a mechanism for mutation if the transfer of material disrupts the coding sequence of the gene or if the transferred material itself contains one or more mutations.

- **gene deletion**
  The total loss or absence of a gene.

- **gene dose**
  The number of copies of a particular gene present in the genome.

- **gene expression**
  The process by which a gene's coded information is converted into the structures present and operating in the cell. Expressed genes include those that are transcribed into mRNA and then translated into protein and those that are transcribed into RNA but not translated into protein (e.g., transfer and ribosomal RNAs); The "turning on" of a gene.Most human genes are active, or turn on, only in certain cells under certain conditions.Genes for eye color are active in eye cells but not in stomach cells.Similarly, some genes may lie dormant for years and then turn on and become malignant late in life.

- **gene expression profiling**
  A technique for classifying cells, such as tumor cells, based on the activity of their genes.Research physicians use the technique in diagnosing disease and in

selecting therapies for patients.Eventually this technique may be useful in the general practice of medicine.

- **gene families**

  Groups of closely related genes that make similar products; A set of genes in one genome all descended from the same ancestral gene. A group of genes that has arisen by duplication of an ancestral gene. The genes in the family may or may not have diverged from each other.

- **gene flow**

  The movement of genes from one population to another by way of interbreeding of individuals in the two populations.

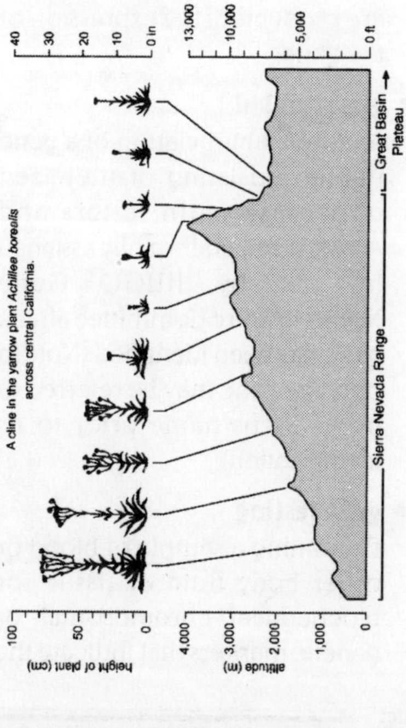


Gradual diffusion of genes from one population to another, as a result of migration and intermarriages.

- **gene fusion**

  The accidental joining of DNA of two genes, such as can occur in a translocation or inversion. Gene fusions can give rise to hybrid proteins or to the misregulation of the transcription of one gene by the cis regulatory elements (enhancers) of another.

- **gene interaction**

  The collaboration of several different genes in the production of one phenotypic character (or related group of characters).

- **gene locus**

  The specific place on a chromosome where a gene is located.

- **gene map**

  A representation of the chromosomal locations of mapped genes, and their arrangement along the length of a chromosome, from p arm through q arm, as deduced from genetic recombination experiments; Determination of the relative positions of genes on a DNA molecule (chromosome or plasmid) and of the distance, in linkage units or physical units, between them.

- **gene markers**

  Landmarks for a target gene, either detectable traits that are inherited along with the gene, or distinctive segments of DNA.

- **gene markers**

  Landmarks for a target gene, either detectable traits that are inherited along with the gene, or distinctive segments of DNA.

- **gene mutation**

  Mutation (point or larger change) that results from changes within the structure of a gene.

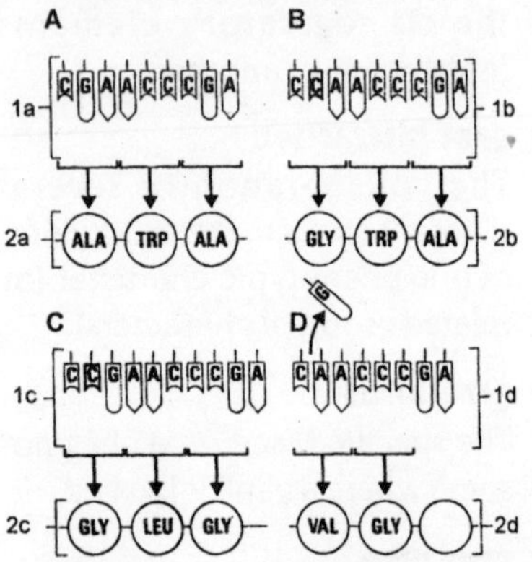


A Normal DNA and polypeptide
B Substitution
C Insertion
D Deletion
1 DNA
1a Normal DNA
1b DNA with base substituted
1c DNA with base inserted
1d DNA with base deleted
2 Polypeptide chains
2a Normal polypeptide chains
2b Mutant polypeptide chains
2c Mutant polypeptide chains
2d Mutant polypeptide chains

- **gene pair**

  The two copies of a particular gene present in a diploid cell (one in each chromosome set).

- **gene pool**

  All the variations of genes in a species; All of the alleles available among the reproductive members of a population from which gametes can be drawn.

- **gene prediction**

  Predictions of possible genes made by a computer program based on how well a stretch of DNA sequence matches known gene sequences.

- **gene product**

  The biochemical material, either RNA or protein, resulting from expression of a gene. The amount of gene product is used to measure how active a gene is; abnormal amounts can be correlated with disease-causing alleles; Genes are transcribed into segments of RNA (ribonucleic acid), which are translated into proteins. Both RNA and proteins are products of the expression of the gene.

- **gene symbol**

  A unique abbreviation of a gene name consisting of italicized uppercase Latin letters and Arabic numbers formally assigned by the by HUGO Gene Nomenclature Committee after a gene has been identified (Note: a putative gene may be referred to by its locus name prior to its identification)

- **gene testing**

  Examining a sample of blood or other body fluid or tissue for biochemical, chromosomal, or genetic markers that indicate the presence or absence of genetic disease; An experimental field of medicine that aims to treat disease by delivering to patients new copies of a gene that is missing or not working properly in their bodies. To date there have been no unqualified successes in gene therapy, and the field has struggled to find safe and effective methods of delivering therapeutic genes to where they are needed in the body.

- **gene transfer**

Incorporation of new DNA into and organism's cells, usually by a vector such as a modified virus. Used in gene therapy; The transfer of genetic material, ranging from a small segment of DNA to the entire genome, from a human cell to another type of cell in culture in order to study the frequency with which known genetic markers are transferred together to the recipient genome; used to determine the physical proximity of genetic markers in the human genome; also used to study gene expression and regulation.

- **generalized transduction**

The ability of certain phages to transduce any gene in the bacterial chromosome. Form of transduction in which any region of the host genome can be transduced.

- **genetic**

Having to do with genes, structures found in every cell of the body. Each gene contains information that directs the activities of cells and controls the way an individual develops.

- **genetic change**

An alteration in a section of a chromosome.

- **genetic code**

The sequence of nucleotides, coded in triplets (codons) along the mRNA, that determines the sequence of amino acids in protein synthesis. A gene's DNA sequence can be used to predict the mRNA sequence, and the genetic code can in turn be used to predict the amino acid sequence.

- The nucleotides (RNA building blocks) **(a)** of mRNA (messenger ribonucleic acid) **(b)** are read in groups of three called codons **(c)**.
- Each codon specifies a particular amino acid **(d)**. This is called the triplet code. Amino acids are the building blocks of proteins **(e)**. As there are twenty amino acids coded for by RNA and sixty-four possible codons, there is more than one codon for each amino acid.
- The codons are read separately and continuously – they do not overlap and there are no gaps between them.
- AUG, which codes for methionine, acts as an intiation ("start") codon **(f)**.

- Three particular codons (UAA, UAG, and UGA) do not specify amino acids, but act as "stop" codons (g).
- The genetic code is almost universal. In most organisms, the same codons specify the same amino acids.

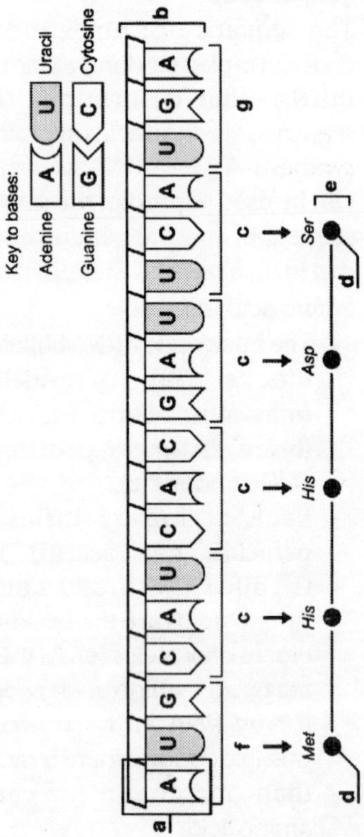


The instructions in a gene that tell the cell how to make a specific protein. A, T, G and C are the "letters" of the DNA code; they stand for the chemicals adenine, thymine, guanine and cytosine, respectively, which are the basic chemical units of DNA. Each gene combines the four chemicals in various ways to spell out 3-letter "words" that specify which amino acid is needed at every step in making a protein. The precise order that spells out these "words" is the genetic code.

- **genetic counseling**

A process, involving an individual or family, comprising evaluation to confirm, diagnose, or exclude a genetic condition, malformation syndrome, or isolated birth defect; discussion of natural history and the role of heredity; identification of medical management issues; calculation and communication of genetic risks; provision of or referral for psychosocial support; The educational process that helps individuals, couples, or families to understand genetic information and issues that may have an impact on them. It helps them comprehend the diagnosis, prognosis, recurrence risks and reproductive choices and to make the best possible adjustment to the condition; A communication process intended to help affected individuals and/or their families to comprehend the diagnosis, prognosis, recurrenece risks and reproductive choices and to make the best possible adjustment to the condition.

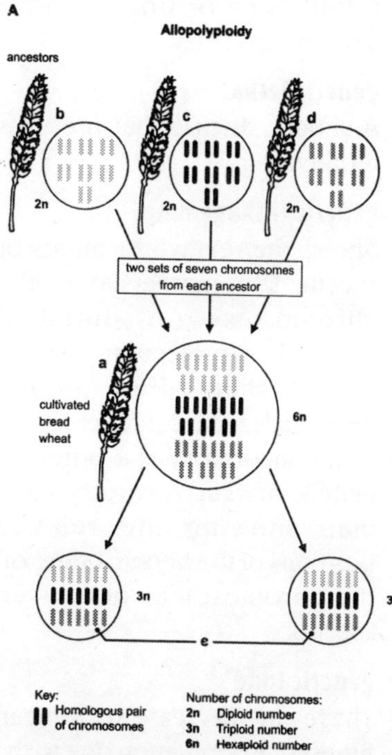


- **genetic counsellor**
  A medical professional (not a physician) specializing in working with patients and families with genetically inherited conditions, like VHL. Genetic counseling may include a discussion and analysis of your family tree and some testing procedures.

- **genetic discrimination**
  Prejudice against those who have or are likely to develop an inherited disorder.

- **genetic disease**
  A disease caused by a genetic mutation that is either inherited or arises spontaneously.

- **genetic dissection**
  The use of mutation and recombination to piece together the various components of a given biological function.

- **genetic drift**
  Random fluctuations in gene frequencies, most evident in small populations.

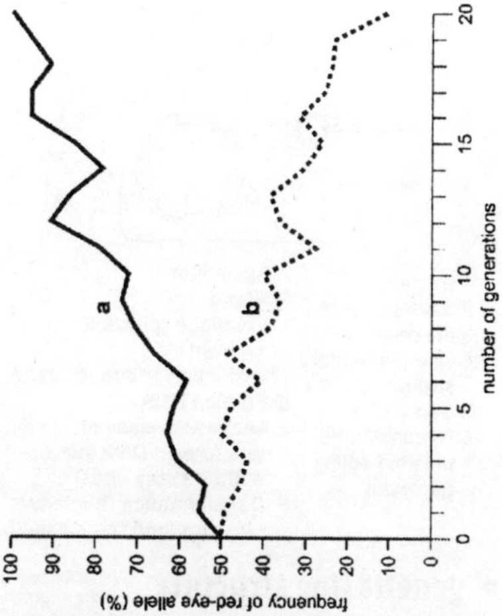


- **genetic engineering**
  Altering the genetic material of cells or organisms to enable them to make new substances or perform new functions; Manufacture, alteration or repair of genetic material by synthetic means; The technology used to genetically manipulate living cells to produce new chemicals or perform new functions; Popular term for recombinant DNA technology.

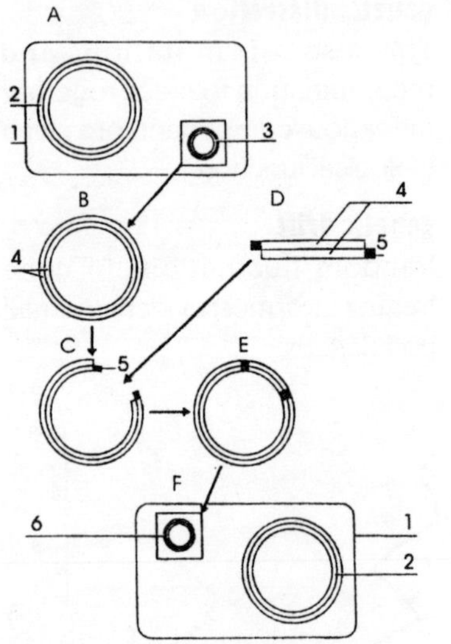


1 Bacterium
2 Bacterial DNA
3 Plasmid
4 Complementary strands of DNA
5 Sticky end
6 Reconstituted plasmid acting as vector

A Bacterium
B Plasid
C Cleavage (plasmid cleaved by restriction endonuclease)
D Foreign DNA
E Annealing (plasmid and foreign DNA join at their sticky ends)
F Transformation (bacterium picks up modifies plasmid)

- **genetic fine structure**
  The structure of the gene analyzed at the level of the smallest units of recombination and mutation (nucleotides).

- **genetic heterogeneity**
  Different mutations causing a similar phenotype; allelic heterogeneity refers to different mutations at the same locus, whereas locus heterogeneity refers to mutations at different loci.

- **genetic illness**
  Sickness, physical disability, or other disorder resulting from the inheritance of one or more deleterious alleles.

- **genetic lethal**
  A genetic disease that prevents fertility.

- **genetic linkage map**
  Shows the relative locations of specific DNA markers along the chromosome. Any inherited physical or molecular characteristic that differs among individuals and is easily detectable in the laboratory is a potential genetic marker; A chromosome map showing the relative positions of the known genes on the chromosomes of a given species.

- **genetic load**
  The relative decrease in the mean fitness of a population due to the presence of genotypes that have less than the highest fitness.

- **genetic map**
  A linear designation of sites within a chromosome or genome, based upon the various frequencies of recombination between genetic markers; Determination of the relative positions of genes on a DNA molecule (chromosome or plasmid); distances are measured in linkage units, i.e., centimorgans (cM), between them; Also known as a linkage map. A chromosome map of a species that shows the position of its known genes and/or markers relative to each other,

rather than as specific physical points on each chromosome. The value of the genetic map is that an inherited disease can be located on the map by following the inheritance of a DNA marker present in affected individuals (but absent in unaffected individuals), even though the molecular basis of the disease may not yet be understood nor the responsible gene identified. Genetic maps have been used to find the exact chromosomal location of several important disease genes, including cystic fibrosis, sickle cell disease, Tay-Sachs disease, fragile X syndrome, and myotonic dystrophy.

- **genetic marker**
  A gene or other identifiable portion of DNA whose inheritance can be followed; Allele, DNA marker or cytogenetic marker used as experimental probe to keep track of an individual, a tissue, a cell, a nucleus, a chromosome, or a gene.

- **genetic mosaic**
  An organism in which different cells contain different genetic sequence. This can be the result of a mutation during development or fusion of embryos at an early developmental stage.

- **genetic polymorphism**
  Difference in DNA sequence among individuals, groups, or populations (e.g., genes for blue eyes versus brown eyes).

- **genetic polymorphism**
  The occurrence together in the same population of more than one allele or genetic marker at the same locus with the least frequent allele or marker occurring more frequently than can be accounted for by mutation alone.

- **genetic predisposition**
  Susceptibility to a genetic disease. May or may not result in actual development of the disease; Increased susceptibility to a particular disease due to the presence of one or more gene mutations associated with an increased risk for the disease and/ or a family history that indicates an increased risk for the disease

- **genetic screening**
  Testing a group of people to identify individuals at high risk of having or passing on a specific genetic disorder.

- **genetic testing**
  Analyzing an individual's genetic material to determine predisposition to a particular health condition or to confirm a diagnosis of genetic disease.

- **genetic variance**
  Phenotypic variance resulting from the presence of different genotypes in the population.

- **genetic variation**
  A phenotypic variance of a trait in a population attributed to genetic heterogeneity.

- **geneticist**

  A geneticist is a scientist specializing in the study of genes and the way they influence our health and in treatment of genetic disorders.

- **genic balance theory**

  The theory of Bridges that the sex of a fruit fly is determined by the relative number of X chromosomes and autosomal sets.

- **genitals**

  The male or female reproductive organs.

- **genito-urinary**

  Relating to the organs of reproduction and urination.

- **genome**

  All the genetic material in the chromosomes of a particular organism; its size is generally given as its total number of base pairs; A collection of genes.The human genome is the collection of human genes, just as the dog genome is the collection of dog genes.All living things have genomes.Plants, animals and bacteria included.A genome contains the biological information for building, running, and maintaining an organism—and for passing life on to the next generation.Nearly every cell in your body contains a complete copy of your genome; so, in fact, you actually have a trillion genomes because scientists believe the human body contains about a trillion cells.The German botanist Hans Winkler coined the term genome in 1920 by combining the words GENE and chromosome.A precise definition of genome is "all the DNA in a cell" because this includes not only genes but also DNA that is not part of a gene, or non-coding DNA; All the genetic material in the chromosomes of a particular organism. The human genome consists of three billion bases, organized in about 100,000 genes on 23 chromosomes; All the genes carried by a single gamete, individual, population or species.

- **genome control maps**

  Would identify all the components of the transcriptional machinery that have roles at any particular promoter and' the contribution that specific components make to coordinate regulation of genes. The map will facilitate modeling of the molecular mechanisms that regulate gene expression and implicate components of the transcription apparatus in functional interactions with gene-specific regulators.

- **genome fingerprint map**

  The collection of all fingerprint clone contigs placed in a genome-wide map.

- **genome map**

  A reconstruction of the entire set of chromosomes for a given organism, showing the relative position of every gene.

- **genome project**
  Research and technology-development effort aimed at mapping and sequencing the genome of human beings and certain model organisms.

- **genome scale metabolic maps**
  Annotated genomic data, along with legacy data on the cell's biochemistry and physiology, can be used to construct genome-scale metabolic maps. The challenge now is to formulate reliable mathematical descriptions of the integrated function of these maps. It has proven difficult, if not impossible, to formulate detailed theory-based models of these genome-scale maps. An alternative approach that is data driven and constraints based will be described. It is an iterative model-building process.

- **genome sequence**
  The sequence of consecutive DNA "letters" spanning all the chromosomes of a cell from start to finish.

- **genomic cartography**
  Fry's research focuses on methods of visualizing large amounts of data from dynamic information sources. The work uses ideas from distributed and adaptive systems to form organic representations that react and respond to the input data. This work is currently directed towards Genomic Cartography which is a study into new methods to represent the data found in the human genome.

- **genomic library**
  A collection of clones made from a set of randomly generated overlapping DNA fragments that represent the entire genome of an organism; A set of cloned fragments representing the entire genome of an organism.

- **genomic mapping**
  While a few technologies for functional analysis on a genomic basis are being developed at present, additional approaches and technologies for genomic interpretation that can be applied efficiently and economically at the level of an entire genome will be required for comprehensive analyses. Informatics will continue to play an important role in achieving all of these goals, as well as in ensuring the maintenance and accessibility of the forthcoming data. The development and application of new technologies for acquisition, management, analysis, and dissemination of genomic data are still required.

- **genomic microarray analysis**
  Array-based comparative genomic hybridization allows the

simultaneous detection of submicroscopic DNA copy number changes at various loci throughout the genome

- **genomics**

The study of genes and their function; The study of large numbers of genes, or genomes.Genetics, by contrast, tends to focus on one gene at a time.

- **genophore**

The chromosome (genetic material) of prokaryotes and viruses.

- **genotype**

The genetic constitution of an organism, as distinguished from its physical appearance (its phenotype); the actual genes carried by an individual (as distinct from phenotype Ñ that is, the physical characteristics into which genes are translated); The specific pair of alleles (copies of the gene) that an individual possesses at a given gene locus or site (two copies of each gene). One of these alleles (copies) is inherited from the mother, the other from the father. Also, the genetic composition of an organism or individual, as distinct from phenotype - that is, the physical characteristics into which genes are translated. In karyotyping, the genotype is designated 46, XX for normal females and 46, XY for normal males. (46 refers to the total number of chromosomes: one pair of each chromosome numbers 1 through 22 plus a pair of sex chromosomes, X and Y); Testing that reveals the specific alleles inherited by an individual; particularly useful for situations in which more than one genotypic combination can produce the same clinical presentation, as in the ABO blood group, where both the AO and AA genotypes yield type A blood

- **genu valgum**

Knock-kneed (genu= knee, valgus= bent inward).

- **genu varum**

Bow-legged (genu= knee, varum= bent outward).

- **germ cell**

Sperm and egg cells and their precursors. Germ cells are haploid and have only one set of chromosomes (23 in all), while all other cells have two copies (46 in all); A sex cell or gamete (egg or spermatozoan).Haldane equation Haldane's law: the generalization that if first generation hybrids are produced between two species, but one sex is absent, rare, or sterile, that sex is the heterogamic sex; The reproductive cells of the body, either egg or sperm cells.

- **germ line**

The continuation of a set of genetic information from one generation to the next.

- **germ line gene therapy**
An experimental process of inserting genes into germ cells or fertilized eggs to cause a genetic change that can be passed on to offspring. May be used to alleviate effects associated with a genetic disease.

- **germ line theory**
A theory to account for the high degree of antibody variability found in population. The germ-line theory suggests that every B lymphocyte has all the genes for every type of immunoglobulin but transcribes only one.

- **germinal mutation**
Mutation occurring in cells that are destined to develop into gametes.

- **germline mosaicism**
Two or more genetic or cytogenetic cell lines confined to the precursor (germline) cells of the egg or sperm; formerly called gonadal mosaicism

- **germline mutation**
The presence of an altered gene within the egg or sperm (germ cell), such that the altered gene can be passed to subsequent generations; A gene change in the body's reproductive cells (egg or sperm) that becomes incorporated in the DNA of every cell in the body; also called Hereditary mutation.

- **gestation**
The length of pregnancy; the developmental time before birth.

- **gestational diabetes mellitus (gdm)**
A type of diabetes mellitus that can occur when a woman is pregnant. In the second half of the pregnancy, the woman may have glucose (sugar) in the blood at a higher than normal level. However, when the pregnancy ends, the blood glucose levels return to normal in about 95 percent of all cases.

- **giemsa stain**
A complex of stains specific for the phosphate groups of DNA.

- **gingival hyperplasia**
Excessive proliferation of gum tissue.

- **glabella**
A smooth prominance.

- **gland**
1. An organ that produces a hormone or other secretion. 2. Glands are groups of cells that make substances enabling body functions. "Glands" generally refer to secreting glands and lymph nodes. Secreting glands manufacture and release chemical substances such as hormones and enzymes. Lymph nodes play an important part in fighting infections; A group of

special cells that make substances so that other parts of the body can work. For example, the pancreas is a gland that releases insulin so that other body cells can use glucose (sugar) for energy.

- **glaucoma**
A disorder in the eye characterized by high pressure inside the eyeball; An eye disease associated with increased pressure within the eye. Glaucoma can damage the optic nerve and cause impaired vision and blindness.

- **gliomia**
A tumor of the brain.

- **globulin**
A category of blood proteins.

- **glottis**
The middle part of the larynx; the area where the vocal cords are located.

- **glucose**
A simple sugar found in the blood. It is the body's main source of energy; also known as dextrose.

- **glucose tolerance test**
A test to see if a person has diabetes. The test is given in a lab or doctor's office in the morning before the person has eaten. A first sample of blood is taken from the person. Then the person drinks a liquid that has glucose (sugar) in it. After one hour, a second blood sample is drawn, and, after another hour, a third sample is taken. The object is to see how well the body deals with the glucose in the blood over time.

- **gluten**
A sticky substance found in wheat flour, indigestible by some people.

- **glycogen**
Form of carbohydrate stored in the liver and muscles vital to human metabolism; A substance made up of sugars. It is stored in the liver and muscles and releases glucose (sugar) into the blood when needed by cells. Glycogen is the chief source of stored fuel in the body.

- **glycogenesis (or glucogenesis)**
The process by which glycogen is formed from glucose.

- **glycosuria**
Having glucose (sugar) in the urine.

- **gonad**
A male reproductive gland; Ovary or testicle, the reproductive organs.

- **gonadal**
Pertaining to the reproductive organs, the ovaries or testicles.

- **gradient**
A gradual change in some quantitative property over a specific distance.

- **graft**
To implant living tissue (skin, muscle, etc.) surgically.

- **grand mal**
  A severe form of epileptic fit.
- **granuloma**
  A tumor like mass or nodule of granulation tissue, with actively growing fibroblasts and capillary buds, due to a chronic inflammatory process associated with an infection or disease.
- **granulomatous**
  Small or granular nodular inflammatory lesions.
- **gravida**
  The number of pregnancies. Commonly see the notation G2P, for example, which means gravida 2 para 1 - two pregnancies with one live birth.
- **gray crescent**
  A cortical region of the newly fertilised egg of frogs and some salamanders that forms just after fertilization on the side opposite sperm penetration.
- **great omentum**
  The great, or gastrocolic, omentum forms, in most mammals, a great sac, which is attached to the stomach and transverse colon, is loaded with fat, and covers more or less of the intestines; the caul.
- **ground state**
  The developmental state of a cell (or group of cells) in the absence of activation of a developmental regulatory switch.
- **group i intron**
  Self-splicing intron that requires an external guanine-containing for splicing; releases the intron in a linear form.
- **group ii intron**
  Self-splicing intron that does not require an external nucleotide for splicing; releases the intron in a lariat form.
- **group selection**
  Selection for traits that would be beneficial to a population at the expense of the individual possessing the trait.
- **g-tube**
  The tube which is inserted into the stomach for feeding, during the surgical procedure called a gastrostomy.
- **guanine**
  One of the four bases that make up the letters ATGC in DNA. Guanine ("G") always pairs with cytosine ("C"); A purine base that pairs with cytosine.
- **guanine (g)**
  A nitrogenous base, one member of the base pair GC (guanine and cytosine) in DNA.
- **guanosine**
  The nucleoside having guanine as its base.
- **guide rna (grna)**
  RNA that guides the insertion of uridines (RNA editing) into mRNAs in trypanosomes. Found in

transcripts from minicircles and maxicircles of DNA in kinetoplasts.

- **gyandromorph**
  Organisms that have both male and female cells and therefore express both male and female characteristics; An individual that is a mosaic of male and female structures. The underlying cause is frequently sex chromosome mosaicism, such that some cells are chromosomal females while others are chromosomal males. Mosaic individuals having simultaneous aspects of both the male and the female phenotype.

- **gynecomastia**
  Abnormal enlargement of breasts in men.

- **gyri**
  Convulsions (wrinkles/crevices) of the surface of the brain.

- **haemangioma**
  An innocent tumour composed of dilated blood vessels.

- **haematoma**
  Collection of blood in the tissues as in bruising.

- **haemoglobin**
  Red pigment in the blood cells carrying oxygen to the tissues; The oxygen-transporting blood cell protein in most animals.

- **haemophilia**
  A disease in which the blood fails to clot. The most common form, primarily affecting males, is caused by a mutation in a gene coding for a clotting protein (factor VIII) inherited as an X-linked recessive phenotype.

- **haemostatic**
  Drug or other agent used to stop severe bleeding.

- **half-chromatid conversion**
  A type of gene conversion that is inferred from the existence of non-identical sister spores in a fungal octad showing a non-Mendelian allele ratio.

- **hamstring**
  Muscles located at the back of the thigh that bend the knee and swing the leg backward from the hip.

- **haplodiploidy**
  The sex-determining mechanism found in some insect groups among which males are haploid and females are diploid.

- **haploid**
  A single set of chromosomes (half the full set of genetic material) present in the egg and sperm cells of animals and in the egg and pollen cells of plants. Human beings have 23 chromosomes in their reproductive cells; Half the diploid or normal number of chromosomes in a somatic cell; the number of chromosomes in a gamete (egg or sperm) cell, which in humans is 23 chromosomes, one chromosome from each chromosome pair.

- **haploidization**
  Production of a haploid from a diploid by progressive chromosome loss.

- **haploinsufficiency**
  The situation in which an individual who is heterozygous for a certain gene mutation or hemizygous at a particular locus, often due to a deletion of the corresponding allele, is clinically affected because a single copy of the normal gene is incapable of providing sufficient protein production as to assure normal function.

- **haplotype**
  A way of denoting the collective genotype of a number of closely linked loci on a chromosome; A collection of variable DNA sequences that tend to be inherited together; A series of known DNA sequences linked on a chromosome. A set of restriction fragment lengths closely linked to one another and to a gene of interest on a particular chromosome.

- **haplotype analysis**
  Molecular genetic testing to identify a set of closely linked segments of DNA; used in linkage analysis or when a given trait is in linkage disequilibrium with a marker or set of markers.

- **haplotype map**
  Francis Collins, director of the NHGRI, speaking at BIO 2001 (San Diego CA, US, June 2001) announced plans for a public-private effort to create a human haplotype map. Creators hope this so- called haplotype map will be a tool for pinning down the genes that contribute to the development of complex diseases such as cancer, diabetes, and mental illness; Is often carried out as part of a genome scan. In a population isolate, the appearance of a rare Mendelian disease is almost always attributable to a single founder gene or mutation. The disease allele can be identified by searching for a common haplotype signature shared among patients. As the ancestral haplotype signature is passed from generation to generation, it is disrupted by recombination. Partial conservation of the haplotype signature in a patient strongly suggests that the disease locus resides in the conserved region of the haplotype.

- **hapmap project**
  An international effort to identify variable DNA sequences across the human genome in different ethnic populations.The project is mapping collections of DNA variations, or haplotypes.When complete, the "Hap Map" will be used to study genetic variations associated with disease and the different responses people have to drugs.

• **hardy-weinberg equilibrium**
The stable frequency distribution of genotypes, AA, Aa, and aa, in the proportions $p^2$, 2pq, and $q^2$ respectively (where p and q are the frequencies of the alleles, A and a) that is a consequence of random mating in the absence of mutation, migration, natural selection, or random drift.

• **hardy-weinberg law**
The concept that both gene frequencies and genotype frequencies will remain constant from generation to generation in an infinitely large, interbreeding population in which mating is at random and there is no selection, migration or mutation.

• **harlequin chromosome**
Sister chromatids that stain differently, so that one appears dark and the other light (harlequin-like).

• **hat medium**
A selection medium for hybrid cell lines; contains hypoxanthine; aminopterin; thymidine. Only cell lines expressing both hypoxanthine phosphoribosyl transferase (HPRT+) and thymidine kinase (TK+) can survive in this medium. Aminopterin inhibits de novo synthesis of nucleosides, while HPRT and TK supply them from hypoxanthine and thymidine.

• **heat-shock protein**
One of a number of proteins appearing in a cell after the cell has been subjected to elevated temperatures.

• **helicase**
A protein that unwinds DNA at replication forks.

• **helix**
External outter ear.

• **helix-turn-helix (hlh) protein**
A protein in which a domain which forms two helices separated by a loop that acts as a sequence-specific DNA binding domain. HLH proteins are thought to act as transcription factors.

• **helix-turn-helix motif**
Configuration, found in some DNA-binding proteins, consisting of a recognition helix and a stabilizing helix separated by a short loop.

• **hemangioblastoma**
An abnormal growth of blood vessels forming a benign tumor; a variety of hemangioma found especially in VHL, in the brain or spinal cord.

• **hemangioma**
An abnormally dense growth of dilated small blood vessels (capillaries), forming a benign tumor. Hemangiomas may occur in the skin or internal organs.

- **hematemesis**
  Vomiting of blood.

- **hemiplegia**
  Paralysis that involves one side of the body in a lateral fashion.

- **hemizygous**
  Having only one copy of a particular gene. For example, in humans, males are hemizygous for genes found on the Y chromosome.

- **hemizygous**
  The situation in which an individual has only one member of a chromosome pair or chromosome segment rather than the usual two; refers in particular to X-linked genes in males who under normal circumstances have only one X chromosome; The condition of loci on the X chromosome of the heterogametic sex of a diploid species. Or more generally when one part of the genome, in a normally diploid species, is present in only one copy.

- **hemizygous gene**
  A gene present in only one copy in a diploid organism for example, X-linked genes in a male mammal.

- **hemodialysis**
  A mechanical method of cleaning the blood for people who have kidney disease.

- **hemophilia**
  A sex-linked disease in humans in which the blood-clotting process is defective.

- **hemorrhagic**
  Referring to hemorrhaging- the loss of large amounts of blood in a short time.

- **hepatic**
  Referring to the liver.

- **hepatomegaly**
  Abnormal enlargement of the liver.

- **hepatosplenomegaly**
  Abnormal enlargement of the spleen and liver.

- **her-2/neu**
  Stands for Human Epidermal Growth factor Receptor-2, a member of the tyrosine kinase family. Multiple copies (amplification) of the HER-2 gene plays a pivotal role in the rapid growth of tumors in 25% to 30% of breast cancers.

- **hereditary**
  Refers to a disease or condition that is passed from parents to child; Transmitted or capable of being transmitted genetically from parent to offspring .

- **hereditary cancer**
  Cancer that occurs due to the inheritance of an altered gene within a family.

- **hereditary mutation**
  A gene change in the body's reproductive cells (egg or sperm) that becomes incorporated in the DNA of every cell in the body; also called germ line mutation.

- **heredity**
  Genetic transmission of traits from parent to offspring; The passing of a trait such as color of the eyes from parent to child. A person "inherits" these traits through the genes; The biological similarity of offspring and parents.

- **heritability**
  A measure of the degree to which the variance in the distribution of a phenotype is due to genetic causes. In the broad sense it is measured by the total genetic variance divided by the total phenotypic variance. In the narrow sense it is measured by the genetic variance due to additive genes divided by the total phenotypic variance.

- **heritability in the narrow sense**
  The proportion of phenotypic variance that can be attributed to additive genetic variance.

- **hermaphrodite**
  Rare condition in which both ovarian and testicular cells exist in the same person; An individual with both male and female genitalia. (1) A plant species in which male and female organs occur in the same flower of a single individual (compare monoecious plant). (2) An animal with both male and female sex organs.

- **hernia**
  A weakness or "rupture" in the wall of an organ, usually through the lower abdominal wall (e.g., umbilical hernia, inguinal hernia).

- **herpes**
  Inflammation of the skin or mucous membrane caused by a virus.

- **heterochromatin**
  Densely staining condensed chromosomal regions, believed to be for the most part genetically inert. Chromatin that remains tightly coiled (and darkly staining) throughout the cell cycle.

- **heterochromia**
  Difference in color of two structures normally alike in color.

- **heteroduplex**
  A DNA double helix formed by annealing single strands from different sources; if there is a sequence difference between the strands, the heteroduplex may show single strand loops or bubbles (unpaired regions); Refers to a region of a double-stranded DNA molecule with non-complementary strands that originated from different duplex DNA molecules.

- **heteroduplex analysis**
  Duplex DNA formed by strands from different sources, referred to as a heteroduplex, will have loops and bubbles in regions where the two DNAs differ. Electron microscopic observation (analysis) of this DNA has been a useful tool in recombinant DNA work.

- **heteroduplex dna model**
  A model that explains both crossing over and gene conversion by assuming the production of a short stretch of heteroduplex DNA (formed from both parental DNAs) in the vicinity of a chiasma.

- **heteroduplex mapping**
  The use of heteroduplex analysis to determine the location of various insertions; deletions; or heterogeneities between two DNA molecules.

- **heterogametic sex**
  The sex with (usually) two heteromorphic (differently shaped) sex chromosomes (for example, X and Y). During meiosis it produces two kinds of gametes in regard to these sex chromo-somes.

- **heterogeneity**
  The phenomenon by which a certain phenotype (or clinical feature) can be produced by different genetic mechanisms; The production of identical or similar phenotypes by different genetic mechanisms.

- **heterogeneous nuclear mrna (hnrna)**
  The original RNA transcripts found in eukaryotic nuclei before post-transcriptional modifications. A diverse assortment of RNA types found in the nucleus, including mRNA precursors (pre-mRNA) and other types of RNA.

- **heterokaryon**
  A cell that contains two or more nuclei from different origins. A cell composed of two different nuclear types in a common cytoplasm.

- **heterokaryon test**
  A test for cytoplasmic organelle mutations (eg. mitochondrial or chloroplast mutations), based on new associations (recombination) of phenotypes in cells derived from genetically marked haploid heterokaryons. Since the heterokaryons are haploid and produce haploid spores by a process that does not involve diploid nuclei normal genetic recombination does not occur. Therefore evidence of recombination is evidence of reassociation by some other means such as reassociation of an organelle with nucleus.

- **heteromorphic chromosomes**
  A chromosome pair with some homology but differing in size, shape, or staining properties. Homologous chromosome pair which are not morphologically identical (e.g., the sex chromosomes).

- **heteromorphism**
  A normal morphologic or staining variant of a chromosome.

- **heteropias**
  Clusters of neurons in abnormal locations, usually in white matter; generally result from a failure of

migration of nerve cells fromthe subependymal region to the cortex. The abnormal faci of neurons may cause seizures.

- **heteroplasmon**
  A cell containing a mixture of genetically different cytoplasms, generally different mitochondria or different chloroplasts.

- **heteroplasmy**
  The situation in which, within a single cell, there is a mixture of mitochondria (energy producing cytoplasmic organelles), some containing mutant DNA and some containing normal DNA; The existence within an organism of genetic heterogeneity within the populations of mitochondria or chloroplasts.

- **heteroploid**
  An individual with an abnormal number of chromosomes (as compared to euploid, which is the normal number of chromosomes).

- **heterotetramer**
  A molecule consisting of four subunits, at least one of which differs from the others.

- **heterothallic**
  A botanical term used for organisms in which the two sexes reside in different individuals.

- **heterothallic fungus**
  A fungus species in which two different mating types must unite to complete the sexual cycle.

- **heterotroph**
  Organism requiring an organic form of carbon as a carbon source.

- **heterotropia**
  When the white and grey matter do not form correctly and the white and grey matter mix up instead of migrate. Usually they move in two distinct layers.

- **heterozygosity**
  The presence of different alleles at one or more loci on homologous chromosomes; A measure of the genetic variation in a population; with respect to one locus, stated as the frequency of heterozygotes for that locus.

- **heterozygote**
  An individual who has two different alleles at a particular locus, one on each chromosome of a pair; one allele is usually normal and the other abnormal; The person only carries one copy of a defective RECESSIVE gene.

- **heterozygote advantage**

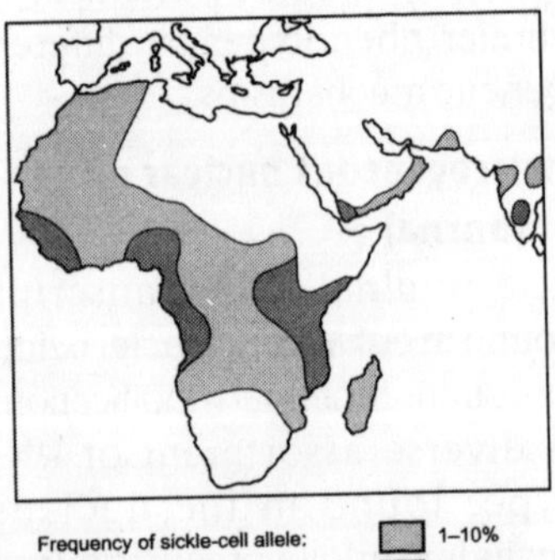

A selection model in which heterozygotes have the highest fitness.

- **heterozygous**

The occurrence of two different alleles at the same chromosome locus.

- **heterozygous dna**

See hybrid DNA.

- **heterozygous gene pair**

A gene pair having different alleles in the two chromosome sets of the diploid individual for example, Aa or, A1A2.

- **heum**

The lowest part or end of the small intestine.

- **hexaploid**

A cell having six chromosome sets, or an organism composed of such cells.

- **hfr**

High frequency of recombination. A strain of bacteria that has incorporated an F factor into its chromosome and can then transfer the chromosome during conjugation. In Escherichia coli, a cell having its fertility factor integrated into the bacterial chromosome; a donor (male) cell.

- **hiatus hernia**

Protrusion of part of the stomach upward through the diaphragm often involved in reflux.

- **hidrotic**

Referring to hydrosis (sweating).

- **high blood pressure**

When the blood flows through the vessels at a greater than normal force. High blood pressure strains the heart; harms the arteries; and increases the risk of heart attack, stroke, and kidney problems. Also called hypertension.

- **high-resolution chromosome studies**

Analysis of the number and structure of the chromosomes when cell division has been arrested and the chromosomes stained at an early stage (pro-metaphase) of mitosis. The chromosomes of a high resolution study appear longer and reveal 700-1200 bands, allowing more detailed analysis of the chromosome structure, as opposed tq the typical 300-600 bands observed with routine metaphase banding.

- **high-resolution genetic maps**

Genetic mapping resolution has been increased through the application of recombinant DNA technology, including in vitro radiation- induced chromosome fragmen-tation and cell fusions (joining human cells with those of other species to form hybrid cells) to create panels of cells with specific and varied human chromosomal components.

- **high-resolution physical mapping**

The two current approaches are termed top- down (producing a macrorestriction map) and bottom- up (resulting in a contig map). With either strategy the maps represent ordered sets of DNA fragments that are generated by cutting genomic DNA with restriction enzymes. The fragments are then amplified by cloning or by polymerase chain reaction (PCR) methods. Electrophoretic techniques are used to separate the fragments according to size into different bands, which can be visualized by direct DNA staining or by hybridization with DNA probes of interest. The use of purified chromosomes separated either by flow sorting from human cell lines or in hybrid cell lines allows a single chromosome to be mapped.

- **high-risk pregnancy**
  A pregnancy is considered high-risk when one of the following occurs; abnormal results are obtained from maternal serum screening or ultrasound, the maternal age is 35 years or older, or there is a family history of genetic disorders.

- **high-throughput sequencing**
  A fast method of determining the order of bases in DNA.

- **highly conserved sequence**
  DNA sequence that is very similar across several different types of organisms.

- **himalayan**
  A mammalian temperature-dependent coat phenotype, generally albino with pigment only at the cooler tips of the ears, feet, and tail.

- **hippocampus**
  An area buried deep in the forebrain that helps regulate emotion and memory.

- **histiocytosis**
  A condition marked by the abnormal appearance of histiocytes (macrophages) in the blood.

- **histocompatibility antigen**
  Antigen that determines acceptance or rejection of a tissue graft by the immune system.

- **histocompatibility gene**
  A gene encoding an histocompatibility antigen.

- **histone**
  A type of basic protein that forms the unit around which DNA is coiled in the nucleosomes of eukaryotic chromosomes. Arginine and lysine rich basic proteins making up a substantial portion of eukaryotic nucleoprotein.

- **hives (urticaria)**
  A skin reaction that results in slightly elevated patches that are redder or paler than the surrounding skin and often are accompanied by itching.

- **hla antigens**

Proteins on the outer part of the cell that help the body fight illness. These proteins vary from person to person. Scientists think that people with certain types of HLA antigens are more likely to develop insulin-dependent diabetes.

- **holandric trait**

Trait controlled by a locus found only on the Y chromosome. Involves father to son transmission.

- **holoenzyme**

The complete enzyme including all subunits. Often used in reference to RNA and DNA polymerases.

- **holoprosencephaly**

Condition in which the cerebral hemispheres fail to divide properly. Some cases are associated with trisomy 13-15 and other chromosomal defects. This condition involves total or partial lack of division of telecephalic vesicles, optic vesicles, and/or olfactory vesicles. Midline facial defects, such as cyclopia (having only one eye in the center of the forhead).

- **homeobox**

A short stretch of nucleotides whose base sequence is virtually identical in all the genes that contain it. Homeoboxes have been found in many organisms from fruit flies to human beings. In the fruit fly, a homeobox appears to determine when particular groups of genes are expressed during development; A consensus sequence of about 180 base pairs discovered in homeotic genes in Drosophila. Also found in other develop-mentally important genes from yeast to human beings. A family of quite similar 180base-pair DNA sequences that encode a polypeptide sequence called a homeo-domain, a sequence-specific DNA binding sequence. While the homeobox was first discovered in all homeotic genes, it is now known to encode a much more widespread DNA-binding motif.

- **homeo-domain**

An approximately sixty-amino acid protein domain translated from the homeo-box. A highly conserved family of protein domain sequences 60 amino acids in length found within a large number of transcription factors that can form a helix-turn-helix structure and bind DNA in a sequence-specific manner.

- **homeologous chromosomes**

Partially homologous chromosomes, usually indicating some original ancestral homology.

- **homeosis**

The replacement of one body part by another. Homeosis can be caused by environmental factors leading to developmental anomalies, or by mutation.

- **homeotic mutations (genes)**
  Mutations (defining genes) with a phenotype in which a given cell develops along a pathway normally followed by a different cell type. Mutations that can change the fate of an imaginal disk in insect development.

- **homogametic sex**
  The sex with homomorphic (similarly shaped) sex chromosomes (for example, XX), producing only one kind of gamete in regard to the sex chromosomes.

- **homolog**
  A member of a chromosome pair in diploid organisms or a gene that has the same origin and functions in two or more species.

- **homologies**
  Similarities in DNA or protein sequences between individuals of the same species or among different species.

- **homologous chromosome**
  Chromosome containing the same linear gene sequences as another, each derived from one parent; The two chromosomes from a particular pair, normally one inherited from the mother and one from the father, containing the same genetic loci in the same order; A pair of chromosomes, one from each parent, carrying genes for the same traits, in the same order. In a karyotype, the members of a homologous pair look alike (e.g., a pair of 1s, 2s, etc.).

- **homologous recombination**
  Breakage and reunion between homologous lengths of DNA mediated in Escherichia coli by products of the genes RecA and RecBCD, and functionally equivalent genes in other organisms.

- **homologue**
  A member of a pair of homologous chromosomes.

- **homology**
  Similarity in DNA or protein sequences between individuals of the same species or among different species.

- **homology map**
  The Davis Human/ Mouse Homology Map, a table comparing genes in homologous segments of DNA from human and mouse sources, sorted by position in each genome. A total of 1793 loci are presented, most of which are genes. The authors did not include pseudogenes, members of multigene families where specific homology relationships could not be determined, nor any other genes for which homology was in doubt. In addition, for 568 of the loci there are provisional

assignments of markers that link the homology map with that of the Gene Map of the Human Genome. These links also provide a rough approximation of the position of markers in the Genethon linkage map. In constructing this table, the authors first ordered genes so as to best maintain order according to both human cytogenetic position and mouse genetic map position. Within these homologous regions, genes were ordered according to the mouse genetic mapping data.

- **homomorphic chromosomes**
Morphologically identical members of a homologous pair of chromosomes.

- **homoplasmy**
The existence within an organism of only one type of plastid; usually referring to genetic identity of mitochondria or chloroplasts; The presence of a single population of mt DNA in the cells of a single individual. This is normal.

- **homotetramer**
A molecule consisting of four identical subunits.

- **homothallic**
A botanical term used for groups whose individuals are not of different sexes.

- **homothallic fungus**
A fungus species in which a single sexual spore can complete the entire sexual cycle.

- **homozygote**
An organism that has two identical alleles of a gene; An individual who has two identical alleles at a particular locus, one on each chromosome of a pair

- **homozygous**
Identical alleles from the individuals who have had children with relatives (see alleles)

- **homozygous gene pair**
A diploid gene pair having identical alleles in both copies for example, AA or, aa.

- **hormone**
Chemical substance produced by an endocrine gland; A chemical released by special cells or glands and transported by the bloodstream to tell other cells or organs what to do. For instance, insulin is a hormone made by the beta cells in the pancreas. When released, insulin tells other cells to use glucose (sugar) for energy.

- **hormone response element (hre)**
An HRE is a cis-regulatory DNA sequence for a hormone that acts by binding to a receptor that can act as a transcription factor, that is a binding site for the hormone-receptor complex.

- **host range**
1. The spectrum of strains of bacterial species that a given strain of phage can infect. 2. The range

of cells that can act as a host to a virus or bacteriophage.

- **hot spot**

A region of a genome exhibiting an increased frequency of some genetic phenomenon such as mutation, recombination and transposition.

- **hotspot mutation region**

DNA sequences of high susceptibility to mutation due to some inherent instability, tendency toward unequal crossing over, or chemical predisposition to single nucleotide substitutions; region where mutations are observed with greater frequency

- **housekeeping genes**

Those genes expressed in all cells because they provide functions needed for sustenance of all cell types.

- **human artificial chromosome (hac)**

A vector used to hold large DNA fragments.

- **human chromosomes**

Chromosome: a very long DNA molecule and associated proteins, that carry portions of the hereditary information of an organism.

a. *Structure of a chromosome (Typical metaphase chromosome)*: A chromo-some is formed from a single DNA molecule that contains many genes. A chromosomal DNA molecule contains three specific nucleotide sequences which are required for replication: a DNA replication origin; a centromere to attach the DNA to the mitotic spindle.; a telomere located at each end of the linear chromosome. The DNA molecule is highly condensed. The human DNA helix occupy too much space in the cell. Small proteins are responsible for packing the DNA into units called nucleosomes.

b. *Stained chromosomes*: Chromosomes are stained with A-T (G bands) and G-C (R bands) base pair specific dyes. When they are stained, the mitotic chromosomes have a banded structure that unambiguously identifies each chromosome of a karyotype. Each band contains millions of DNA nucleotide pairs which do not correspond to any functional structure. Adapted from K.F. Jorgenson, J.H. van de Sande, and C.C. Lin, Chromosoma 68:287-302, 1978.

c. *Karyotype of a male*: The human haploid genome contains 3,000,000,000 DNA nucleotide pairs, divided among twenty two (22) pairs of autosomes and one pair of sex chromosomes.

- **human gene therapy**

Insertion of normal DNA directly into cells to correct a genetic defect.

- **human genome**

The full collection of genes needed to produce a human being; The complete set of human genes - approximately 100,000 total - which together contain information covering every aspect of human physical development and function.

- **human genome initiative**

Collective name for several projects begun in 1986 by DOE to create an ordered set of DNA segments from known chromosomal locations, develop new computational methods for analyzing genetic map and DNA sequence data, and develop new techniques and instruments for detecting and analyzing DNA. This DOE initiative is now known as the Human Genome Program. The joint national effort, led by DOE and NIH, is known as the Human Genome Project.

- **human genome project**

An international research effort (led in the United States by the National Institutes of Health and the Department of Energy) aimed at identifying and ordering every base in the human genome.

- **huntington disease**

A disease characterized by irregular, spasmodic involuntary movements of the limbs and facial muscles, mental deterioration and death, usually within 20 years of the onset of symptoms.

- **huntington's disease**

An adult-onset disease characterized by progressive mental and physical deterioration; it is caused by an inherited dominant gene mutation; A late but variable age onset lethal human disease of nerve degeneration. Inherited as an autosomal dominant phenotype. Shows imprinting individuals inheriting HD from their father show significantly earlier onset than those inheriting a maternal allele. Shows genetic anticipation, in that the severity increase and age of onset decreases in affected individuals of later generations in a pedigree. The HD gene, encoding a protein called huntingtin, has been cloned.

- **h-y antigen**

The histocompatibility Y-antigen, a protein found on the cell surfaces of male mammals.

- **hybrid**

The offspring of genetically different parents; (1) A heterozygote. (2) A progeny individual from any cross involving parents of differing genotypes. Offspring of unlike parents. (3) A duplex polynucleotide formed by hybridization of two single stranded polynucleotides of different origin.

- **hybrid cell**
  A cell formed by fusion of two cells of different origin in which the two nuclei have merged into one. Can be cloned to produce hybrid cell lines.
- **hybrid dna**
  DNA whose two strands have different origins.
- **hybrid dysgenesis**
  A syndrome of effects including sterility, mutation, chromosome breakage, and male recombination in the hybrid progeny of crosses between certain laboratory and natural isolates of Drosophila.
- **hybrid plasmid**
  A plasmid that contains an inserted piece of foreign DNA.
- **hybrid vector/hybrid vehicle**
  An episome or plasmid containing an inserted piece of foreign DNA.
- **hybrid zone**
  Geographical region in which previously isolated populations that have evolved differences come into contact and form hybrids.
- **hybridization**
  The process of joining two complementary strands of DNA or one each of DNA and RNA to form a double-stranded molecule; The pairing of a single-stranded, labeled probe (usually DNA) to its complementary sequence; The binding of complementary sequences of DNA through specific base-pairing of Adenine with Thymine and Guanine with Cytosine.
- **hybridization in situ**
  Finding the location of a gene or gene product by adding specific radioactive or chemically tagged probes for the gene and detecting the location of the radioactivity or chemical on the chromosome or in the cell after hybridization.
- **hybridize**
  (1) To form a hybrid by performing a cross. (2) To anneal nucleic acid strands from different sources.
- **hybridoma**
  A cell resulting from the fusion of a spleen cell and myeloma cell. These cells can be cloned and maintained indefinitely in cell culture and produce monoclonal antibodies.
- **hydramnios**
  Amniotic fluid that accumulates progressively throughout pregnancy.
- **hydranencephaly**
  Cerebral hemispheres are replaced by thin-walled sacs filled with CSF; results from massive destruction after the 12th week of gestation from vascular infections or traumatic disorders. Transillumination of the skull occurs.

- **hydrocephalus**

Abnormal increase of cerebrospinal fluid within the skull; An abnormally large amount of fluid in the skull. A condition marked by dilatation of the ventricles of the brain.

- **hydrogen bond**

A weak bond involving the sharing of an electron with a hydrogen atom; hydrogen bonds are important in the specificity of base pairing in nucleic acids and in the determination of protein shape.

- **hydronephrosis**

Blockage of the urinary tract. A dilation of the branches and pelvic cavity of the kidney.

- **hydroxyapatite**

A form of calcium phosphate that binds double-stranded DNA.

- **hyper**

Prefix meaning excessive or increased.

- **hyperammonaemia**

State where ammonia is present in the blood.

- **hyperbilirubinemia**

An excess of bilirubin in the blood.

- **hypercalcinemia**

Excretion of abnormally large amount of calcium in the urine, as in hypoparathyroidism.

- **hyperextensibility**

Extend beyond normal limits.

- **hyperextensible**

Able to extend beyond the normal limit.

- **hyperglycemia**

Too high a level of glucose (sugar) in the blood; a sign that diabetes is out of control. Many things can cause hyperglycemia. It occurs when the body does not have enough insulin or cannot use the insulin it does have to turn glucose into energy. Signs of hyperglycemia are a great thirst, a dry mouth, and a need to urinate often. For people with insulin-dependent diabetes, hyper-glycemia may lead to diabetic ketoacidosis.

- **hyperinsulinism**

Too high a level of insulin in the blood. This term most often refers to a condition in which the body produces too much insulin. Researchers believe that this condition may play a role in the development of noninsulin-dependent diabetes and in hypertension.

- **hyperlipidemia**

Too high a level of fats (lipids) in the blood.

- **hypermobile**

Increased range of movement of joints as in young children or those with Marfan's or Ehlers-Danlos, or a degenerative joint disorder.

- **hypermorph**

A mutant with more than the normal amount of some gene product.

- **hypernephroma**
  A tumor of the kidney which contains cancer cells. These may also be referred to as renal cell carcinoma (RCC).
- **hyperosmolar coma**
  A coma (loss of consciousness) related to high levels of glucose (sugar) in the blood and requiring emergency treatment. A person with this condition is usually older and weak from loss of body fluids and weight. The person may or may not have a previous history of diabetes. Ketones (acids) are not present in the urine.
- **hyperpigmentation**
  Excess of pigmentation (coloring) in the tissues.
- **hyperplasia**
  Over-production of cells.
- **hyperploid**
  Aneuploid containing a small number of extra chromosomes.
- **hypertelorism**
  Abnormal increased distance between two paired organs, such as unusually wide-set eyes with flattened bridge of the nose. May also refer to other farther apart than normal physical traits.
- **hypertension**
  Increased blood pressure; Blood pressure that is above the normal range.
- **hyperthermia**
  Very high body temperature.
- **hypertonia**
  Increased degree of tone or tension in muscles.
- **hypertonic**
  Having a greater degree of tension or pressure.
- **hypertonicity**
  Increased pressure of body fluids.
- **hypertrophic**
  Increase in the normal size.
- **hypertrophy**
  Over growth or thickening of part of an organ.
- **hypervariable locus**
  locus with many alleles; especially those whose variation is due to variable numbers of tandem repeats.
- **hypervariable region**
  The part of a variable region that actually determines the specificity of an immunoglobulin.
- **hypha (plural hyphae)**
  A thread-like structure (composed of cells attached end to end) that forms the main tissue in many fungus species.
- **hypo**
  Prefix meaning inadequate or insufficient.
- **hypoglycemia**
  Too low a level of glucose (sugar) in the blood. This occurs when a person with diabetes has injected too much insulin, eaten too little

food, or has exercised without extra food. A person with hypoglycemia may feel nervous, shaky, weak, or sweaty, and have a headache, blurred vision, and hunger. Taking small amounts of sugar, sweet juice, or food with sugar will usually help the person feel better within 10-15 minutes.

- **hypogonadism**
  Increased secretion of gonadal hormones.

- **hypomorph**
  A mutant with less than the normal amount of some gene product.

- **hypophosphatemia, hypophosphatasia**
  Low amount of alkaline phosphatase in the blood.

- **hypoplasia**
  Defective or incomplete development of any tissue. Lingual hypoplasia: Incomplete development of the tongue. Mandibular hypoplasia; Micrognathia or unusually small lower jaw, usually accompanied by recession of the chin.

- **hypoplasia, hypoplastic**
  The incomplete or under-development of a tissue or organ. Poorly formed or small.

- **hypoploid**
  Aneuploid with a small number of chromosomes missing.

- **hypospadias**
  A congenital deformity in which the urethra opens on the lower surface of the penis; A defect of the urethra; an abnormal urethral opening on the underside (ventral surface), rather than the tip, of the penis in males.

- **hypostatic gene**
  A gene whose expression is masked by an epistatic gene.

- **hypotelorism**
  Decreased distance between the eyes.

- **hypotension**
  Low blood pressure or a sudden drop in blood pressure. A person rising quickly from a sitting or reclining position may have a sudden fall in blood pressure, causing dizziness or fainting.

- **hypothesis**
  A tentative question that accounts for a set of facts and can be tested by further investigation.

- **hypotonia**
  1. Low, or poor muscle tone (floppy muscles). 2. Damage to any part of the brain, usually including the cerebellum and basal ganglia, resulting in decreased stiffness of the extremities and trunk.

- **hypoxia**
  Oxygen deficiency caused by reduced oxygen carrying capacity such as in aspiration.

- **hypsarrythmia**
A type of infantile convulsion.

- **ichthyosis**
Any of several hereditary or congenital skin conditions; skin of affected individuals has a dry, scaly appearance.

- **identical twin**
Twins produced by the division of a single zygote; both have identical genotypes; Twins that develop from a simple fertilized egg in a single placental sack. Such twins are the same sex and usually resemble one another closely.

- **identity by descent**
The state of two alleles when they are identical copies of the same ancestral allele (autozygous).

- **idiogram**
A photograph or diagram of the chromosomes of a cell arranged in an orderly fashion. See karyotype.

- **idiopathic**
Disorder of unknown cause.

- **idiotypic variation**
Variation unique to an individual immunoglobulin molecule produced by the variable region of immunoglobulin genes.

- **idling reaction**
The production of guanosine tetraphosphate (3' ppGpp 5', magic spot) by the stringent factor when a ribosome encounters an uncharged tRNA in the A site.

- **iliac**
Pertaining to the ileus; an obstruction of the bowel.

- **iliostomy**
Surgical incision creating an artificial opening into the ileum, the lower part of the small intestine.

- **immune**
Resistant to, or free from the possibility of acquiring, an infection.

- **immune system**
The complex group of cells and organs that defends the body against infection and disease; The cells and tissues involved in recognizing and attacking foreign substances within the body of an animal.

- **immunity**
The ability of an organism to resist infection.

- **immunoglobulin (ig)**
A general term for the kind of globular blood proteins that constitute antibodies. A tetrameric protein composed of two identical light chains and two identical heavy chains. Specific proteins produced by derivatives of B lymphocytes that interact with and help protect an organism from specific antigens.

- **immunoglobulin gene**

A gene encoding one of the protein chains (light or heavy) of an immunoglobulin. The germline genes are activated by a special recombination process that joins a number of different gene segments together. In the case of immunoglobulin light chains there are three segments (V variable, J joining and C constant). In the case of immunoglobulin heavy chains there are four segments (V variable, D diversity, J joining and C constant). There are many different V segments (light chains ~300, heavy chains ~500), 4 J segments in both light and heavy chain genes, 12 D segments in the heavy chain gene and 1 C segment in light chain genes, 5 C segments in heavy chain gene. The recombination process appears to be able to join any V with any J (light chain) or any V to D to J (heavy chain). The total number of possible immunoglobulins (i.e., the number of possible light chains times the number of possible heavy chains) that can be generated by this mechanism is thus several 10s of millions (300 x 4 x 500 x12 x 4 = 28800000). It is certain that the number is greater than this because the recombination events themselves are not precise and random loss of nucleotides from each recombining end occurs.

- **immunohistochemistry**

The use of antibodies or antisera as histological tools for identifying patterns of antigen distribution within a tissue or an organism. An antibody (or mixture of antibodies) that binds to a specific protein or other antigen is tagged with a fluorescent chemical or an enzyme that can convert a substrate to a visible dye. The tagged antibody is incubated with the tissue and after washing unbound antibody away the bound antibody distribution is revealed by fluorescence microscopy or incubation with a chromogenic substrate. It is assumed that antibody distribution reflects antigen distribution.

- **immunotherapy**

Using the immune system to treat disease, for example, in the development of vaccines. May also refer to the therapy of diseases caused by the immune system.

- **impaired glucose tolerance (igt)**

Blood glucose (sugar) levels higher than normal but not high enough to be called diabetes. People with IGT may or may not develop diabetes. Other names (no longer used) for IGT are "borderline," "subclinical," "chemical," or "latent" diabetes.

- **imperforatè anus**

Absence of an anal opening- must be repaired surgically may require prior colostomy.

- **impotence**

The loss of a man's ability to have an erect penis and to emit semen. Some men may become impotent after having diabetes for a long time because the nerves or blood vessels have become damaged. Sometimes the problem has nothing to do with diabetes and may be treated with counseling.

- **imprinted gene**

A gene that behaves one way when inherited from the father and another way when inherited from the mother.For example, the paternal copies of some imprinted genes are never "turned on," or activated.

- **imprinting**

A phenomenon in which the disease phenotype depends on which parent passed on the disease gene. For instance, both Prader-Willi and Angelman syndromes are inherited when the same part of chromosome 15 is missing. When the father's complement of 15 is missing, the child has Prader-Willi, but when the mother's complement of 15 is missing, the child has Angelman syndrome; The process by which maternally and paternally derived chromosomes are uniquely chemically modified leading to different expression of a certain gene or genes on those chromosomes depending on their parental origin

- **imprinting**

A biochemical phenomenon that determines, for certain genes, which one of the pair of alleles, the mother's or the father's, will be active in that individual; Refers to the modification of a gene as it is transmitted through the father or the mother. One mechanism may be the methylation (inactivation) of a gene. A biochemical phenomenon that determines, for certain genes, which one of the pair of alleles, the mother's or the father's, will be active in that individual; Modification of a gene or allele through the methylation process. Imprinting of specific genes occurs differently due to the maternal or paternal origin of each chromosome.

- **in situ hybridization**

Use of a DNA or RNA probe to detect the presence of the complementary DNA sequence in cloned bacterial or cultured eukaryotic cells.

- **in vitro**

Studies performed outside a living organism such as in a laboratory; In an experimental situation outside the organism. Biological or chemical work done in the test tube (literally in glass) rather than in living systems; Refers to a biologic or biochemical phenomenon that occurs outside of a living organism.

- **in vitro mutagenesis**
  The production of either random or specific mutations in a piece of cloned DNA. Typically, the DNA will then be reintroduced into a cell or an organism to assess the results of the mutagenesis.

- **in vivo**
  Studies carried out in living organisms; Refers to a biologic or biochemical phenomenon that occurs within a living organism.

- **inborn**
  Acquired or occuring prior to birth.

- **inborn errors of metabolism**
  Inherited diseases resulting from alterations in genes that code for enzymes. Inborn errors of metabolism are now often referred to as congenital metabolic diseases or inherited metabolic diseases, and these terms are considered synonymous.

- **inbred mouse strain**
  A strain of mice that has been maintained by successive brother to sister matings over many generations, e.g., BALB/c and C57BL/6 mice strains.

- **inbreeding**
  The mating of genetically related individuals. Mating between relatives.

- **inbreeding coefficient (f)**
  The probability of homozygosity by descent (having common ancestors). The probability that a zygote obtains copies of the same ancestral gene from both its parents because they are related.

- **inbreeding depression**
  A depression of vigour or yield due to inbreeding.

- **incestuous**
  A mating between blood relatives who are more closely related than the law of the land allows.

- **incidence**
  How often a disease occurs; the number of new cases of a disease among a certain group of people for a certain period of time.

- **incisor**
  Any of the four front teeth in either the upper or lower jaw.

- **inclusion**
  Educational program where the child is included as much as possible in a regular classroom with typical children Program is adapted for success of the student.

- **inclusive fitness**
  The expansion of the concept of the fitness of a genotype to include benefits accrued to relatives of an individual since relatives share parts of their genomes. Hence an apparently altruistic act toward a relative may in fact enhance the fitness of the individual performing the act.

- **incomplete autosomal dominant**
  An inheritance pattern in which the phenotypes observed lie on a

continuum (differing in degree or kind) depending on whether one or two mutated alleles are present

- **incomplete dominance**

The situation in which both alleles of a heterozygote influence the phenotype. The phenotype is usually intermediate between the two homozygous phenotypes. The situation in which a heterozygote shows a phenotype somewhere (but not exactly half-way) intermediate between the corresponding homozygote phenotypes.

- **incomplete penetrance**

The gene for a condition is present in an individual but is not obviously expressed in all individuals in the family that carry the gene.

- **independent assortment**

During meiosis each of the two copies of a gene is distributed to the germ cells independently of the distribution of other genes; Mendel's second rule describing the independent segregation of alleles of different unlinked or remotely linked loci.

- **index case**

The affected individual who brings the family to the attention of the geneticist, also known as the proband or propositus.

- **indicanuria**

Increased urinary excretion of indican, formed during the putrefaction of protein.

- **individualized education plan (iep)**

A written plan that identifies a child's strengths, weaknesses, education and related service needs. Must be reviewed at least annually. Federal Mandate.

- **individualized family service plan (ifsp)**

A written plan to document the family and child's strengths, needs, and the services to be provided to meet those needs. It is developed by the family and a team of early intervention professionals.

- **inducer**

An environmental agent that triggers transcription from an operon; A molecule that induces the expression of a gene.

- **inducible operon**

A gene system, often encoding a coordinated group of enzymes involved in a catabolic pathway, is inducible if an early metabolite in the pathway causes activation, usually by interaction with and inactivation of a repressor, of transcription of the genes encoding the enzymes.

- **induction**

1. The relief of repression for a gene or set of genes under negative control by a repressor. 2. Regarding temperate phages, the process causing a prophage to become virulent. 3. In

development, an interaction between two cell lineages to alter the developmental fate of one or both of them.

- **inductive interaction**
  The interaction between two groups of cells in which a signal passed from one group of cells causes the other group of cells to change their developmental state (or fate).

- **industrial melanism**
  The darkening of several species of moths during the recent period of industrialization in many countries by the spread of a gene controlling elevated melanin synthesis.

- **inexetensible**
  Unable to extend or straighten.

- **infectious transfer**
  The rapid transmission of free episomes (plus any host chromosomal genes they may carry) from donor to recipient cells in a bacterial population.

- **inflammation**
  A by-product of the immune response, the body's protective reaction of tissue to injury or infection, characterized by redness, pain, swelling, heat, and sometimes impaired function.

- **informativeness**
  In linkage analysis, the ability to distinguish between maternally-inherited and paternally-inherited DNA markers (polymorphisms) within or near a given gene of interest.

- **informed consent**
  An individual willingly agrees to participate in an activity after first being advised of the risks and benefits; Permission given by an individual to proceed with a specific test or procedure, with an understanding of the risks, benefits, limitations, and potential implications of the procedure itself and its results.

- **in-frame mutation**
  A mutation that does not cause a shift in the triplet reading frame; such mutations can, however, lead to the synthesis of an abnormal protein product.

- **infusion**
  1. Product that results when a drug or herb is steeped to extract its medicinal properties, sometimes referred to as a tea. 2. Slow and/or prolonged intravenous delivery of a drug or fluids.

- **inguinal**
  Relating or belonging to the groin.

- **inguinal hernia**
  Condition in which a loop of the intestine enters the groin-most often repaired surgically.

- **inherit**
  In genetics, to receive genetic material from parents through biological processes.

- **inheritance pattern**
  The way in which a gene or trait is passed through generations of a family.

- **inherited**
  Passed through generations of a family, from parents to children.

- **initiation codon**
  The mRNA sequence AUG, which specifies methionine, the first amino acid used in the translation process. (Occasionally GUG, valine, is recognized as an initiation codon).

- **initiation complex**
  The complex formed for initiation of translation. It consists of the 30S ribosomal subunit; mRNA; N-formyl-methionine tRNA; and three initiation factors .

- **initiation factor**
  A protein that associates with the small subunit of a ribosome when protein synthesis begins.

- **initiation factors (if1, if2, if3)**
  Proteins (prokaryotic with eukaryotic analogues) required for the proper initiation of translation.

- **initiator protein**
  Protein that recognizes the origin of replication on a replicon and takes part in primosome construction.

- **inosine**
  A rare base that is important at the wobble (3rd) position of some tRNA anticodons.

- **insertion**
  A chromosome abnormality in which material from one chromosome is inserted into another non-homologous chromosome; a mutation in which a segment of DNA is inserted into a gene or other segment of DNA, potentially disrupting the coding sequence.

- **insertion mutagenesis**
  Change in gene activity due to an insertion (of DNA) event that either changes the gene directly or disrupts control mechanisms.

- **insertion sequence (is)**
  A mobile piece of bacterial DNA (several hundred nucleotide pairs in length) that is capable of inactivating a gene into which it inserts. Small simple transposons.

- **insertional mutagenesis**
  The production of a mutation by insertion of one or more copies of a transgene into a host genome.

- **insertional translocation**
  The insertion of a segment from one chromosome into another non-homologous chromosome.

- **inside marker**
  The middle locus of three linked loci.

- **insulin**
  A hormone produced by the pancreas; A hormone that helps the body use glucose (sugar) for energy. The beta cells of the pancreas (in areas called the islets

of Langerhans) make the insulin. When the body cannot make enough insulin on its own, a person with diabetes must inject insulin made from other sources, i.e., beef, pork, human insulin (recombinant DNA origin), or human insulin (pork-derived, semisynthetic).

- **insulin reaction**

Too low a level of glucose (sugar) in the blood; also called hypoglycemia. This occurs when a person with diabetes has injected too much insulin, eaten too little food, or exercised without extra food. The person may feel hungry, nauseated, weak, nervous, shaky, confused, and sweaty. Taking small amounts of sugar, sweet juice, or food with sugar will usually help the person feel better within 10-15 minutes.

- **insulin resistance**

Many people with noninsulin-dependent diabetes produce enough insulin, but their bodies do not respond to the action of insulin. This may happen because the person is overweight and has too many fat cells, which do not respond well to insulin. Also, as people age, their body cells lose some of the ability to respond to insulin. Insulin resistance is also linked to high blood pressure and high levels of fat in the blood. Another kind of insulin resistance may happen in some people who take insulin injections. They may have to take very high doses of insulin every day (200 units or more) to bring their blood glucose (sugar) down to the normal range. This is also called "insulin insensitivity.

- **insulin shock**

A severe condition that occurs when the level of blood glucose (sugar) drops quickly. The signs are shaking, sweating, dizziness, double vision, convulsions, and collapse. Insulin shock may occur when an insulin reaction is not treated quickly enough.

- **insulin-dependent diabetes mellitus (iddm)**

A chronic condition in which the pancreas makes little or no insulin because the beta cells have been destroyed. The body is then not able to use the glucose (blood sugar) for energy. IDDM usually comes on abruptly, although the damage to the beta cells may begin much earlier. The signs of IDDM are a great thirst, hunger, a need to urinate often, and loss of weight. To treat the disease, the person must inject insulin, follow a diet plan, exercise daily, and test blood glucose several times a day. IDDM usually occurs in children and adults who are under age 30. This type of diabetes used to be known as "juvenile diabetes," "juvenile-onset diabetes," and "ketosis-prone diabetes." It is also called type I diabetes mellitus.

- **insulinoma**
  A tumor of the beta cells in areas of the pancreas called the islets of Langerhans. Although not usually cancerous, such tumors may cause the body to make extra insulin and may lead to a blood glucose (sugar) level that is too low.

- **intellectual property rights**
  Patents, copyrights, and trademarks.

- **intensive intermittent claudication**
  Pain in the muscles of the leg that occurs off and on, usually while walking or exercising, and results in lameness (claudication). The pain results from a narrowing of the blood vessels feeding the muscle. Drugs are available to treat this condition.

- **intercalary heterochromatin**
  Heterochromatin, other than centromeric heterochromatin, dispersed throughout eukaryotic chromosomes.

- **intercalating agent**
  A chemical that can insert itself between the stacked bases at the centre of the DNA double helix, possibly causing a frameshift mutation.

- **interchromosomal recombination**
  Recombination resulting from independent assortment.

- **interfamilial variability**
  Variability in clinical presentation of a particular disorder among affected individuals from different families

- **interference**
  One crossover event inhibits the chances of another crossover event. Also known as positive interference. Negative interference increases the chance of a second crossover; A measure of the independence of crossover events from each other, calculated by subtracting the coefficient of coincidence from one.

- **interference competition**
  A form of competition that involves a fight or other active interaction among organisms.

- **intergenic dna**
  The untranscribed DNA of unknown function that makes up a large proportion of the total DNA.

- **intergenic suppression**
  A mutation at a second locus that apparently restores the wild-type phenotype to a mutation at a first locus.

- **interkinesis**
  The abbreviated interphase that occurs between meiosis I and II. No DNA replication occurs here.

- **international snp map working group**
  Identifies and localizes 1.42 millions SNPs in the human genome.

- **interphase**
  The period in the cell cycle when DNA is replicated in the nucleus; followed by mitosis; The cell cycle stage between nuclear divisions, when chromosomes are extended and functionally active. The metabolically active non-dividing stage of the cell cycle.

- **interrupted mating**
  A technique used to map bacterial genes by determining the sequence in which donor genes enter recipient cells. A gene mapping technique in which bacterial conjugation is disrupted after specified time intervals.

- **intersex**
  An organism with external sexual characteristics that have attributes of both sexes.

- **interstitial region**
  The chromosomal region between the centromere and the site of a rearrangement.

- **intra uterine growth retardation (iugr)**
  The failure of the fetus to grow at the expected rate during pregnancy.

- **intra-allelic complementation**
  The restoration of activity or partial activity (complementation) to an enzyme made of identical subunits (polypeptides encoded by one gene) in a heterozygote of two different mutant alleles of that gene.

- **intrachromosomal recombination**
  Recombination resulting from crossing over between two linked gene pairs.

- **intraepithelial**
  Within the layer of cells that forms the surface or lining of an organ.

- **intrafamilial variability**
  Variability in clinical presentation of a particular disorder among affected individuals within the same immediate or extended family.

- **intragenic marker**
  An identifiable, polymorphic region of DNA (i.e., marker) located within a gene (i.e., intragenic), as opposed to a flanking marker, which is located on either side of a gene. Intragenic markers are used in linkage analysis to track the coinheritance of the gene in question.

- **intragenic suppression**
  A second mutation within a mutant gene that results in an apparent restoration of the original phenotype.

- **intraocular pressure**
  The pressure of fluid within your eyeball.

- **intraperitoneal**
  Within the peritoneal cavity, the area that contains the abdominal organs.

- **intron**

DNA sequence that interrupts the protein-coding sequence of a gene; an intron is transcribed into RNA but is cut out of the message before it is translated into protein. Non-coding sequence of DNA removed from mature messenger RNA prior to translation.

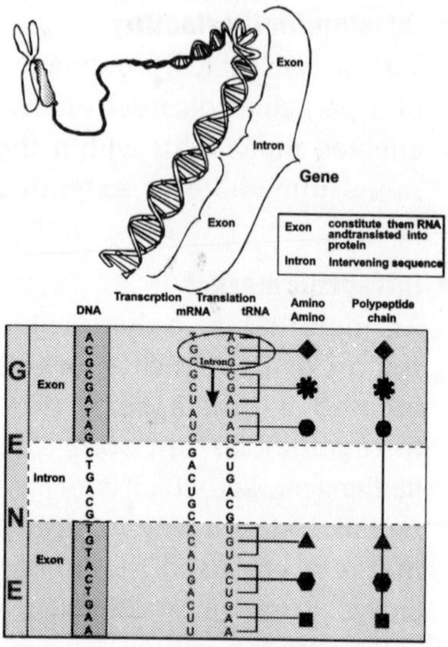


A DNA segment of largely unknown function within a gene that specifically interupts the coding (exon) sequences of that gene. Introns are transcribed as part of the normal gene primary transcript, but intron sequences are not found in the functional mRNA. Intron sequences are removed from the primary transcript by a splicing mechanism.

- **intronic mutation**

A mutation (usually a base substitution) within an intron that creates an alternative splice site that competes with the normal splice sites during RNA processing. Such a mutation results in a proportion of mature messenger RNA with improperly spliced intron sequences.

- **intubated**

A tube inserted as a mechanical aid to provide body function.

- **invasive**

Describes medical procedures which require entering or "invading" your body.

- **inversion**

A chromosomal rearrangement in which a segment of a chromosome has inverted from end to end, and re-inserted into the chromosome at the same breakage site. Balanced inversions (in which no net loss or gain of genetic material occurs) are usually not associated with phenotypic abnormalities, however, in some cases, gene disruptions at the breakpoints can cause adverse phenotypic effects, including some known genetic diseases. Unbalanced inversions (in which loss or gain of chromosome material occurs) nearly always yield an abnormal phenotype; A chromosomal mutation involving the removal of a chromosome segment, its rotation through 180 degrees, and its reinsertion in the same location. The replacement of a section of a chromosome in the reverse orientation.

- **inverted repeat (ir) sequence**
A sequence found in identical (but inverted) form, for example, at the opposite ends of a transposon. A nucleotide sequence found at two sites on the same double helix but in opposite orientation.

- **involuntary**
Not controlled through will; Occuring without conscience control or direction.

- **iojap**
A locus in maize that produces variegation.

- **ionizing radiation**
Radiation, such as X-rays and gamma rays (high energy photons), that causes atoms to release electrons and become ions.

- **iridocyclitis**
Inflammation of the iris and ciliary body in the eye.

- **islet cell transplantation**
Moving the beta (islet) cells from a donor pancreas and putting them inta person whose pancreas has stopped producing insulin. The beta cells make the insulin that the body needs to use glucose (sugar) for energy. Although transplanting islet cells may one day help people with diabetes, the procedure is still in the research stage.

- **islets of langerhans**
Special groups of cells in the pancreas. They make and secrete hormones that help the body break down and use food. Named after Paul Langerhans, the German scientist who discovered them in 1869, these cells sit in clusters in the pancreas. There are five types of cells in an islet: beta cells, which make insulin; alpha cells, which make glucagon; delta cells, which make somatostaton; and PP cells and D1 cells, about which little is known.

- **isoaccepting trna**
The various types of tRNA molecule carrying a specific amino acid.

- **isochromosome**
A metacentric chromosome produced during mitosis or meiosis when the centromere splits transversely instead of longitudinally; the arms of such chromosome are equal in length and genetically identical, however, the loci are positioned in reverse sequence in the two arms; A chromosome with two genetically and morphologically identical arms; A structural chromosome rearrangement caused by the division of a chromosome along an axis perpendicular to the usual axis of division; results in chromosomes with either two short arms or two long arms.

- **isodisomy**
  The presence of two identical homologues of a transmitted chromosome from only one of the parents. Junk DNA with no apparent function.

- **isoelectric focusing**
  Method of mutation detection by which proteins are separated according to the pH at which their net charge is zero (isoelectric point); often used in conjunction with a western blot to allow identification of wild-type versus mutant protein products. A DNA sequence alteration resulting in an amino acid substitution can change the isoelectric point of a protein.

- **isoenzyme**
  An enzyme performing the same function as another enzyme but having a different set of amino acids. The two enzymes may function at different speeds.

- **isoforms**
  The protein products of different versions of messenger RNA created from the same gene by employing different promoters, which causes transcription to skip certain exons. Since the promoters are tissue-specific, different tissues express different protein products of the same gene.

- **isolated**
  An abnormality that occurs in the absence of other systemic involvement

- **isoschizomer**
  Restriction endonuclease that recognizes the same target DNA sequence and cleaves it in the same way.

- **isotope**
  One of several forms of an element having the same atomic number but differing atomic masses.

- **isozyme**
  A different electrophoretic form of the same multi-subunit enzyme. Unlike allozymes isozymes are due to differing subunit configurations rather than allelic differences.

- **jaundice**
  A yellowish stain or tint.

- **joint**
  The point of juncture between two or more bones where movement occurs.

- **joint contractures**
  Permanently flexed positions.

- **junctional diversity**
  Variability in immunoglobulins caused by differences in the exact crossover point during V-J, V-D, and D-J joining.

- **junk dna**
  Stretches of DNA that do not code for genes; most of the genome consists of so-called junk DNA which may have regulatory and

other functions. Also called non-coding DNA; DNA in the genome that is not directly involved in making proteins or other molecules.About 98 percent of the human genome consists of non-coding DNA.The term "junk" reflects the outdated belief that this DNA accumulated over the course of evolution and no longer serves a purpose in humans.But it's now clear that some non-coding DNA controls the activity of genes and may have other functions.

- **juvenile**
  A minor, or child; referring to children.

- **juvenile onset diabetes**
  Former term for insulin-dependent or type one diabetes. See: Insulin-dependent diabetes mellitus.

- **kappa particle**
  Bacteria-like particle that gives a Paramecium the killer phenotype.

- **karyokinesis**
  The process of nuclear division.

- **karyotype**
  A photomicrograph of an individual's chromosomes arranged in a standard format showing the number, size, and shape of each chromosome type; used in low-resolution physical mapping to correlate gross chromosomal abnormalities with the characteristics of specific diseases; A photographic representation of the chromosomes of a single cell, cut and arranged in pairs based on their size and banding pattern according to a standard classification; The chromosome complement of an individual arranged in a standard order from large to small. (Numbering the largest chromosome 1, and so on with chromosome 22 the shortest); A photomicrograph of an individual's chromosomes arranged in a standard format showing the number, size, and shape of each chromo some type.

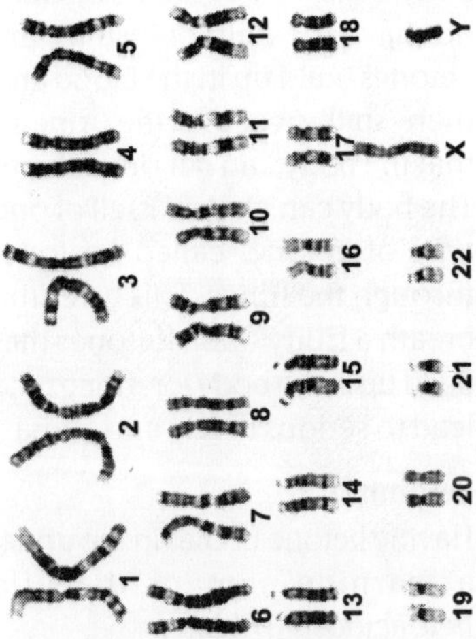

- **karyotyping (standard)**
  A visual display of all chromosomes present in a cell, usually by arrangement in matched pairs. Used to detect structural and numerical abnormalities in chromosomes.

• **keratopachydermia**
A syndrome of congenital deafness with hyperkeratosis of the skin of the palms, soles, elbows, and knees in childhood, and band-like constrictions of the fingers.

• **keratopathy**
Corneal dystrophy (an eye disorder).

• **ketone bodies**
Chemicals that the body makes when there is not enough insulin in the blood and it must break down fat for its energy. Ketone bodies can poison and even kill body cells. When the body does not have the help of insulin, the ketones build up in the blood and then "spill" over into the urine so that the body can get rid of them. The body can also rid itself of one type of ketone, called acetone, through the lungs. This gives the breath a fruity odor. Ketones that build up in the body for a long time lead to serious illness and coma.

• **ketonuria**
Having ketone bodies in the urine; a warning sign of diabetic ketoacidosis (DKA).

• **ketosis**
A condition of having ketone bodies build up in body tissues and fluids. The signs of ketosis are nausea, vomiting, and stomach pain. Ketosis can lead to ketoacidosis.

• **kidney**
One of a pair of organs in back of the abdominal cavity which filter waste materials out of the blood and pass them out of the body as urine.

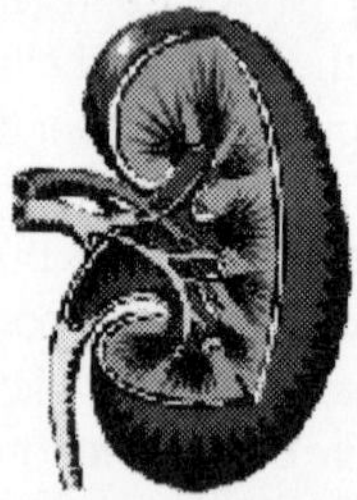

Two organs in the lower back that clean waste and poisons from the blood. The kidneys are shaped like two large beans, and they act as the body's filter. They also control the level of some chemicals in the blood such as hydrogen, sodium, potassium, and phosphate.

• **kidney disease**
Any one of several chronic conditions that are caused by damage to the cells of the kidney. People who have had diabetes for a long time may have kidney damage. Also called nephropathy.

• **kilobase**
Unit of DNA sequence equal to 1000 base pairs of nucleotides.

• **kin selection**
The mode of natural selection that acts on an individual's inclusive fitness.

- **kindred**
  An extended family; term often used in linkage studies to refer to large families

- **kinetochore**
  The chromosomal attachment point for the spindle fibers located within the centromeres; A structure at the centromere to which the spindle fibers are attached.

- **klinefelter syndrome**
  A genetic abnormality that is caused by an extra X chromosome in a male, and is typically identified as 47, XXY. An endocrine condition caused by a an extra X-chromosome (47,XXY); characterized by the lack of normal sexual development and testosterone, leading to infertility and adjustment problems if not detected and treated early.

- **knockout**
  Deactivation of specific genes; used in laboratory organisms to study gene function; The process by which genes are made inactive in a laboratory. Scientists often use knockouts in mice in order to study what effect the inactivity of a given gene will have on the animal.

- **kussmaul breathing**
  The rapid, deep, and labored breathing of people who have ketoacidosis or who are in a diabetic coma. Kussmaul breathing is named for Adolph Kussmaul, the 19th century German doctor who first noted it. Also called "air hunger".

- **labia**
  Lips; commonly refers to the lips of the femal external genitalia.

- **labia major**
  The two folds of the female genatalia forming the borders of the external (outside) genetalia.

- **labile diabetes**
  A term used to indicate when a person's blood glucose (sugar) level often swings quickly from high to low and from low to high. Also called brittle diabetes.

- **lability**
  Unstableness, unsteadiness.

- **labor**
  Periodic rhythmical contraction of the uterus which opens the cervix and leads to the birth of a baby.

- **labyrinth**
  Portion of the inner ear responsible for balance.

- **lac operon**
  An inducible operon including three loci involved in the uptake and breakdown of lactose in Escherichia coli. The lac operon in E.Coli is an example of that dual control. Glucose and lactose levels control the initiation of trans-

cription of the lac operon, i.e. whether the lac operon is switched "ON" or "OFF".

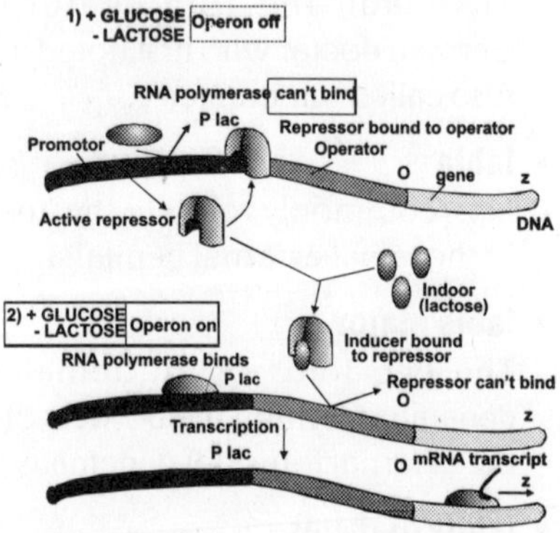


- **lacrimal gland**

  Gland of the eye that secretes tears.

- **lactate or lactic acid**

  A chemical that is formed when sugars are broken down for energy without the presence of adequate oxygen. Lactic acid cannot be used by the body and will accumulate in blood and urine. Lactic acid causes the muscle pain when one runs too fast for too long. In people with mitochondrial disorders, lactic acid forms when the oxidative capacity (ability to burn foods using oxidative phosphorylation) of the person is impaired.

- **lactic acidosis**

  The buildup of lactic acid in the body. The cells make lactic acid when they use glucose (sugar) for energy. If too much lactic acid stays in the body, the balance tips and the person begins to feel ill. The signs of lactic acidosis are deep and rapid breathing, vomiting, and abdominal pain. Lactic acidosis may be caused by diabetic ketoacidosis or liver or kidney disease.

- **lacunae**

  Small pits or depression in an organ or tissue.

- **lagging strand**

  In DNA replication, the strand that is synthesized apparently in the 3' to 5' direction, but actually in the 5' to 3' direction by ligating short fragments synthesized individually. Strand of DNA being replicated discontinuously.

- **lagging strand of dna**

  The new strand of a DNA replicating in the 3' to 5' direction. It is synthesized in short fragments in the 5'to 3' direction that are subsequently joined together.

- **lambda dgal**

  A lambda phage carrying a gal(galactose) bacterial gene and defective (d) for some phage function.

- **lamina**

  Flattened part of the vertebral arch, the ring of bone which, with the vertebral body, surrounds and encloses the spinal cord within that segment of the vertebral column.

- **laminectomy**
  Surgical removal of the lamina of a vertebra.

- **laminotomy**
  Surgical shaving of bone from the lamina of a vertebra.

- **lampbrush chromosomes**
  Chromosomes of amphibian oocytes having loops suggestive of a lampbrush. Large chromosomes found in amphibian eggs, with lateral DNA loops, extending from chromomeres, producing a brushlike appearance under the microscope.

- **lanugo**
  Fine, downy hair appearing on the skin of a fetus.

- **laparoscopy**
  A technique for performing a surgical procedure through slits in the skin using special surgical probes, rather than making one large incision. Depending on the position of the tumor and the extensiveness of the procedure, use of this technique may or may not be possible.

- **laryngeal webbing**
  When a membrane grows between the true vocal cords. It's presence results in a voice disorder that not only affects phonation, but can cause a blockage of the airway. These people experience shortness of breath and a higher-pitched than usual voice with some hoarseness. These webs must be surgically removed, followed by subsequent voice therapy.

- **laryngotracheal cleft**
  An opening between the voicebox and the windpipe.

- **larynx**
  The portion of the throat that contains the vocal mechanism.

- **laser treatment**
  The surgical use of a minutely focused ligh to deliver a microscopic cauterization, or burn.

- **latent diabetes**
  Former term for impaired glucose tolerance. See also: Impaired glucose tolerance.

- **lateral**
  The side of the body or body part that is farther from the middle or center (median) of the body. Typically, lateral refers to the outer side of the body part, but it is also used to refer to the side of a body part. For example, when referring to the knee, lateral would mean the side of the knee that is farthest from the opposite knee. The opposite of lateral is medial.

- **lateral inhibition**
  The signal produced by one cell that prevents adjacent cells from acquiring their fate.

- **lawn**
  A continuous layer of bacteria on the surface of an agar medium.

- **lcfa**
  Long chain fatty acids, which make up the vast majority of fats we consume in our diet.

- **leader peptide gene**
  A small gene within the attenuator control region of repressible amino acid operons. Translation of a specific leader peptide tests for the concentration of a specific amino acid or set of amino acids in the cell. If the concentration is high transcription is terminated in the attenuator, if low continued leading to the production of enzymes for amino acid synthesis and hence more amino acid.

- **leader sequence**
  The sequence at the 5' end of an mRNA that is not translated into protein. The length of untranslated mRNA from the 5' end to the initiation codon AUG.

- **leader transcript**
  The mRNA transcribed by the attenuator region of repressible amino acid operons. The transcript is capable of several alternative stem-loop structures dependent on translation of a short leader peptide gene.

- **leading strand**
  Strand of DNA being replicated continuously. In DNA replication, the strand that is made in the 5' to 3' direction by continuous polymerization at the 3' growing tip.

- **leaky mutant**
  A mutant (typically an auxotroph) that results from a partial rather than a complete inactivation of the wild-type function.

- **left ventricle**
  The largest and most muscular chamber of the heart concerned with the pumping of oxygen-rich blood from the lungs (via the left atrium) to all the other tissues of the body, via the aorta.

- **leigh disease or syndrome**
  Subacute Necrotizing Encephalomyelopathy.

- **lens**
  The clear structure in the eye that focuses light rays on the retina.

- **leptomeninges**
  The pia mater (highly vascular membrane) and arachnoid mater (spider-like membrane) of the brain.

- **leptonema (leptotene stage)**
  The first stage of prophase 1 of meiosis in which chromosomes become distinct.

- **lesion**
  Injury or loss of function; Any localized abnormal structural change, such as an angioma. A broad term, including wounds, sores, ulcers, tumors, cataracts and any other tissue damage; A damaged area (a mutant site) in a gene, a chromosome, or a protein.

- **lesser curve**
  The right side of the stomach from the cardia (entrance at the end of the esophagus or gullet) to the pylorus (exit into the duodenum or beginning of the small bowel).
- **lethal factor**
  An abnormality of the genome that leads to death in utero, e.g., numerous chromosomal anomalies.
- **lethal gene**
  A gene whose expression results in the death of the individual expressing it.
- **lethal-equivalent alleles**
  Alleles whose summed effect is that of lethality for example, four alleles each of which would be lethal 25% of the time (or to 25% of their bearers), are equivalent to one lethal allele.
- **leucine zipper**
  Configuration of a DNA-binding protein in which leucine residues on two protein alpha-helices interdigitate in zipper fashion to stabilize the protein.
- **leukemia**
  Cancer that begins in developing blood cells in the bone marrow.
- **leukocytosis**
  More than normal leukocytes in the blood.
- **leukopenia**
  Fewer than normal leukocytes in the blood.
- **level of significance**
  The probability value in statistics used to reject the null hypothesis.
- **lhon**
  Leber Hereditary Optic Neuropathy.
- **library**
  An unordered collection of clones (i.e., cloned DNA from a particular organism) whose relationship to each other can be established by physical mapping.
- **li-fraumeni syndrome**
  A family predisposition to multiple cancers, caused by a mutation in the p53 tumor-suppressor gene.
- **ligament**
  Thick band of fibrous tissue connecting bones and joints.
- **ligand**
  A molecule that can bind to a receptor and thereby induce a signal in the cell, e.g., a hormone.
- **ligand-receptor interaction**
  Interaction between a molecule (usually of an extracellular origin) and a protein on or within a target cell. One type of ligand-receptor interaction can be between steroid hormones and their cytoplasmic or nuclear receptors. Another can be between secreted polypeptide ligands and trans-membrane receptors.
- **ligase**
  An enzyme that can rejoin a broken phosphodiester bond in a nucleic acid.

- **limited joint mobility**
  A form of arthritis involving the hand; it causes the fingers to curve inward and the skin on the palm to tighten and thicken. This condition mainly affects people with IDDM.

- **line**
  Long interspersed element; a type of large repetitive DNA segment found throughout the genome of Eukaryotes; A group of identical pure-breeding diploid or polyploid organisms, distinguished from other individuals of the same species by some unique phenotype and genotype.

- **linear tetrad**
  A tetrad that results from the occurrence of the meiotic and postmeiotic nuclear divisions in such a way that sister products remain adjacent to one another in an ordered manner constrained within an ascus.

- **lingual frenulum**
  Band of tissue which joins the floor of the mouth to the bottom of the tongue.

- **linkage**
  The proximity of two or more markers (e.g., genes, RFLP markers) on a chromosome; the closer the markers, the lower the probability that they will be separated during DNA repair or replication processes (binary fission in prokaryotes, mitosis or meiosis in eukaryotes), and hence the greater the probability that they will be inherited together.

- **linkage analysis (synonym indirect DNA analysis)**
  Testing DNA sequence polymorphisms (normal variants) that are near or within a gene of interest to track within a family the inheritance of a disease-causing mutation in a given gene; A gene-hunting technique that traces patterns of heredity in large, high-risk families, in an attempt to locate a disease-causing gene mutation by identifying traits that are co-inherited with it.

- **linkage disequilibrium**
  Where alleles occur together more often than can be accounted for by chance. Indicates that the two alleles are physically close on the DNA strand.

- **linkage equilibrium**
  When the observed frequencies of haplotypes in a population agrees with haplotype frequencies predicted by multiplying together the frequency of individual genetic markers in each haplotype.

- **linkage group**
  A group of gene loci known to be linked; a chromosome. There are as many linkage groups as there are homologous pairs of chromosomes.

- **linkage map**

A map of the relative positions of genetic loci on a chromosome, determined on the basis of how often the loci are inherited together. Distance is measured in centimorgans (cM); An abstract map of chromosomal loci, based on recombinant frequencies; A chromosome map showing the relative positions of genetic markers of a given species, as determined by linkage analysis; not the same as a physical, or gene, map, which uses linkage analysis, cytogenetic examination, and physical techniques to generate the map.

Linkage (or genetic) maps give the relative location of genes on a chromosome.

**PRINCIPLES**

- The genes have a known order along a chromosome.
- The "distance" (degree of linkage) between genes is statistically measured by how often recombination occurs between them.
- Recombination occurs when homologous (matching) chromosomes exchange corresponding segments. This happens during meiosis – the cell divsion that creates gametes (sex cells) such as ova and sperm.

**1. Parental (P) generation**: Two flies are crossed. One is heterozygous (has nonmatching alleles) for both traits, so it has a gray body and red eyes. The other parent is homozygous (has matching alleles) for the recessive genes, so it has a black body and purple eyes.

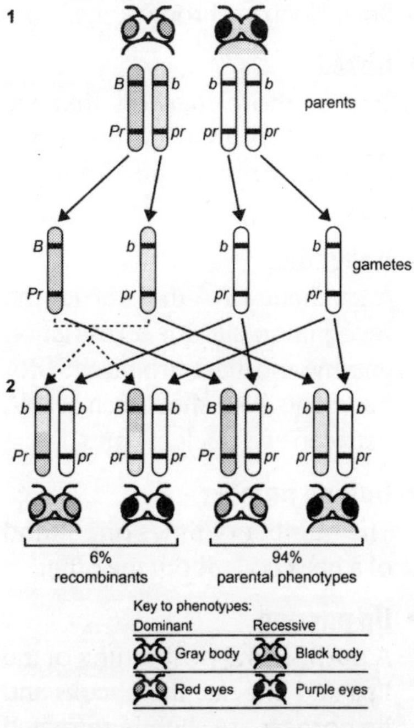


**2 First (F1) generation**: Without recombination occurring, half of the F1 offspring would have gray bodies and red eyes and the other half would have black bodies and purple eyes. These characteristics are the same as the parental phenotypes (appearances). In this case, however, recombination does occur. As a result:

- 94% of the flies have the parental phenotypes, but

- 6% have either black bodies and red eyes or gray bodies and purple eyes.

These flies must be recombinants.

- **linkage phase**

The arrangement of alleles of linked loci on chromosomes.

- **linked**

Two or more markers that are close enough together on a chromosome to be inherited together.

- **linker dna**

A synthetic DNA that carries the recognition site for a restriction enzyme and that can bind two DNA fragments. Also, the stretch of DNA between two nucleosomes.

- **linking number**

The number of times one strand of a helix coils about the other.

- **lip pursing**

A purse-string positioning of the lips and cheeks; the cheeks and lip corners are slightly retracted for abnormal stability while the central portions of the lips are semi-protruded and appear to be puckering.

- **lipid**

Descriptive term for a fat or fat-like substance found in the blood, such as cholesterol. The body stores fat as energy for future use just like a car that has a reserve fuel tank. When the body needs energy, it can break down the lipids into fatty acids and burn them like glucose (sugar).

- **lipodystrophy**

Lumps or small dents in the skin that form when a person keeps injecting the needle in the same spot. Lipodystrophies are harmless. People who want to avoid them can do so by changing (rotating) the places where they inject their insulin. Using purified insulins may also help.

- **lipomas**

Small nodules of fat under the skin.

- **liver**

A large organ in the upper right side of the abdominal cavity which secretes bile and is active in regulating various parts of the process of digesting food and using it to best advantage in the body.

- **lligase**

An enzyme that functions in DNA repair.

- **lobe**

1. A subdivision of an organ, divided by fissures, connective tissue or other natural boundaries. 2. A rounded projecting portion, such as the lobe of the ear; Round or protruding parts.

- **localize**

Determination of the original position (locus) of a gene or other marker on a chromosome.

- **localizome mapping**

  One can imagine comprehensive mapping projects of the "localizome", with the goal of recording not only where all proteins of a proteome can be found but also when.

- **locu ceruleus**

  An area of the brain involved in attention.

- **locus**

  Any genomic site, whether functional or not, that can be mapped through formal genetic analysis.

- **locus heterogeneity**

  The situation in which mutations in genes at different chromosomal loci cause the same phenotype

- **locus name**

  An informally assigned abbreviation used in the process of mapping to designate a putative gene prior to gene identification; once the gene is identified. The locus name is generally replaced by a formally assigned gene symbol (which often differs from the locus name).

- **lod score**

  A measure of the likelihood of two loci being within a measurable distance of each other; Logarithm of the odd score; a measure of the likelihood of two loci being within a measurable distance of each other.

- **lod score method**

  A technique (logarithmic odds) for determining the most likely recombination frequency between two loci from pedigree data.

- **long-range restriction mapping**

  Restriction enzymes are proteins that cut DNA at precise locations. Restriction maps depict the chromosomal positions of restriction-enzyme cutting sites. These are used as biochemical "signposts," or markers of specific areas along the chromosomes. The map will detail the positions where the DNA molecule is cut by particular restriction enzymes.

- **lordosis**
  - Exaggerated forward curvature of the lower spine causing swayback.
  - An abnormal extension deformity: A curvature of the spine also known as Saddle Back or Hollow Back.

- **loss of heterozygosity (synonym loh)**

  At a particular locus heterozygous for a deleterious mutant allele and a normal allele, a deletion or other mutational event within the normal allele renders the cell either hemizygous (one deleterious allele and one deleted allele) or homozygous for the deleterious allele.

- **low birth weight**
  A term applied to babies that weigh 5 1/2 pounds (2,500 grams) or less at birth. Low birth weight infants are of two different types: those who are born too small because they are born to soon, and those who are born on time, but are too small for their gestational age.

- **low forceps delivery**
  Childbirth using obstetric forceps applied to the head of the fetus after it has descended into the lower vagina.

- **low total ridge count**
  Abnormal fingerprints.

- **lte**
  Larynx-Trachea-Esopagus (larngo / tracheal / esophageal).

- **lte cleft**
  Abnormal fissure in the LTE area which failed to close during development, may cause problems with swallowing or breathing.

- **lte defect**
  A type of defect involving the larynx, trachea, and esophagus. Many different types of abnormalities may be involved.

- **lumbar**
  Pertaining to the lower back; Relating to the lumbus or part of the back and sides between the ribs and pelvis.

- **lumen**
  The channel within a tubular structure.

- **lungs**
  The two organs of respiration that bring air and blood into close contact so that oxygen can be added to and carbon dioxide removed from the blood.

- **lymph node-positive**
  Breast cancer that has spread to the underarm lymph nodes.

- **lymphangiectatic**
  Relating to lymphatiectasis - the dilation of the lymphatic vessels.

- **lymphatic system**
  The tissues and organs, including the bone marrow, spleen, thymus, and lymph nodes, that produce and store cells that fight infection and disease. This system also has channels that carry lymph.

- **lymphedema**
  Abnormal accumulation of lymph fluid in the tissues of the body; Swelling due to obstruction of lymphatic vessels or lymph nodes forming an accumulation of large amounts of lymph in the area.

- **lymphoma**
  Cancer of the lymph nodes and spleen that causes excessive production of lymphocytes.

- **lyon hypothesis**
  The hypothesis, named after Mary Lyon who stated it, suggesting that doseage compensation in mammals is by inactivation of all but one X chromosome in cells with more

than one X chromosome. The Barr body, visible in some female mammalian cells, is an inactivated X chromosome.

- **lyonization (synonym X-chromosome inactivation)**
  The phenomenon in females by which one X chromosome (either maternally derived or paternally derived) is randomly inactivated in early embryonic cells, with fixed inactivation in all descendant cells; first described by the geneticist Mary Lyon.

- **lyonization**
  The random inactivation of loci on one of a pair of X chromosomes. In each cell, only one X chromosome is active. This process of inactivation occurs early in fetal development and explains the variable expressivity of X-linked traits in females; A term used for the phenomenon of X inactivation, which was first proposed by the geneticist Mary Lyon.

- **lysate**
  The contents released from a lysed cell.

- **lysis**
  The breaking open of a cell by the destruction of its wall or membrane. The rupture and death of a bacterial cell upon the release of phage progeny.

- **lysogenic**
  The state of a bacterial cell that has an integrated phage (prophage) in its chromosome.

- **lysogenic bacterium**
  A bacterial cell capable of spontaneous lysis due, for example, to the release of a prophage from the bacterial chromosome.

- **lysosomes**
  Intracellular particles particularly abundant in the liver and kidney.

- **macromolecule**
  A large polymer such as DNA, RNA, protein, lipid or polysaccharide.

- **macrophage**
  Large cells found throughout the body, particularly in the spleen, that have the ability to ingest other substances such as "old" red blood cells; also important in the immune response.

- **macrorestriction map**
  Map depicting the order of and distance between sites at which restriction enzymes cleave chromosomes; Describes the order and distance between enzyme cutting (cleavage) sites. In top- down mapping, a single chromosome is cut (with rare-cutter restriction enzymes) into large pieces, which are ordered and subdivided; the smaller pieces are then mapped further. The resulting macro- restriction maps depict the order of and distance between sites at which rare-cutter enzymes cleave. This approach yields maps with more continuity and fewer gaps

between fragments than contig maps, but map resolution is lower and may not be useful in finding particular genes; in addition, this strategy generally does not produce long stretches of mapped sites. Currently, this approach allows DNA pieces to be located in regions measuring about 100,000 bp to 1 Mb.

- **macrosomia**

Larger-than-normal birth weight (usually more than 9 ¾ pounds, or 4,500 grams); Abnormally large; in diabetes, refers to abnormally large babies that may be born to women with diabetes.

- **macrostomia**

Increased width of the mouth, resulting from failure of union of the maxillary and mandibular processes, with extension of the oral orifice toward the ear.

- **macrovascular disease**

A disease of the large blood vessels that sometimes occurs when a person has had diabetes for a long time. Fat and blood clots build up in the large blood vessels and stick to the vessel walls. Three kinds of macrovascular disease are coronary disease, cerebrovascular disease, and peripheral vascular disease.

- **macula**

The central area of the retina.

- **macular edema**

A swelling (edema) in the macula, an area near the center of the retina of the eye that is responsible for fine or reading vision. Macular edema is a common complication associated with diabetic retinopathy.

- **magnetic resonance imaging (m.r.i.)**

A noninvasive diagnostic procedure using radio waves and magnetic fields to provide a highly detailed map of an interior structure of the body, such as the brain. MRI depicts detailed internal anatomy by exploiting the interaction of the magnetic properties of atoms with an external magnetic field; An imaging technique where magnetic energy is used to examine tissues in your body, and the information is used by a computer to create an image. There is no radiation exposure. The resulting images look very much like X-rays, but include images of soft tissues (like blood vessels) as well as hard tissues (like bones). Claustrophobia can be an issue, since this procedure requires lying still in a tunnel-like structure for at least half an hour. Calming drugs can be used, or there are new machines that have a more open, cage-like structure, and various attempts are being made to shorten the time required.

- **major histocompatibility complex (mhc)**

A group of highly polymorphic genes whose products appear on the surface of cells imparting the property of self (belonging to that organism). A genetic region found in all mammals whose products are primarily responsible for the rapid rejection of tissue grafts between indiviuals, and function in signalling between lymphocytes and cells expressing antigen.

- **malabsorption**
  Defective absorption of fluids.

- **malar**
  Relating to the cheek bones.

- **malignant**
  Describes any disease which progresses rapidly, spreading to other parts of the body and eventually leading to death.

- **malignant cancerous**
  Cancer cells can spread through the blood or lymphatic system to start new cancers in other parts of the body.

- **malleus**
  The outermost of three tiny bones, connecting the eardrum to the vibration-sensitive structures of the inner ear and thereby amplifying and transmitting sound waves.

- **malocclusion**
  Refers to an abnormal fit of the upper and lower dental structures.

- **mandible**
  The mandible is the bone of the lower jaw. The joint where the mandible meets the upper jaw at the temporal bone is called the temporomandibular joint.

- **mandibular**
  Referring to the lower jaw.

- **mandibulofacial**
  Referring to the lower jaw and face.

- **manifesting carrier**
  An individual who has, at a particular locus, a recessive, disease-causing allele on one chromosome and a normal allele on the other chromosome and who manifests some symptoms of the disorder; generally refers to female carriers of an X-linked recessive mutation who are clinically affected, although the phenotype is usually less severe as compared to males with the same mutation.

- **manx**
  Tailless phenotype in cats, caused by an autosomal dominant mutation that is lethal when homozygous.

- **map unit (m.u.)**
  The distance between two linked gene pairs where 1 percent of the products of meiosis are recombinant. A unit of distance in a linkage map. The distance equal to 1% recombination between two loci.

- **mapped gene**
  A gene or phenotype whose relative position on a segment of

DNA or on a chromosome has been established.

- **mapping**
The determination of the relative positions of genes within the chromosomes or of restriction sites along a DNA molecule. The process of determining the position of a locus on the chromosome relative to other loci; The study of the position of genes on chromosomes.

- **mapping function**
The mathematical relationship between measured map distance and actual recombination frequency. A formula expressing the relationship between distance in a linkage map and recombinant frequency.

- **mapping population**
The group of related organisms used in constructing a genetic map.

- **marfan syndrome**
Autosomal dominant condition of connective tissue; affects the skeletal, ocular and cardio-vascular systems.

- **marfan's syndrome**
A human disorder of the connective tissue expressed as a range of symptoms, including very long limbs and digits, and heart defects; inherited as an autosomal dominant phenotype. Mutations in a gene called fibrillin.

- **marker**
An identifiable segment of DNA (e.g., RFLP, VNTR, microsatellite) with enough variation between individuals that its inheritance and co-inheritance with alleles of a given gene can be traced; used in linkage analysis; A gene or DNA fragment with a known location on a chromosome that is associated with a certain disease; it can be used as a point of reference when looking for disease-causing mutations; An identifiable physical location on a chromosome (e.g., restriction enzyme cutting site, gene) whose inheritance can be monitored; Any genetic element (locus, allele, DNA sequence or chromosome feature) which can be readily detected by phenotype, cytological or molecular techniques, and used to follow a chromosome ,or chromosomal segment during genetic analysis.

- **marker chromosome**
A small chromosome containing a centromere occasionally seen in tissue culture, often in a mosaic state (present in some cells but not in others). A marker chromosome may be of little clinical significance or, if it contains material from one or both arms of another chromosome, may create an imbalance for whatever genes are present; assessment to establish clinical significance, particularly if found in a fetal karyotype, is often difficult.

- **marker retention**
  A technique used in yeast to test the degree of linkage between two mitochondrial mutations.

- **mass spectrometry**
  An instrument used to identify chemicals in a substance by their mass and charge.

- **mate-killer**
  A phenotype of Paramecium induced by intracellular bacteria-like mu particles.

- **maternal contamination**
  The situation which occurs in prenatal testing in which a sample of chorionic villus, amniotic fluid, or umbilical blood becomes contaminated with maternal (usually blood) cells, which can confound interpretation of the results of genetic analysis

- **maternal effect**
  The effect of the maternal parent's genotype on the phenotype of her offspring.

- **maternal effect lethal**
  A recessive mutation that is viable in zygotes, but in which homozygous mutant mothers produce inviable offspring.

- **maternal inheritance**
  A type of uniparental inheritance in which all progeny have the genotype and phenotype of the female parent.

- **mating type**
  In many species of microorganisms individuals can be divided into two types. Mating can take place only between individuals of opposite mating types due to the interaction of cell surface components. The equivalent in lower organisms of the sexes in higher organisms; the mating types typically differ only physiologically and not in physical form.

- **matroclinal**
  Traits transmitted from the mother.

- **matroclinous inheritance**
  Inheritance in which all offspring have the phenotype of the mother.

- **maturity-onset diabetes**
  Former term for noninsulin-dependent or type II diabetes.

- **maxam-gilbert method**
  A method for determining the exact nucleotide sequence via a chemical degradation process.

- **maxilla**
  Upper jaw bone, the portion of skull holding the upper teeth.

- **maxilliary hypoplasia**
  Underdeveloped upper jaw bone.

- **mean**
  The arithmetic average; the sum of the data divided by the sample size.

- **mean fitness of the population w(bar)**

  The sum of the fitnesses of the genotypes of a population weighted by their proportions; hence a weighted mean fitness.

- **meatus**

  The outer opening of a passageway of the body.

- **meconium**

  A newborn's first bowel discharge, which is usually black or green; Material in the intestines of a fetus which forms the first stools of a newborn infant. Causes problems if it is inhaled during baby's delivery.

- **meconium aspiration**

  A situation where meconium (greenish fecal matter, the first bowel movement of a fetus) filled amniotic fluid is breathed into the infant's lungs during the birth process. There may or may not be subsequent anoxia resulting in brain damage. Meconium aspiration is rare in babies born at less than 34 weeks gestation, and may be as high as 40 percent in post term babies, A cause of respiratory problems and pneumonia in newborns, occurs as a result of passage of meconium into the amniotic fluid during fetal distress during labor and delivery.

- **media**

  The middle, muscular layer in the wall of an artery.

- **medial**

  The side of the body or body part that is nearer to the middle or center (median) of the body. For example, when referring to the knee, medial would mean the side of the knee that is closest to the other knee The opposite of medial is lateral.

- **medial compartment**

  The inner of the two joint areas between the thigh-bone (femur) and shin-bone (tibia).

- **medial meniscus**

  The cartilage lining the inner upper end of the shin-bone (tibia).

- **mediastinum**

  The area that separates the lungs from each other. It contains the heart and its large veins and arteries, the trachea (wind-pipe), the esophagus, the thymus gland, and lymph nodes.

- **medical geneticist**

  A medical doctor who specializes in the diagnosis and treatment of inherited diseases.

- **medical informatics**

  An emerging discipline that melds the data analysis tools of computing with medical information and the provision of health-care services.

- **medium**

  Any material on (or in) which experimental cultures are grown.

- **medulla**
The central part of the structure of an organ; Any soft marrow-like structure, especially in the center of a part.

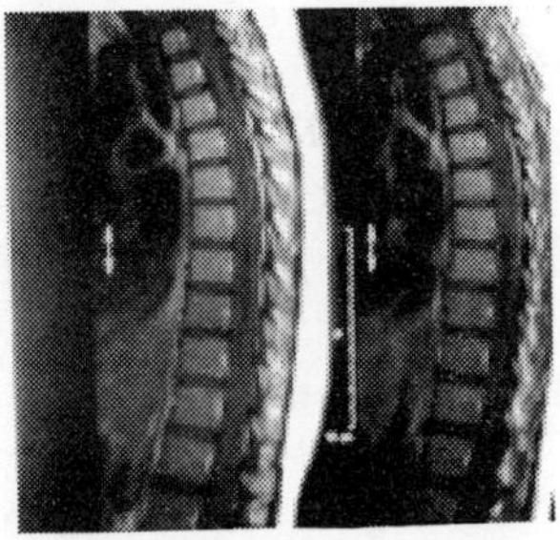

- **medulla oblongata**
The tapering caudal position of the hind brain.

- **megabase (mb)**
Unit of length for DNA fragments equal to one million nucleotides and roughly equal to one cM.

- **megalencephaly**
Brain much larger than normal. This condition amy or may nont be associated with mental retardation.

- **meiocyte**
Cell in which meiosis occurs.

- **meiosis**
The process of two consecutive cell divisions in the diploid progenitors of sex cells. Meiosis results in four rather than two daughter cells, each with a haploid set of chromosomes; A special type of cell division that occurs when mature eggs and sperm are formed. Through the process of meiosis the number of chromosomes present in a cell is decreased by half. In humans the diploid number of chromosomes is 46. This is decreased to 23 during meiosis; Nuclear division forming gametes wherein the number of chromosomes is reduced from the diploid to the haploid number; resulting cells normally contain one member of each pair of homologous chromosomes. Results in four rather than two daughter cells, each with a haploid set of chromosomes; Two successive nuclear divisions (with corresponding cell divisions) that produce haploid gametes (in animals) or haploid sexual spores (in plants and fungi) having one-half of the genetic material of the original cell. The nuclear and cell division process in diploid eukaryotes that results in four haploid gametes or spores having one member of each original pair of homologous chromosomes only per nucleus.

- **meiospore**
Cell that is one of the products of meiosis in plants.

- **melanin**
Dark brown/black shapeless pigments found in melanotic tumours, the hair, skin, part of the brain and the choroid coat of the eye.

- **melanocytes**
  Cells in the skin that produce and contain the pigment called melanin.

- **melanoma**
  A cancer that begins in skin cells called melanocytes and spreads to internal organs, Cancer of the cells that produce pigment in the skin. Melanoma usually begins in a mole or skin cells called melanocytes and spreads to internal organs.

- **melting of dna**
  Denaturation of duplex DNA by heat or increased pH leading to strand separation.

- **membrane**
  Thin elastic tissue which covers the surface of certain organs and lines the cavities of the body.

- **mendelian disorder (also called single-gene disorder)**
  A disease caused by a single gene that is inherited in a straightforward manner from parent or parents to child.Huntington's disease and cystic fibrosis are examples.The term "Mendelian" refers to Gregor Mendel, an Austrian who did pioneering work on genes and traits in ordinary garden peas by showing that a single trait, such as color, can be determined by a single gene. Compared to "complex diseases," Mendelian disorders are relatively rare.

- **mendelian inheritance**
  One method in which genetic traits are passed from parents to offspring. Named for Gregor Mendel, who first studied and recognized the existence of genes and this method of inheritance; A trait obeying Mendel's first law of independent segregation of the alleles at the same locus conveyed by each parent.

- **mendelian ratio**
  A ratio of progeny phenotypes reflecting the operation of Mendel's laws.

- **mendel's first law**
  The two members of a gene pair segregate from each other during meiosis; each gamete has an equal probability of obtaining either member of the gene pair.

- **mendel's second law**
  The law of independent assortment; unlinked or distantly linked segregating gene pairs assort independently at meiosis.

- **meninges**
  The three membranes that cover the spinal cord and brain.

- **meningocele**
  Hernia of the meanings of the spinal cord or brain.

- **meningomyocele**
  Hernia of some portion of the spinal cord and its meanings.

- **meniscus**
  A crescentic cartilage (gristle) lying on either side (medial and

lateral) of the upper end of the tibia (shin bone), cushioning the joint with the femur (thigh bone).

- **mental retardation**

Intellectual functioning at least two standard deviations below the norm. According to the new definition by the American Association on Mental Retardation (AAMR), an individual is considered to have mental retardation based on the following three criteria: intellectual functioning level (IQ) is below 70-75; significant limitations exist in two or more adaptive skill areas; and the condition is present from childhood.

- **merozygote**

A bacterial cell having a second copy of a particular chromosomal region in the form of an exogenote. A partially diploid Escherichia coli cell formed from a complete chromosome (the endogenote) plus a fragment (the exogenote).

- **mesentery**

Fold in the abdominal lining that connects the intestine to the back of the abdominal wall; contains the arteries and veins that supply the intestines.

- **mesocolon**

The fold of peritoneum, or mesentery, attached to the colon, that holds the lower colon the back abdominal wall.

- **messenger rna (mrna)**

RNA that serves as a template for protein synthesis; The template for protein synthesis. Each set of three bases, or codons, in mRNA orders the production of a certain protein. The structure of mRNA is the same as one strand of DNA; A single-stranded molecule of ribonucleic acid that directs protein production; An RNA molecule transcribed from the DNA of a gene, and from which a protein is translated by the action of ribosomes. The basic function of the nucleotide sequence of mRNA is to determine the amino acid sequence in proteins.

- **metabolic disorder**

1. A condition or disease related to dysfunction in the chemical processes and activities of the body. 2. Defects in the body's ability to process substances and nutrients normally. Lack of treatment for people with metabolic errors will result in mental retardation and in some cases death. In many of these conditions the primary treatment is diet. These conditions are rare and should be treated at centers that specialize in these disorders. Also referred to as "inborn errors".

- **metabolism**

Physical and chemical processes by which food is transformed into energy and tissues are broken down into waste products. It is a two-part process: One part is called catabolism — when the body uses food for energy. The other is called anabolism — when the body uses food to build or mend cells; The total metabolism are all biochemical processes of an organism. The cell metabolism includes all chemical processes in a cell. The Dynamic Energy Budget theory aims to quantify the metabolic organisation of individual organisms; many species are unicellular. Insulin is necessary for the metabolism of food.

- **metacarpal**

Referring to the metacarpus, the five bones in the palm of the hand between the carpus and finger bones.

- **metacentric chromosome**

A chromosome having its centromere in the middle.

- **metafemale**

A fruit fly with an X chromosome: Autosome ratio greater than unity.

- **metagon**

An RNA necessary for the maintenance of mu particles in Paramecium.

- **metamale**

A fruit fly with X chromosome: Autosome ratio below 0.5.

- **metamere**

Segmental repeat unit in higher animals.

- **metaphase**

The stage of mitosis or meiosis in which spindle fibers are attached to kinetochores and the chromosomes are positioned in the equatorial plane of the cell. An intermediate stage of nuclear division when chromosomes align along the equatorial plane of the cell spindle.

**Mitosis**

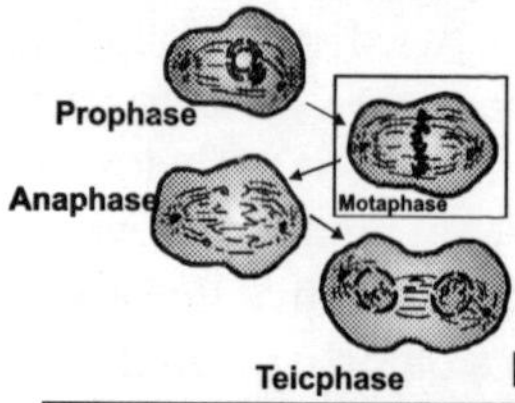


**Metaphase**

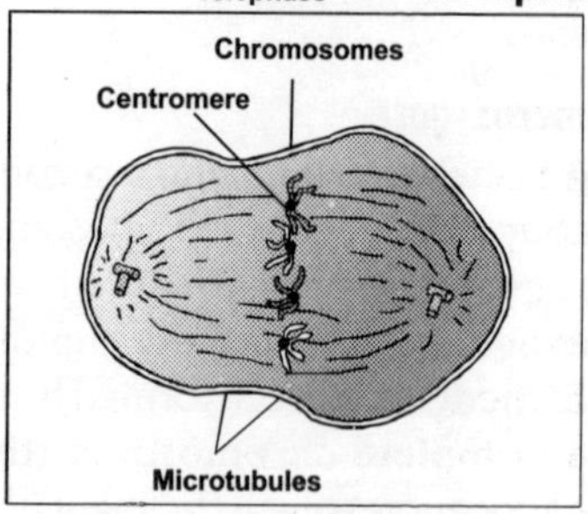


- **metaphase plate**

The plane of the equator of the spindle into which chromosomes are positioned during metaphase.

- **metaphyseal, metaphyses**

Referring to a conical section near the end of long bones, such as the arm and leg bones.

- **metastasis**

The migration of cancerous cells to other parts of the body.

• **metastasize**
To spread from one part of the body to another. When cancer cells metastasize and form secondary tumors, the cells in the metastatic tumor are like those in the original tumor.

• **metatarsals**
Bones just behind the toes.

• **methylation**
The attachment of methyl groups to DNA at cytosine bases; correlated with reduced transcription of the gene and thought to be the principal mechanism in X-chromosome inactivation and imprinting

• **methylation**
Addition of a methyl group (-CH3) to DNA or RNA. Modification of a molecule by the addition of a methyl group.

• **methylation analysis**
Testing that evaluates the methylation status of a gene (attachment of methyl groups to DNA cytosine bases); genes that are methyalted are not expressed; methylation plays a role in X-chromosome inactivation and imprinting

• **methylmalonic acidemia**
A group of conditions characterized by the inability to metabolize methylmalonic acid or by a defect in the metabolism of Vitamin B12.

• **metopic synostosis**
The metopic suture (found in the forhead) is one of several "joints" between the bony plates that form the skull. Synostosis refers to the premature fusion of theses bony plates.

• **microaneurysm**
A small swelling that forms on the side of tiny blood vessels. These small swellings may break and bleed into nearby tissue. People with diabetes sometimes get microaneurysms in the retina of the eye.

• **microarrary technology**
After microaaray a new way of studying how large numbers of genes interact with each other and how a cell's regulatory networks control vast batteries of genes simultaneously.

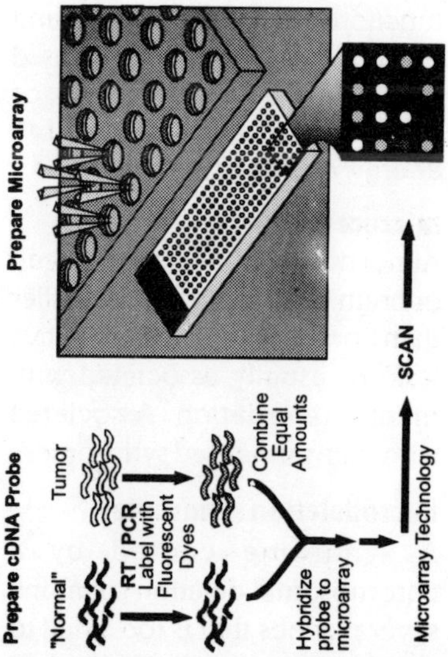

The method uses a robot to precisely apply tiny droplets containing functional DNA to glass slides. Researchers then attach fluorescent labels to DNA from the cell they are studying. The labeled probes are allowed to bind to complementary DNA strands on the slides. The slides are put into a scanning microscope that can measure the brightness of each fluorescent dot; brightness reveals how much of a specific DNA fragment is present, an indicator of how active it is. A method of determining how a cell can control the expression of large numbers of genes simultaneously. Up to 10,000 different cDNA segments are spotted on to a glass slide, making a DNA "chip".

- **microbial genetics**
  The study of genes and gene function in bacteria, archaea, and other microorganisms. Often used in research in the fields of bioremediation, alternative energy, and disease prevention.

- **microcephaly**
  Abnormal smallness of the head or brain case. Brain much smaller than normal without degenerative lesions; usually associated with mental retardation. Associated with many inherited syndromes.

- **microdeletion syndrome**
  A syndrome caused by a chromosomal deletion spanning several genes that is too small to be detected under the microscope using conventional cytogenetic methods. Depending on the size of the deletion, other techniques, such as FISH or other methods of DNA analysis can sometimes be employed to identify the deletion

- **micrognathia**
  Abnormally small (lower) jaw.

- **microinjection**
  A technique for introducing a solution of DNA into a cell using a fine microcapillary pipet.

- **micromelia**
  Abnormally small or short limb.

- **micronuclei**
  Chromosome fragments that are not incorporated into the nucleus at cell division.

- **microphthalmia, microthalmia**
  Abnormal smallness of the eye or eyes.

- **micropthalmos**
  An abnormally small eyeball.

- **micrornas**
  Small molecules found in plants and animals that may regulate the activity of genes.

- **microsatellite**
  (synonym satellite DNA, short tandem repeats) Repetitive segments of DNA two to five nucleotides in length (dinucleotide /trinucleotide / tetranucleotide / pentanucleotid e repeats), scattered throughout the genome

in non-coding regions between genes or within genes (introns), often used as markers for linkage analysis because of the naturally occurring high variability in repeat number between individuals. These regions are inherently unstable and susceptible to mutations.

- **microsatellite instability (synonym MSI, replication error phenotype, RER)**
The presence of a discrepancy between the size of microsatellites in DNA from tumor tissue compared to nontumor tissue from the same person, resulting from mutations in a gene in the DNA mismatch repair pathway (MMR) that would normally correct these errors.

- **microsatellite instability testing (synonym MSI testing)**
It is used to identify tumors caused by defective mismatch repair by comparing the number of nucleotide repeats in a panel of microsatellite markers in normal tissue with the number from tumor tissue from the same individual. Microsatellite stability (MSS) is present if the same number of repeats is present in each marker in both the tumor and the normal tissue. Microsatellite instability (MSI) is present if the number of repeats in the tumor and the normal tissue differs.

- **microstomia**
Abnormal smallness of the mouth.

- **microthalmia, microphthalmia**
Abnormal smallness of the eye or eyes.

- **microtubules**
Hollow cylinders made of the protein tubulin that form, among other things, the spindle fibers.

- **microvascular disease**
Disease of the smallest blood vessels that sometimes occurs when a person has had diabetes for a long time. The walls of the vessels become abnormally thick but weak, and therefore they bleed, leak protein, and slow the flow of blood through the body. Then some cells, for example, the ones in the center of the eye, may not get enough blood and may be damaged.

- **midbrain**
The uppermost of the three segments of the brainstem, primarily serving as an intermediary between the rest of the brain and the spinal cord.

- **middle cerebral artery**
One of three sets of paired arteries supplying oxygen-rich blood to the cerebral hemispheres and originating from the Circle Of Willis near the termination of the internal carotid artery.

- **midline**
The middle of the body; head in midline refers to the head in alignment with the spine. Center

of the body or median plane of the body.

- **midparent value**
The mean of the values of a quantitative phenotype for two specific parents.

- **midtrimester**
The middle three months of pregnancy.

- **migration**
Movement of individuals between otherwise reproductively isolated populations.

- **mimicry**
A phenomenon in which an individual; gains an advantage by looking like the individuals of a different species.

- **minimal genome**
The smallest number of genes an organism needs to stay alive in a particular environment.A goal of research on the minimal genome is to design synthetic micro-organisms that can perform useful tasks such as generating biological forms of energy.

- **minimal medium**
A culture medium for micro-organisms that contains the minimal necessities for growth of the wild-type. A medium containing only inorganic salts, a carbon source, and water.

- **minimal promoter**
The minimal elements of a promoter, including the TATA box and transcription initiation site, which is inactive unless regulatory elements that enhance promoter activity are placed upstream; used to test candidate sequences for enhancer activity.

- **mismatch**
The presence in one chain of double-stranded DNA of a base that is not complementary to the corres-ponding base in the other chain. Also known as mispairing.

- **mismatch repair**
A form of excision repair initiated at the sites of mismatched bases in DNA.

- **mismatch repair mechanism (synonym mismatch repair)**
The DNA 'proof-reading' system controlled by certain genes that identifies, excises, and corrects errors in the pairing of the bases during DNA replication. Mutations in the genes responsible for this mechanism can lead to certain genetic diseases and some forms of cancer.

- **missense mutation**
A single base pair substitution that results in the translation of a different amino acid at that position; A change in the base sequence of a gene that alters or eliminates a protein.

- **mitochondria**
A part of the cell (organelle) that is responsible for energy production. The organelle consists

of two sets of membranes, a smooth continuous outer coat and an inner membrane arranged in tubules or in folds that form plate-like double membranes (cristae); the principal energy source of the cell, containing the cytochrome enzymes of terminal electron transport and the enzymes of the citric acid cycle, fatty acid oxidation, and oxidative phosphorylation. Responsible for converting nutrients into energy as well as many other specialized tasks; A small, intracellular, spherical to rod-shaped cytoplasmic organelle, enclosed by Z membranous spaces; the inner membrane is folded, forming a series of projections called cristae. Mitochondria are the principal sites of ATP synthesis; they contain enzymes of the tricarboxylic acid cycle and enzymes for fatty acid oxidation, oxidative phos-phorylation, and many other biochemical pathways. They contain their own nucleic acids and ribosomes, replicate independently, and code for the synthesis of some of their own proteins.

- **mitochondrial cytopathy**

Disease process characterized by mitochondrial dysfunction. The preferred general term for referring to mitochondrial diseases.

- **mitochondrial dna**

The genetic material found in mitochondria, the organelles that generate energy for the cell. Not inherited in the same fashion as nucleic DNA; The mitochondrial genome consists of a circular DNA duplex, with 5 to 10 copies per organelle.

- **mitochondrial encephalopathy**

Disease process characterized by mitochondrial dysfunction in the brain.

- **mitochondrial inheritance**

Mitochondria, cytoplasmic organelles that produce the energy source ATP for most chemical reactions in the body, contain their own distinct genome; mutations in mitochondrial genes are responsible for several recognized syndromes and are always maternally inherited since ova contain mitochondria, whereas sperm do not.

- **mitochondrion**

A eukaryotic organelle that is the site of ATP synthesis and of the citric acid cycle. The eukaryotic cellular organelle in which the Krebs cycle and electron transport reactions take place.

- **mitosis**

The process of nuclear division in cells that produces daughter cells that are genetically identical to each other and to the parent cell.

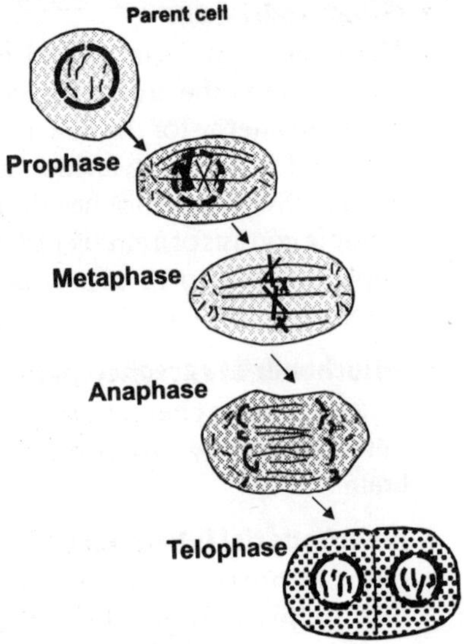


- **mitotic crossover**
  A crossover resulting from the pairing of homologous chromosomes in a diploid during mitosis.

- **mitral regurgitation**
  Backflow of oxygen-rich blood from the larger and more muscular left ventricle back into the smaller left atrium of the heart (and thus to the lungs) because of malfunctioning of the mitral valve due to pathological distortion of one or more of its components.

- **mitral valve**
  Heart valve that allows blood to move from the left atrium into the left ventricle and prevents the reverse flow.

- **mitral valve prolapse**
  Bulging of the leaflets of the mitral valve into the left atrium during the heart's contraction.

- **mixed codon family**
  Group of four codons sharing their first two bases but coding for more than one amino acid.

- **mobile elements**
  DNA sequences that are capable of inserting themselves into other locations in the genome.

- **mobility-shift assay**
  An assay used to detect specific protein binding to DNA. Such binding creates complexes that migrate more slowly during gel electrophoresis than free DNA. Also known as gel-shift assay.

- **mode**
  The single class in a statistical distribution having the greatest frequency.

- **mode of inheritance**
  (synonym inheritance pattern, pattern of inheritance) The manner in which a particular genetic trait or disorder is passed from one generation to the next. Autosomal dominant, autosomal recessive, X-linked dominant, X-linked recessive, multifactorial, and mitrochondrial inheritance are examples

- **model organism (also called animal model)**
  A creature, like the mouse or the fruit fly, used in the laboratory to study biology.Many genes in humans are found in other

species, and biologists study model organisms to learn about how these genes might operate in the human body.

- **model organisms**
A laboratory animal or other organism useful for research.

- **modeling**
The use of statistical analysis, computer analysis, or model organisms to predict outcomes of research.

- **modifier gene**
A gene that affects the phenotypic expression of another gene.It is a segment of DNA found on a chromosome that codes for a particular protein; a unit of heredity.

- **molars**
The grinding or chewing teeth, located at the back of both jaws.

- **molecular biology**
The study of the structure, function, and makeup of biologically important molecules.

- **molecular chaperone**
A protein that aids in the folding of a second protein. The chaperone prevents proteins from taking conformations that would be inactive.

- **molecular cloning**
The isolation of a DNA sequence and obtaining multiple copies of that sequence often in a bacteria (recombinant DNA) but can also be replicated in vitro (by the polymerase chain reaction method).

- **molecular evolutionary clock**
A measurement of evolutionary time in nucleotide substitutions per year.

- **molecular farming**
The development of transgenic animals to produce human proteins for medical use.

- **molecular genetic testing (synonym DNA testing, DNA-based testing, molecular testing)**
Testing that involves the analysis of DNA, either through linkage analysis, sequencing, or one of several methods of mutation detection

- **molecular genétics**
The study of macromolecules important in biological inheritance.

- **molecular genetics**
The study of the molecular processes underlying gene structure and function.

- **molecular genetics**
The study of the structure and function of genes at the molecular level.

- **molecular hybridization**
The ability of a single-stranded DNA or RNA to anneal to its complementary single strand by Watson-Crick base pairing.

- **molecular imprinting**
  The phenomenon in which there is differential expression of a gene depending on whether it was maternally or paternally inherited. Paternal imprinting means that an allele inherited from the father is not expressed in offspring. Maternal imprinting means that an allele inherited from the mother is not expressed in offspring.

- **molecular medicine**
  The treatment of injury or disease at the molecular level. Examples include the use of DNA-based diagnostic tests or medicine derived from DNA sequence information.

- **molecule**
  A molecule is generally an aggregate of at least two atoms in a definite arrangement held together by special forces. Generally, a molecule is considered the smallest particle of a pure chemical substance that still retains its composition and chemical properties. Even for some pure chemical substances existing as liquids or solids (such as metals, molten salts, crystals, etc.) such a definition may not always be possible, and it must recognized that such substances are composed of atoms, but not recognizable molecules.

- **mongoloid**
  Resembling a person of the mongolian race, as in Down Syndrome.

- **monocistronic mrna**
  An mRNA that codes for only one protein.

- **monoclonal**
  A group of cells that consist of a single clone, i.e., all cells are derived from the same single ancestral cell.

- **monoclonal antibody**
  The unique immunoglobulin molecule (antibody) produced by a clone of cells derived from a fusion of a B lymphocyte with a myeloma cell.

- **monocytes**
  Largest single cells with a nucleus seen in normal blood.

- **monoecious plant**
  A plant species in which male and female organs are found on the same plant but in different flowers (for example maize).

- **monogenic**
  Describing a single gene or mendelian trait.

- **monogenic disorder**
  A disorder caused by mutation of a single gene.

- **monohybrid**
  Offspring of parents that differ in only one genetic characteristic. Usually implies heterozygosity at a single locus under study.

- **monohybrid cross**
  A cross between two individuals identically heterozygous at one gene pair for example, Aa x Aa.

- **mononeuropathy**
  A form of diabetic neuropathy affecting a single nerve. The eye is a common site for this form of nerve damage. See also: Neuropathy.

- **monoplegia**
  Paralysis that involves one limb.

- **monoploid**
  A cell having only one chromosome set (usually as an aberration) or an organism composed of such cells.

- **monosomic**
  A diploid cell missing a single chromosome. A cell or individual that is basically diploid but that has only one copy of one particular chromosome type and thus has chromosome number 2n - 1.

- **monosomy**
  Possessing only one copy of a particular chromosome instead of the normal two copies.

- **monozygotic**
  Refers to twins derived from a single fertilized egg.

- **monozygotic twinning**
  Single egg twinning (identical twins).

- **morbid map**
  A diagram showing the chromosomal location of genes associated with disease.

- **morbidity rate**
  The sickness rate; the number of people who are sick or have a disease compared with the number who are well.

- **morphogen**
  A protein present in embryonic tissues in a concentration gradient that induces a developmental process.

- **morphogenetic**
  The changes that occur in the process of embryonic development.

- **morphological species concept**
  Organisms are classified in the same species if they appear identical by morphological (anatomical) criteria.

- **mortality rate**
  The death rate; the number of people who die of a certain disease compared with the total number of people. Mortality is most often stated as deaths per 1,000, per 10,000, or per 100,000 persons.

- **mosaic**
  A chimera; a tissue containing two or more genetically distinct cell types, or an individual composed of such tissues. Individual made up of two or more genetically distinct cell lines. Mosaic is the art of decoration with small pieces of colored glass, stone or other material. It may be a technique of decorative art, an aspect of interior decoration or of cultural significance as in a cathedral.

- **mosaicism**
  A single embryo that has two or more cell types of different chromosomal makeup. Such abnormalities can arise from defects in embryonic development or can emerge artificially when fetal cells are grown in a laboratory prior to analysis. The presence of two or more cell lines (cell populations) which differ from each other in genotype or chromosome number.

- **motility**
  Power to move spontaneously/ involuntarily

- **motor**
  Relating to movement.

- **motor development**
  The increasing ability to use muscles.

- **mri**
  Magnetic Resonance Imaging which provides clear images of interior parts of the body, especially the brain

- **mrna**
  Messenger RNA; an RNA molecular that functions during translation to specify the sequence of amino acids in a nascent polypeptide.

- **mu particle**
  Bacteria-like particle found in the cytoplasm of Paramecium that have the mate-killer phenotype.

- **mu phage**
  A kind (species) of phage with properties similar to those of insertion sequences, being able to insert, transpose, and cause chromosome rearrangements and mutations.

- **mucosa**
  A mucous lining of various tubular organs.

- **mullerian mimicry**
  A form of mimicry in which noxious species evolve to resemble each other.

- **multicolor fish (m-fish)/ spectral karyotyping(™) (sky(™))**
  SKY and M-FISH utilize "whole chromosome paint" DNA probes, which are labeled with a unique fluorescent color for each of the 24 human chromosomes. The technique visualizes and thus identifies chromosomal material in marker chromosomes and subtle translocations whose origin cannot be determined by other cytogenetic techniques.

- **multifactorial**
  A trait that is determined by the interaction between a number of genes and environmental factors.

- **multifactorial inheritance**
  (synonym polygenic) The combined contribution of one or more often unspecified genes and environmental factors, often

unknown, in the causation of a particular trait or disease

- **multihybrid**
  An organism heterozygous at numerous loci.
- **multimeric structure**
  A structure composed of several identical or different subunits held together by weak bonds.
- **multinomial expansion**
  The terms generated when a multinomial is raised to a power.
- **multipara**
  A woman who has given birth to more than one baby.
- **multiple allelism**
  The existence of several known alleles of a gene.
- **multiple gestation**
  More than one fetus developing in the uterus.
- **multiple polyposis**
  A disease characterized by numerous polyps in the colon and rectum. May also be referred to as familial polyposis.
- **multiple-factor hypothesis**
  A hypothesis to explain quantitative variation by assuming the interaction of a large number of genes (polygenes) each with a small additive effect on the character.
- **multiple-hit hypothesis**
  The proposal that a single cell must receive a series of mutational events in order to become malignant or cancerous.
- **multiplexing**
  A laboratory approach that performs multiple sets of reactions in parallel (simultaneously); greatly increasing speed and throughput.
- **multiplicity of infection (moi)**
  The average number of phage particles that infect a single bacterial cell in a specific experiment.
- **multipoint mapping**
  A type of genetic mapping in which the recombination frequencies among three or more loci are estimated simultaneously.
- **murine**
  Organism in the genus Mus. A rat or mouse.
- **murmur**
  Sounds made by turbulent blood moving through the chambers and valves of the heart or through the blood vessels near the heart, may signify a structural defect in the heart or valves.
- **muscle wasting**
  Loss of muscle bulk because of disuse or pathological process.
- **muscles**
  Bundles of specialized cells that can contract and relax to create movement for the body itself and the organs within it.

- **muscular dystrophy (md)**

  A group of genetic degenerative myopathies characterized by weakness and muscle atrophy without nervous system involvement. The three main types are pseudohypertrophic, limb-girdle and facioscapulohumeral.

- **musculoskeletal**

  Includes the bones, joints, and surrounding soft tissue such as the skin, muscles, ligaments, and joint capsules.

- **mutability**

  The ability to change.

- **mutable normal allele**

  In disorders caused by nucleotide repeat expansion, an abnormally large allele that is not associated with clinical symptoms but that can expand into a reduced penetrance allele or a full penetrance allele when transmitted to offspring. Mutable normal alleles are larger than normal alleles and smaller than reduced penetrance alleles and full penetrance alleles.

- **mutagen**

  An agent that causes a permanent genetic change in a cell. Does not include changes occurring during normal genetic recombination; An agent that is capable of increasing the mutation rate .

- **mutagenicity**

  The capacity of a chemical or physical agent to cause permanent genetic alterations.

- **mutant**

  An organism or cell carrying a mutation. An alternative phenotype to the wild-type; the phenotype produced by a non-wildtype allele.

- **mutant allele**

  An allele differing from the allele found in the standard or wild type organism.

- **mutant screening**

  The process of screening for mutations showing abnormalities in a certain structure or in a particular function, as a preparation for genetic analysis of that strucutre or function.

- **mutant site**

  The damaged or altered area within a mutated gene.

- **mutation**

  Any heritable change in DNA sequence; Any alteration in a gene from its natural state; may be disease-causing or a benign, normal variant; A permanent structural alteration in DNA. In most cases such DNA changes either have no effect or cause harm. Occasionally, however, a mutation can improve an organism's chance of surviving and passing the beneficial change on to its descendants. A permanent, heritable change in a gene or chromosome structure. (1) The process producing a gene or a chromosome differing from the wild-type. (2) The gene or chromosome that results from such a process.

**Types of mutation**

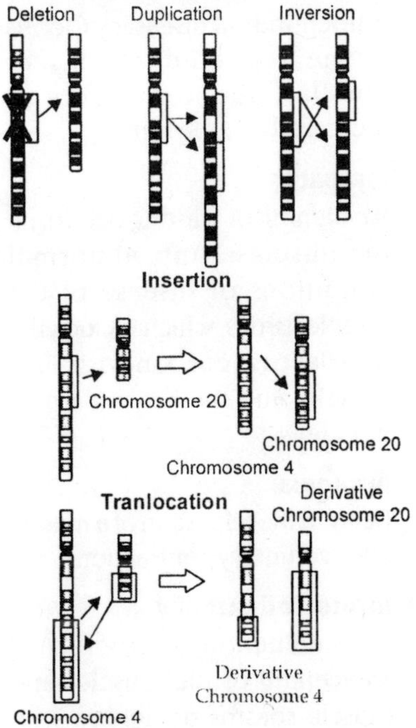


- **mutation analysis (synonym targeted mutation analysis)**
  Testing for the presence of a specific mutation (e.g., Glu6Val for sickle cell anemia), a specific type of mutation (e.g., the trinucleotide repeat expansion associated with spinocerebellar ataxia type 1, deletions associated with Duchenne muscular dystrophy), or set of mutations (e.g., a panel of mutations for cystic fibrosis), as opposed to complete gene sequencing or mutation scanning, which detect most mutations in the tested region

- **mutation breeding**
  Use of mutagens to develop variants that can increase agricultural yield.

- **mutation event**
  The actual occurrence of a mutation in time and space.

- **mutation frequency**
  The frequency of mutations in a population.

- **mutation rate**
  The number of mutation events per gene per unit of time (for example, per cell generation). The proportion of mutations per cell division in bacteria or single-celled organisms or the proportion of mutations per gamete in higher organisms.

- **mutational dissection**
  The study of the components of a biological system through a study of mutations affecting that system.

- **mutational load**
  Genetic load caused by mutation.

- **mutator mutation**
  Mutation of DNA polymerase that increases the overall mutation rate.

- **muton**
A term coined by Benzer for the smallest mutable site within a cistron. The smallest part of a gene that can be involved in a mutation event; now known to be a single nucleotide pair.

- **myelin**
Fatty sheath which encloses certain nerve fibres in the central nervous system.

- **myelinization**
Acquirement of fat like substance forming a sheath for nerve fibers.

- **myelogram**
A diagnostic procedure which creates an image of the spinal cord. A dye is injected into the spinal canal, and X-ray pictures are taken of the spinal cord.

- **myelomeningocele**
Spina Bifida in association with the protrusion of the spinal cord and its membranes.

- **myocardial infarction**
Also called a heart attack; results from permanent damage to an area of the heart muscle. This happens when the blood supply to the area is interrupted because of narrowed or blocked blood vessels.

- **myocardium**
The heart muscle.

- **myoclonic**
A type of muscle contraction.

- **myoclonus**
A single spasm or twitching of a muscle. Myoclonus can be a single event (twitch) or repeated events. Myoclonus can be a normal event (the jerks that occur when we fall asleep) or an abnormal event (those that occur while awake, or those associated with seizures or mitochondrial diseases). Clonus is the repeated spasms of muscles, due to a seizure or increased muscle tone.

- **myopathy**
Weakening or wasting occurring in muscles; Any abnormal conditions or disease of the muscle tissues, which include the muscles over our bones (skeletal muscle) and the heart (cardiac muscle).

- **myotonia**
Delay in the relaxation of a muscle after voluntary contraction.

- **myotonic dystrophy**
A combination of progressive weakening of the muscles and muscle spasms or rigidity, with difficulty relaxing a contracted muscle; inherited as an autosomal dominant trait.

- **nares**
Nostrils, openings of the nose.

- **narp**
Neuropathy Ataxia and Retinitis Pigmentosa.

- **nasal hypoplasia**
  Underdevelopment of the nose.
- **nasofrontal duct**
  Channel connecting the frontal sinus with the cavity of the nose.
- **nasogastric tube (n.g. tube)**
  A plastic tube with a number of openings at the lower end, passed through the nose into the stomach for the purpose of decompressing gas and draining accumulated liquids.
- **nasopharynx**
  The area of the upper throat behind the nose.
- **natural selection**
  The process in nature whereby one genotype leaves more offspring than another genotype because of superior life history attributes (fitness)such as survival or fecundity.
- **nausea**
  Nausea is the urge to vomit. It can be brought by many causes including, systemic illnesses, such as influenza, medications, pain, and inner ear disease.
- **nearest-neighbour analysis**
  A technique of transferring radioactive atoms between adjacent nucleotides in DNA used to demonstrate that the two strands of DNA run in opposite directions.
- **necrobiosis lipoidica diabeticorum**
  A skin condition usually on the lower part of the legs. The lesions can be small or extend over a large area. They are usually raised, yellow, and waxy in appearance and often have a purple border. Young women are most often affected. This condition occurs in people with diabetes, or it may be a sign of diabetes. It also occurs in people who do not have diabetes.
- **necrosis**
  Process of cell death that results from massive disruption of normal cellular homeostasis, that is so disruptive that the cells cannot repair themselves and then die. This is a common form of cell death following injury to tissue.
- **negative assortative mating**
  Preferential mating between phenotypically different partners.
- **negative control**
  Transcription regulation mediated by factors that block, turn down or turn off transcription.
- **negative interference**
  The phenomenon whereby a crossover in a particular region enhances the occurrence of other apparent crossovers in the same region of the chromosome.
- **negative predictive value**
  The likelihood that an individual with a negative test result is actually unaffected and/or does not have the particular gene mutation in question.

- **n-end rule**
The life span of a protein is determined by its amino-terminal (N-terminal) amino acid.

- **neo-darwinism**
The merger of classical Darwinian evolution with population genetics.

- **neomorph**
Mutant showing a novel substance or structure not found in wild-types.

- **neonatal**
The first four weeks after a child's birth.

- **neoplasia**
Literally, new growth, grown from a single cell, not transplanted from another place.

- **neoplasm**
Any new or abnormal growth; specifically a new growth of tissue in which the growth is uncontrolled and progressive. Malignant neoplasm are distinguished from benign in that the former show a greater degree of anaplasia and have the properties of invasion and metastasis. Also called a tumor.

- **neovascularization**
The term used when new, tiny blood vessels grow in a new place, for example, out from the retina.

- **nephrectomy**
Removal of all (total) or some (partial) of one kidney.

- **nephro**
Relating to the kidneys.

- **nephrologist**
A doctor who sees and treats people with kidney diseases.

- **nephropathy**
Disease of the kidneys caused by damage to the small blood vessels or to the units in the kidneys that clean the blood. People who have had diabetes for a long time may have kidney damage.

- **nerve**
A nerve is a bundle of fibers that uses electrical and chemical signals to transmit sensory and motor information from one body part to another.

- **nerve conduction studies**
Tests to determine nerve function; can detect early neuropathy.

- **nerve root**
A sheaf of nerve fibres entering and leaving a segment of the spinal cord.

- **nervous system**
The nervous system is the body tissue that records and distributes information in the body using electrical and chemical transmission. It has two parts. The "central" nervous system is comprised of the brain and spinal cord. The "peripheral" nervous system is the nerve tissue that transmits sensation and motor information back and forth from the body to the central nervous system.

- **neural tube**
  A structure in early fetal life that develops into the brain, spinal cord, spinal nerves and spine.

- **neural tube defect**
  A congenital abnormality of the spinal cord or brain resulting from the abnormal closure of the neural groove early in embryogenesis (e.g., spina bifida, anencephaly).

- **neurocutaneous**
  A group of conditions that combine skin and sensory or nervous difficulties.

- **neurofibromatosis**
  One of the most common single gene conditions affecting the human nervous system; in most cases, "cafe au lait" spots, are the only symptom; inherited as an autosomal dominant trait, with 50% being new mutations.

- **neurofibromin**
  The protein product of the neurofibromatosis type 1 gene.

- **neurological**
  Referring to the nervous system (the brain, spinal cord, and nerves, and their function.).

- **neurologist**
  A doctor who sees and treats people nonsurgically who have problems of the nervous system, the brain, spinal cord and peripheral nerves.

- **neuromuscular**
  Pertaining to the nerves and muscles.

- **neuron**
  A complete nerve cell.

- **neuropathy**
  Group of symptoms caused by abnormalities in sensory or motor nerves. Symptoms include tingling and numbness in hands or feet, followed by gradually progressive muscular weakness. The three major forms of nerve damage are: peripheral neuropathy, autonomic neuropathy, and mononeuropathy. The most common form is peripheral neuropathy, which mainly affects the feet and legs.

- **neurospora**
  A pink mold, commonly found growing on old food.

- **neurosurgeon**
  A physician specializing in the surgical treatment of the nervous system, the brain, spinal cord, and nerves.

- **neurotransmitter**
  Chemicals that act as messengers between cells in the brain and nervous system; they transmit impulses across the gap from a neuron to another neuron, a muscle, or a gland.

- **neutral gene hypothesis**
  The hypothesis that most genetic variation in natural populations is

not maintained by selection because most alleles have equal fitness.

- **neutral mutation**
  (1) A mutation that has no effect on the Darwinian fitness of its carriers. (2) A mutation that has no phenotypic effect.

- **neutral petite**
  A petite yeast that produces all wild-type progeny when crossed with wild-type.

- **neutrophils**
  The larger and physiologically most numerous class of infection-fighting white blood cells, characteristically even more numerous in generalised bacterial infections.

- **nevus**
  A mole or birthmark; Malformation of the skin which may be colored by hypo-pigmentation or increased vascularization (more blood vessels) Skin blemishes such as mole, birthmarks, beauty marks.

- **new mutation**
  An alteration in DNA sequence that appears for the first time in a family as the result of a mutation in one of the parent's germ cell.

- **newborn screening**
  Testing done within days of birth to identify infants at increased risk for a specific genetic disorder so that treatment can begin as soon as possible; when a newborn screening result is positive, further diagnostic testing is usually required to confirm or specify the results and counseling is offered to educate the parents.

- **nicking**
  Nuclease action to sever the sugar-phosphate backbone in one DNA strand but not the other at one specific site.

- **nitrocellulose filter**
  A type of filter used to bind DNA for hybridization.

- **nitrogen base**
  Type of molecule that forms an important part of nucleic acid, composed of a nitrogen-containing ring structure. Hydrogen bonds between bases in opposing complementary strands link the two strands of a DNA double helix.

- **nitrogenous base**
  A nitrogen-containing molecule having the chemical properties of a base. DNA contains the nitrogenous bases adenine (A), guanine (G), cytosine (C), and thymine (T).

- **nodular**
  Node-like, a know or swelling.

- **non-coding dna**
  One of the two identical strands that make up the DNA double helix. The non-coding strand, or antisense strand, is a mirror-image of the coding strand, but does not carry the information

needed to order the production of proteins.

- **non-coding dna (also called junk dna)**

DNA in the genome that is not directly involved in making proteins or other molecules.About 98 percent of the human genome consists of non-coding DNA.The term "junk" reflects the belief that the DNA, which is often repetitive, no longer serves a purpose in humans.But it's now clear that some non-coding DNA controls the activity of genes and may have other functions.

- **non-consangineous**

This means that the parents of the proband were not related.

- **nondisjunction**

Failure of paired chromosomes to separate (into each daughter cell) during cell division; The failure of a pair of homologous chromosomes to separate properly during meiosis. The failure of homologues (at meiosis) or sister chromatids (at mitosis) to separate properly to opposite poles, that is two chromosomes or chromatids go to one pole and none to the other.

- **non-histone protein**

The protein remaining in chromatin after the histones are removed. The scaffold structure is made of nonhistone proteins.

- **noninsulin-dependent diabetes mellitus (niddm)**

The most common form of diabetes mellitus; about 90 to 95 percent of people who have diabetes have NIDDM. Unlike the insulin-dependent type of diabetes, in w hich the pancreas makes no insulin, people with noninsulin-dependent diabetes produce some insulin, sometimes even large amounts. However, either their bodies do not produce enough insulin or their body cells are resistant to the action of insulin (see Insulin Resistance). People with NIDDM can often control their condition by losing weight through diet and exercise. If not, they may need to combine insulin or a pill with diet and exercise. Generally, NIDDM occurs in people who are over age 40. Most of the people who have this type of diabetes are overweight. Noninsulin-dependent diabetes mellitus used to be called "adult-onset diabetes," "maturity-onset diabetes," "ketosis-resistant diabetes," and "stable diabetes." It is also called type II diabetes mellitus.

- **noninvasive blood glucose monitoring**

A way to measure blood glucose without having to prick the finger to obtain a blood sample. Several noninvasive devices are currently being developed.

- **nonketotic coma**

A type of coma caused by a lack of insulin. A nonketotic crisis means: (1) very high levels of glucose (sugar) in the blood; (2) absence of ketoacidosis; (3) great loss of body fluid; and (4) a sleepy, confused, or comatose state. Nonketotic coma often results from some other problem such as a severe infection or kidney failure.

- **non-linear tetrad**

A tetrad in which the meiotic products are in no particular order.

- **non-mendelian ratio**

An unusual ratio of progeny phenotypes that does not reflect the simple operation of Mendel's laws; for example, mutant:wild-type ratios of 3:5, 5:3, 6:2, or 2:6 in tetrads indicate that gene conversion has occurred.

- **non-parental ditype (npd)**

A spore arrangement in Ascomycetes that contains only the two recombinant-type ascospores (assuming two segregating loci). A tetrad type containing two different genotypes, both of which are recombinant.

- **nonpenetrance**

Lack of clinical expression of the mutant phenotype in an individual with the appropriate genotype.

- **non-recombinant**

In mapping studies the offspring that have alleles arranged as in the original parents are non-recombinants.

- **nonsense codon**

One of the mRNA sequences (UAA, UAG, UGA) that signals the termination of translation. A codon for which no normal tRNA molecule exists. The presence of a nonsense codon causes termination of translation (ending polypeptide chain synthesis). There are three nonsense codons are called amber (UAG) ochre (UAA) and opal (UGA).

- **nonsense mutation**

A single base pair substitution that prematurely codes for a stop in amino acid translation (stop codon); A substitution of one of the bases of DNA that results in a stop codon; a mutation in which a codon is changed to a stop codon, resulting in a truncated protein product.

- **nonsense suppressor**

A mutation in the anticodon of tRNA that alters the anticodon so it is now complementary to a nonsense codon allowing the tRNA to insert its cognate amino acid at this nonsense codon during translation.

- **non-verbal**

Unable to communicate with the spoken word; does not mean non-communicative; person may use sign language, pointing, or body language to communicate.

- **noonan syndrome**
A condition characterized by short stature and ovarian or testicular dysfunction, mental deficiency, and lesions of the heart.

- **norm of reaction**
The pattern of phenotypes produced by a given genotype under different environmental conditions.

- **normal distribution**
Any of a family of bell-shaped frequency curves whose relative position and shape are defined on the basis of the mean and standard deviation.

- **normal saline**
Salt solution at the same concentration as in the body fluids.

- **normal sinus rhythm**
Regular rhythm of the heart, at regular rates (depending whether resting or mildly exercising), originating in electrical control by the usual (sino-atrial node) pacemaker of the heart.

- **northern analysis**
A technique for transferring electrophoretically resolved RNA segments from an agarose gel to a nitrocellulose filter paper sheet via capillary action.

- **northern blot**
A gel-based laboratory procedure that locates mRNA sequences on a gel that are complementary to a piece of DNA used as a probe; The separation of sequences or fragments of RNA, partially digested by endonucleases, on an electrophoretic gel; Transfer of electrophoretically separated RNA molecules from a gel onto an absorbent sheet, which is then immersed in a labeled probe that will hybridize to an RNA of interest to reveal its presence.

- **nosology**
Study of the classification of a syndrome or disease.

- **novel mutation**
A distinct gene alteration that has been newly discovered; not the same as a 'new' or 'de novo' mutation

- **nuchal cord**
Umbilical cord is wrapped around the fetus's neck before birth or at delivery.

- **nuclear family**
A pair of biologic parents and their children.

- **nuclear medicine**
Medical procedures for diagnosis and treatment which involve some sort of radioactive isotope.

- **nuclear transfer**
A laboratory procedure in which a cell's nucleus is removed and

placed into an oocyte with its own nucleus removed so the genetic information from the donor nucleus controls the resulting cell. Such cells can be induced to form embryos. This process was used to create the cloned sheep "Dolly".

- **nuclear transplantation**
  The technique of placing a nucleus from another source into an enucleated cell.

- **nuclease**
  One of the several classes of enzymes that degrade nucleic acid. An enzyme that can degrade DNA or RNA by breaking phosphodiester bonds.

- **nuclease hypersensitive site**
  Region of eukaryotic chromosome DNA that is specifically vulnerable to nuclease attack perhaps because it is not wrapped in histone as nucleosomes.

- **nucleic acid**
  A large molecule composed of nucleotide subunits.

- **nucleoid**
  A DNA mass within a chloroplast or mitochondrion.

- **nucleolar organizer**
  The chromosomal region around which the nucleolus forms, a site of tandem repeats of the rRNA gene. A region (or regions) of the chromosome set physically associated with the nucleolus and containing rRNA genes.

- **nucleolar organizing region**
  A part of the chromosome containing rRNA genes.

- **nucleolus**
  The globular nuclear organelle formed at the nucleolar organizer. Site of ribosome construction. An organelle found in the nucleus, containing rRNA and multiple copies of the genes coding for rRNA.

- **nucleoprotein**
  The substance of eukaryotic chromosomes consisting of proteins and nucleic acids.

- **nucleoside**
  A sugar-base compound that is a nucleotide precursor. Nucleotides are nucleoside phosphates. A nitrogen base linked to a sugar molecule.

- **nucleosome**
  A nu body; the basic unit of eukaryotic chromosome structure; a ball of eight histone molecules wrapped about by two coils of about 220 base pairs of DNA. Arrangement of DNA and histones forming regular spherical structures in eukaryotic chromatin.

- **nucleotide**
  A subunit of DNA or RNA consisting of a nitrogenous base (adenine, guanine, thymine, or cytosine in DNA; adenine, guanine, uracil, or cytosine in RNA), a phosphate molecule, and a sugar molecule (deoxyribose in DNA and ribose

in RNA). Thousands of nucleotides are linked to form a DNA or RNA molecule.

**Deoxyribonucleic Acid (DNA)**

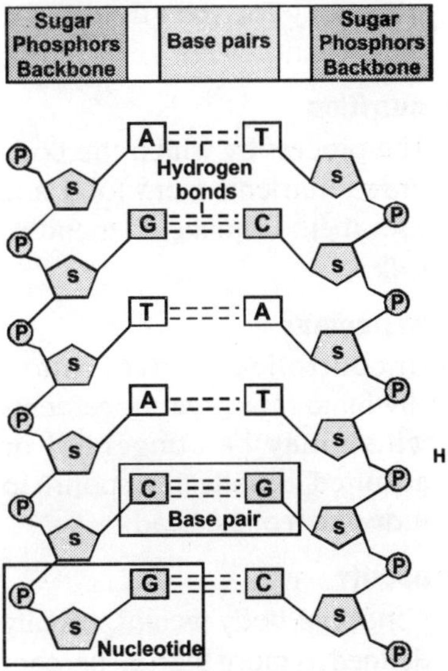


Constituent components of DNA and RNA. Each nucleotide has three parts: a nitrogen-containing base, a five-carbon sugar, and a phosphate group. The bases are adenine, cytosine, guanine, thymine (in DNA), and uracil (in RNA).

- **nucleotide mapping**

  Two- dimensional separation and analysis of nucleotides.

- **nucleotide pair**

  A pair of complementary nucleotides (one in each strand of DNA) that are joined by hydrogen bonds.

- **nucleotide-pair substitution**

  The replacement of a specific nucleotide pair by a different pair; often mutagenic.

- **nucleus**

  The cellular organelle in eukaryotes that contains most of the genetic material. The information center of a cell. The genetic information of most living things is physically located in the nucleus of a cell, which contains chromosomes, where genes are found.

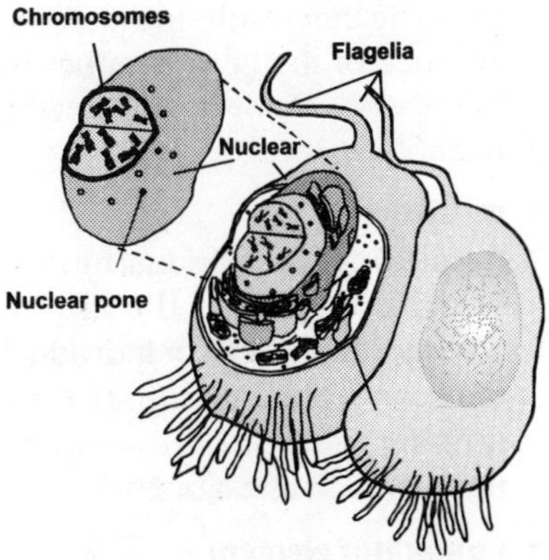


- **nucleus basalis of meynert**

  A small group of cholinergic nerve cells in the forebrain and connected to areas of the cerebral cortex.

- **nude mice**

  Immunologically deficient mice used to permit growth of tumor cells from mouse and other species, such as human.

- **null allele**
A mutation that results in either no gene product or the absence of function at the phenotypic level. An allele whose effect is either an absence of normal gene product at the molecular level or an absence of normal function at the phenotypic level.

- **null hypothesis**
The statistical hypothesis that states that there are no differences between observed and expected data.

- **null mutation**
An allele that results in either the absence of the gene product or the absence of any function at the phenotypic level.

- **nullisomic**
A diploid cell or individual missing both copies of the same chromosome. A cell or individual with one chromosomal type missing, with a chromosome number such as n-1 or 2n-2.

- **numerator element**
Genes on the X chromosome in Drosophila that regulate the sex switch (sxl) to the on condition (femaleness). Refers to the numerator of the X/A (number of X chromosomes/autosomes) genic balance equation.

- **nurse cell**
A sister cell of an oocyte in insects. Nurse cells produce the bulk of the cytoplasmic contents of the mature oocyte.

- **nutrients**
Proteins, carbohydrates, fats, vitamins, and minerals. These are provided by food and are necessary for growth and the maintenance of life.

- **nutrition**
The process by which the body draws nutrients from food and uses them to make or mend its cells.

- **nystagmus**
Uncontrolled, involuntary rhythmic rapid eye movements which may be congenital or acquired. Usually in response to movement of the head.

- **obesity**
Abnormal body weight, usually defined as more than 20 percent above average for age, height and bone structure.

- **obligate carrier (synonym obligate heterozygote)**
An individual who may be clinically unaffected but who must carry a gene mutation based on analysis of the family history; usually applies to disorders inherited in an autosomal recessive or X-linked recessive manner.

- **obligate heterozygote (synonym obligate heterozygote)**
An individual who may be clinically unaffected but who must carry a gene mutation based on

analysis of the family history; usually applies to disorders inherited in an autosomal recessive and X-linked recessive manner

- **obstetrician**
  A doctor who sees and gives care to pregnant women and delivers babies.

- **obstetrics**
  Branch of medicine concerned with pregnancy and childbirth.

- **occipital**
  Pertaining to the back of the head.

- **occipital lobe**
  Area at the back of the brain that receives and processes visual information.

- **occipitoposterior position**
  The baby's face is directed to the front of the birth canal and results in diameters of the baby's head that may be too large to pass through the birth passage unless the position of the head can be corrected.

- **occiput**
  The back of the head.

- **occlusion**
  The action of closing up or of being closed up.

- **occulta**
  A concealed or hidden feature.

- **occupational therapy**
  Treatment in which the activities of daily life are incorporated to meet the specific needs of the individual patient, may include sensory integration.

- **ochre codon**
  The codon UAA, a nonsense codon.

- **ocipital**
  Referring to the occiput bone in the back of the head, or the lower back lobes of the brain where vision is processed; the back of the head.

- **octad**
  An ascus containing eight ascospores, produced in species in which the tetrad normally undergoes a postmeiotic mitotic division.

- **oedema**
  Swelling of the body caused by abnormal acculation of fluid in the tissues of the body.

- **oesophageal sphincter**
  A circular band of muscle where the esophagus is attached to the stomach.

- **oesophagram**
  X-ray image made of the esophagus using a water-soluable feeding solutionto determine the swallowing dysfunction.

- **oesophagus**
  The canal down which solids and fluids pass from the mouth to reach the stomach.

- **oestrogen**
  Hormone which stimulates the function of the female reproductive organs.

- **okazaki fragment**
  Segment of newly replicated DNA produced during discontinuous DNA replication.

- **olfactory**
  Pertaining to sense of smell.

- **oligogenic**
  A phenotypic trait produced by two or more genes working together.

- **oligogenic diseases**
  Diseases or traits that result from the effects of relatively few genes, some of which have rather large effects.

- **oligonucleotide**
  A molecule usually composed of 25 or fewer nucleotides; used as a DNA synthesis primer.

- **oligoprobe**
  A short DNA probe whose hybridization is sensitive to a single base, mismatch.

- **omentum**
  A free fold of the peritoneum, or one serving to connect viscera, support blood vessels, etc..

- **oncogene**
  A gene, one or more forms of which is associated with cancer. Many oncogenes are involved, directly or indirectly, in controlling the rate of cell growth; A gene that contributes to the production of a cancer. Oncogenes are generally mutated forms of normal cellular genes (proto-oncogenes). A gene capable, when activated, of transforming a cell. Oncogenes are found in the oncogenically activated state in retroviruses and transformed cells and in their normal non-oncogenically activated state in non-transformed cells in which they are called proto-oncogenes.

- **oncologist**
  A physician specializing in treatment of various forms of cancer.

- **one-gene-one-enzyme hypothesis**
  Hypothesis of Beadle and Tatum that one gene controls the production of one enzyme. Later modified to the concept that one cistron controls the production of one polypeptide.

- **oogenesis**
  The process of ovum formation in female animals.

- **oogonia**
  Cells in females that produce primary oocytes by mitosis.

- **opal codon**
  The codon UGA, a nonsense codon.

- **open reading frame**
  All exons of a gene that contribute to the protein product(s) of the gene.

- **open reading frame (orf)**
  The sequence of DNA or RNA located between the start-code

sequence (initiation codon) and the stop-code sequence (termination codon).

- **operator**
  A DNA region at one end of an operon that acts as the binding site for repressor protein. A DNA sequence that is recognized by a repressor protein or repressor-corepressor complex. When the operator is complexed with the repressor, transcription is prevented.

- **operon**
  A set of genes transcribed under the control of an operator gene. A set of adjacent structural genes in bacteria whose mRNA is synthesized in one piece, together with the adjacent regulatory signals that affect transcription of the structural genes. A sequence of adjacent bacterial genes all under the transcriptional control of the same operator.

- **ophthalmologist**
  A doctor who sees and treats people with eye problems or diseases.

- **ophthalmoplegia**
  Weakness or paralysis of muscles of the eye.

- **optic nerve**
  Nerve that carries visual impulses from the retina to the brain.

- **optical mapping**
  An enabling technology for whole genome analysis which involves the capture of individual DNA molecules, obtained directly from genomic DNA, followed by digestion in situ by selected restriction endonucleases. The resulting fragments are then visualized directly to produce detailed optical restriction maps. This methodology allows patterns of sequence variation to be detected across entire genomes, without the need for DNA amplification, and, unlike other genomewide scanning methods, provides detailed haplotype information by analyzing individual DNA molecules. OpGen will provide optical mapping services to three main markets — i.e., genome sequencing projects, cancer diagnostics, and genetic association studies.

- **optometrist**
  An optometrist, or doctor of optometry (O.D.) is a professionally trained person who has attended a college of optometry, studying the science of measuring focal lengths and correcting visual acuity with the aid of glasses and contact lenses. An optometrist is not a physician and has not attended medical school. Optometrists are prepared to recognize eye diseases they may see in the course of examining a patient, but they are not licensed to diagnose or treat eye diseases.

- **orf (open reading frame)**
  A section of a sequenced piece of DNA that begins with an initiation (methionine ATG) codon and ends with a nonsense codon. ORFs all have the potential to encode a protein or polypeptide, however many may not actually do so.

- **organelle**
  A subcellular structure having a specialized function for example the mitochondrion, the chloroplast, or the spindle apparatus; Membrane-bound intracellular, cytoplasmic structures having specialized functions, e.g., mitochondria, plastics, Golgi apparatus, lysosomes.

- **organogenesis**
  The production of organ systems during animal embryogenesis.

- **origin of replication**
  The point of specific sequence at which DNA replication is initiated.

- **orofacial**
  Pertaining to the mouth and face.

- **oropharynx**
  The area of the throat at the back of the mouth.

- **orthopnea**
  Difficulty breathing except in an upright position.

- **osseous**
  Boney, in consistancy or structure.

- **ossicle**
  A small bone, in this case in the middle ear.

- **osteochondritis**
  Inflammation of bone and cartilage.

- **osteogenesis imperfecta**
  A condition also known as brittle bone disease; characterized by a triangular shaped face with yellowish brown teeth, short stature and stunted growth, scoliosis, high pitched voice, excessive sweating and loose joints.

- **otitis media**
  Otitis media (also known as glue ear) is an inflammation of the middle ear segment of the ear. It is usually associated with a buildup of fluid and frequently causes an earache. The fluid may or may not be infected. The typical progress of otitis media is: the tissues surrounding the Eustachian tube swell due to an infection and/or severe congestion. The Eustachian tube remains blocked most of the time.

- **otosclerosis**
  A new formation of spongy bone that results in progressively increasing deafness.

- **outbred mouse strains**
  Strains of mice propagated by nonstandardized matings. These mice retain substantial genetic variability.

- **outbreeding**
  The mating of genetically unrelated individuals.

- **outside markers**
  Loci on either side of another locus or specified region.

- **ovarian**
  Relating to the ovaries, the female reproductive organs containing the ova (eggs).

- **ovary**
  An ovary or "egg sac" is one of a pair of reproductive glands in women. The ovaries produce the ovum or female egg which is transferred through the fallopian tube for fertilization by the sperm. The ovary also produces both the hormones estrogen and progesterone.

- **overdominance**
  A relationship in which the phenotypic expression of the heterozygote is greater than that of either homozygote.

- **overt diabetes**
  Diabetes in the person who shows clear signs of the disease such as a great thirst and the need to urinate often.

- **oxygen**
  A gas present in air that is vital to life.

- **p (peptidyl) site**
  The site on the ribosome occupied by the peptidyl-tRNA just before peptide bond formation.

- **p element**
  A Drosophila transposable element that has been used as a tool for insertion mutagenesis and for germline transformation.

- **p henotype**
  The outward physical characteristics of an organism.

- **p1-derived artificial chromosome (pac)**
  One type of vector used to clone DNA fragments (100- to 300-kb insert size; average, 150 kb) in Escherichia coli cells. Based on bacteriophage (a virus) P1 genome.

- **p53**
  A gene responsible for regulating the growth cycle of a cell. A mutation to this gene can cause certain types of cancer.

- **p53**
  A 53KDa protein the product of a tumour suppressor gene. The loss of this protein due to mutation is a primary event in the formation of many types of cancer (breast, colon, lung, leukaemia, liver). P53 is involved in regulating the activity of some other genes (eg. P21, a cell division kinase inhibitor). It also prevents cells entering cell division. P53 levels are increased after DNA is damaged by UV and ionizing radiation and cells are arrested in cell division until either the damage is repaired or they die by apoptosis (programmed cell death).

- **p53 (tumor-suppressor genes)**
  Genes that normally restrain cell growth but, when missing or inactivated by mutation, allow cells to grow uncontrolled.

- **pac**
  The artificial chromosome vector derived from the temperate bacteriophage, P1, used for cloning 100- to 200-kb DNA fragments.

- **pacemaker**
  A group of cells, known as the sinoatrial node, that are located in the atrium of the heart and serve to regulate the rate and rhythm of the heart. An artificial cardiac pacemaker is an electrical device used to simulate the natural process by generating electrical impulses.

- **pachygyria**
  Very broad thick gyri; often associated with mental retardation.

- **pachynema (pachytene stage)**
  The stage of prophase one of meiosis in which chromatids are first distinctly visible.

- **palate**
  The roof of the mouth. The front portion is bony (hard palate), and the back portion is muscular (soft palate); The bony and muscular partition between the mouth and nasal cavity.

- **palindrome**
  A sequence of letters, words, phrases, or nucleotides that reads the same regardless of direction, for instance what Adam said to Eve "Madam I'm Adam". The DNA sequence of type II restriction endonuclease recognition sites (e.g. EcoRI 5'GAATTC3') and the binding sites of many other DNA binding proteins (eg. catabolite activator protein (CAP) binding site 5'GTGAGTTAGCTCAC3') are not true palindromes but in double stranded form are similar and have two-fold rotational symetry; In molecular biology, a nucleotide sequence in which the 5'to 3' sequence of 1 strand of a segment of DNA is the same as that of its complementary strand. The sites of many restriction enzymes are palindromes.

- **palliative**
  Treatment undertaken not to cure but to improve a problem or condition.

- **palmar**
  Referring to the palm of the hand.

- **palpebral**
  Referring to the eyelids.

- **palpebral fissures**
  The gap between the upper and lower eyelids.

- **palsy**
  An alternative term for paralysis.

- **pancreas**

A small organ that lies behind the lower part of the stomach. The pancreas makes insulin needed to convert glucose to energy. The pancreas also makes enzymes that help the body digest food. Cells concentrated in areas known as Islets of Langerhans have specific functions. Alpha cells make glucagon, which raises the blood levels of glucose in the blood; beta cells make insulin; delta cells make somatostatin. There are also the PP cells and the D1 cells, about which little is known. A gland near the stomach which secretes digestive enzymes into the intestine and also secretes the hormone insulin into the blood as needed to regulate the level of sugar in the blood. Spread all over the pancreas are areas called the islets of Langerhans. The cells in these areas each have a special purpose. The alpha cells make glucagon, which raises the level of glucose in the blood; the beta cells make insulin; the delta cells make somatostatin. There are also the PP cells and the D1 cells, about which little is known.

- **pancreas transplant**

A surgical procedure that involves replacing the pancreas of a person who has diabetes with a healthy pancreas that can make insulin. The healthy pancreas comes from a donor who has just died or from a living relative. A person can donate half a pancreas and still live normally. At present, pancreas transplants are usually performed in persons with insulin-dependent diabetes who have severe complications. This is because after the transplant the patient must take immuno-suppressive drugs that are highly toxic and may cause damage to the body.

- **pancreatectomy**

A procedure in which a surgeon takes out the pancreas.

- **pancreatitis**

Inflammation (pain, tenderness) of the pancreas; it can make the pancreas stop working. It is caused by drinking too much alcohol, by disease in the gallbladder, or by a virus.

- **panmictic**

Referring to unstructured (random-mating) populations.

- **papilla**

A nipple-like projection or structure.

- **papilledema**

Swelling around the optic nerve, usually due to pressure on the nerve by a tumor.

- **para**

The number of live births. Commonly see the notation G2P, for example, which means gravida 2 para 1 - two pregnancies with one live birth.

- **paracentric inversion**
  An inversion in which the breakpoints are confined to one arm of a chromosome; the inverted segment does not span the centromere.

- **paraesophageal hernia**
  A hernia involving the diaphragm next to the esophagus.

- **paralogous genes**
  Two genes or clusters of genes at different chromosomal locations in the same organism that have structural similarities indicating that they derived from a common ancestral gene.

- **paralysis**
  Complete or partial inability to move a part of the body.

- **paramecin**
  A toxin liberated by a killer Paramecium.

- **parameters**
  Measurements of attributes of a population.

- **paranasal sinuses**
  Airspaces in the base of the skull in communication with the air passages of the nose.

- **paraparesis**
  Weakness below the waist, including the legs.

- **parapatric speciation**
  Speciation in which the evolution of reproductive isolating mechanisms occurs when a population enters a new niche or habitat within the range of the parent species.

- **paraplegia**
  Paralysis that involves the legs only.

- **parasympathetic**
  Division of the autonomic (automatic) nervous system. Parasympathetic nerves control functions of digestion, heart and lung activity, constriction of eye pupils and many other normal functions of the body.

- **parentage testing (synonym maternity testing, paternity testing)**
  The process through which DNA sequences from a particular child and a particular adult are compared to estimate the likelihood that the two individuals are related, DNA testing can reliably exclude but cannot absolutely confirm an individual as a biological parent.

- **parental ditype (pd)**
  A tetrad type containing two different genotypes, both of which are parental. A spore arrangement in Ascomycetes that contains only the two non-recombinant-type ascospores.

- **parental empowerment**
  Parents taking charge, assuming responsibility and exercising appropriate and rationale power

in a situation. (i.e.: obtaining a second opinion, requesting copies of laboratory reports, requesting or rejecting a muscle biopsy).

- **parenteral**
  Brought into the body in some other way than the digestive tract, as by subcutaneous or intravenous injection.

- **parent-of-origin studies**
  An analysis used to determine whether a particular chromosome or segment of DNA was inherited from an individual's mother or father; helpful in the diagnosis of disorders in which imprinting or uniparental disomy is a possible underlying etiological mechanism.

- **paresthesia**
  Abnormal sensations occurring spontaneously or in response to stimulation. Paresthesias may include prickling, tingling, burning, or tickling feelings; numbness; "pins and needles"; or cramp-like sensations. Various neurologic movement disorders may be characterized by paresthesias, including restless legs syndrome (RLS), paroxysmal kinesigenic dyskinesia (PKD), and paroxysmal non-kinesigenic dyskinesia (PNKD).

- **parietal**
  Relating to the wall of any cavity, or the parietal bone.

- **parietal lobe**
  Area of the brain that lies in front of the occipital lobe that is important in processing information from the sense of touch and bringing together sensory information.

- **paronychia**
  Infection around a fingernail bed.
  paroöxysmal nocturnal dyspnea
  Episodic shortness of breath at night.

- **part h**
  A section of IDEA that mandates states to have early intervention programs for children with special needs.

- **parthenogenesis**
  The development of an individual from an egg without fertilization; The production of offspring by a female with no genetic contribution from a male. The development of an individual from an unfertilized egg that did not arise by meiotic chromosome reduction.

- **partial digest**
  A restriction digest that has not been allowed to go to completion and thus contains pieces of DNA with some restriction endonuclease sites that have not yet been cleaved.

- **particulate inheritance**
  The model proposing that genetic information is transmitted from

one generation to the next in discrete units (particles) so that the character of the offspring is not a smooth blend of essences from the parents.

- **pascal's triangle**
  A triangular array of numbers made up of the coefficients of the binomial expansion.

- **patent**
  In genetics, conferring the right or title to genes, gene variations, or identifiable portions of sequenced genetic material to an individual or organization.

- **patent ductus arteriosus (pda)**
  Congenital heart defect which may close or "heal itself" spontaneously.

- **path diagram**
  A modified pedigree showing only the direct line of descent from common ancestors.

- **pathogen**
  An organism that causes disease in another organism.

- **pathogenic agent**
  A disease-causing organism. It could be anything from a virus, bacteria, to a multicellular organism such as a parasitic worm.

- **patroclinous inheritance**
  Inheritance in which all off-spring have the nucleus-based phenotype of the father.

- **pattern formation**
  The developmental processes by which the complex shape and structure of higher organisms occurs.

- **pcr- polymerase chain reaction**
  A procedure that produces millions of copies of a short segment of DNA through repeated cycles of: 1) denaturation, 2) annealing, and 3) elongation; PCR is a very common procedure in molecular genetic testing and may be used to 4) generate a sufficient quantity of DNA to perform a test (e.g., sequence analysis, mutation scanning), or 2) may be a test in and of itself (e.g., allele-specific amplification, trinucleotide repeat quantification).

  1. When double-stranded DNA (a) is heated up to 95° C (203° F), the two strands separate.
  2. Two types of chemically synthesized, short DNA strands called primers (b) are added. These primers are complementary to one part of each DNA strand and become attached by base pairing.
  3. When the DNA is cooled, the primers allow the enzyme (biological catalyst) DNA polymerase (c) to synthesize two new strands complementary to the regions "downstream" of each of the primers.

4. If this heating, cooling, and polymerization (synthesis) sequence is repeated over and over, the number of copies of the original DNA molecule doubles with each cycle. After 30 cycles, there will be over one billion double-stranded DNA molecules.

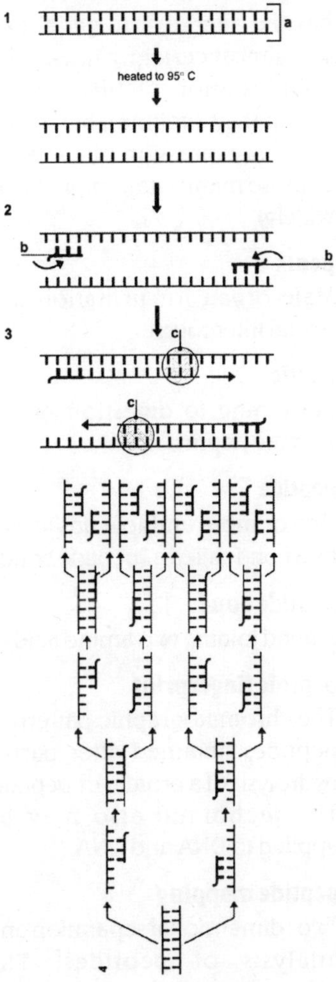


- **pearson syndrome**
  1. A severe disease occuring in infancy affecting bone marrow and pancreas function.
  2. Infants with Pearson syndrome may develop KSS as they get older.

- **pectoral**

  Pertaining to the chest.

- **pectoral muscles**

  Muscles that overlay the chest wall and help to support the breasts.

- **pectus carinatum**

  Convex chest (bowed out) opposite of pectus excavatum.

- **pectus excavatum**

  Sunken,concave or hollow chest. (Pectus-chest; excavatum-hollow, caved in or dug out).

- **pediatric endocrinologist**

  A doctor who sees and treats children with problems of the endocrine glands; diabetes is an endocrine disorder.

- **pedigree**

  A family tree diagram that shows how a particular genetic trait or disease has been inherited; A diagram of the genetic relationships and medical history of a family using standard symbols and terminolog; A multi-generational family tree using symbols to denote lineage and genetic information. A graphic representation of a person's family created using a standardized set of symbols.

- **pelvic**
  Having to do with the pelvis, the lower part of the abdomen, located between the hip bones.

- **pelvic floor muscles**
  A group of muscles at the base of the pelvis. They help support the bladder, urethra, rectum and (in women) vagina and uterus.

- **pelvic girdle**
  The bony ring composed of the two hip bones laterally and in front, and the sacrum and coccyx behind.

- **pelvic pouch**
  Surgically-fashioned artificial rectum.

- **pelvis**
  The ring of bones that link the spine and hip bones, and protects abdominal organs such as the uterus in women.

- **penetrance**
  The probability of a gene or genetic trait being expressed. "Complete" penetrance means the gene or genes for a trait are expressed in all the population who have the genes. "Incomplete" penetrance means the genetic trait is expressed in only part of the population. The percent penetrance also may change with the age range of the population; A term indicating the likelihood that a given gene will actually result in disease. The frequency with which individuals carrying a given gene will show the clinical manifestations associated with the gene. The probability that a gene will make any effect of its alteration evident. The VHL gene has almost complete penetrance (if someone has the altered VHL gene, they will almost certainly have some manifestation of VHL disease within their lifetime), but widely variable expression (the severity of those manifestations will vary widely).

- **penis**
  Male organ for urination and sexual intercourse.

- **peptic**
  Pertaining to digestion or the enzyme pepsin.

- **peptide**
  Two or more amino acids joined by a bond called a "peptide bond."

- **peptide bond**
  A bond joining two amino acids.

- **peptide fingerprint**
  The chromatographic pattern of peptides obtained after partial hydrolysis of a protein or peptide. The technique also may be applied to DNA and RNA.

- **peptide mapping**
  Two-dimensional separation and analysis of peptides. The

characteristic pattern of fragments formed by the separation of a mixture of peptides resulting from hydrolysis of a protein or peptide.

- **peptide maps**
One way to research the structure of a protein is to seek to identify the specific sequence of amino acids which form the protein. Tr. at 202-3. An initial approach is to cut the protein into fragments, called peptides, using enzymes or chemicals which reliably divide the chain at predictable points. Tr. at 523. These fragments can be isolated and analyzed to create "peptide maps," which show the pattern of pieces from these breaks as a unique "fingerprint." ... A peptide map does not disclose the precise order of the amino acids in a protein, although it may point to areas of difference between similar proteins.

- **peptidyl transferase**
The enzymatic centre in the ribosome responsible for peptide bond formation during translation.

- **percutaneous umbilical blood sampling**
A procedure in which a blood sample is withdrawn from the umbilical cord while the fetus is still in the uterus. Used mainly for rapid chromosome analysis or to evaluate fetuses at risk for certain blood disorders.

- **perforation**
Process of making a hole, or the hole itself.

- **pericardium**
Membranous sac enclosing the heart.

- **pericentric inversion**
An inversion in which the breakpoints occur on both arms of a chromosome. The inverted segment spans the centromere.

- **perinatal**
Pertaining to or occurring in the period of time shortly before and after the birth of an infant (28 weeks gestation to 1-4 months of age).

- **periodic**
Recurring at regular intervals.

- **periodontal**
Pertaining to the area immediately around a tooth.

- **periodontist**
A specialist in the treatment of diseases of the gums.

- **perioral**
Around the mouth.

- **periosteum**
Fibrous tissue that encases bone.

- **peripheral**
On the surface of an organ or of the body.

- **peripheral dysostosis**
Abnormally short and malformed bones of the hands and feet.

- **peripheral nervous system**
  The parts of the nervous system that are outside the brain and spinal cord.

- **peripheral neuropathy**
  Nerve damage, usually affecting the feet and legs; causing pain, numbness, or a tingling feeling. Also called "somatic neuropathy" or "distal sensory polyneuropathy.

- **peripheral vascular disease**
  Disease in the large blood vessels of the arms, legs, and feet. People who have had diabetes for a long time may get this because major blood vessels in their arms, legs, and feet are blocked and these limbs do not receive enough blood. The signs of PVD are aching pains in the arms, legs, and feet (especially when walking) and foot sores that heal slowly. Although people with diabetes cannot always avoid PVD, doctors say they have a better chance of avoiding it if they take good care of their feet, do not smoke, and keep both their blood pressure and diabetes under good control.

- **peritoneal dialysis**
  A way to clean the blood of people who have kidney disease.

- **permissive condition**
  Environmental condition under which a conditional mutation shows the wild-type phenotype.

- **permissive temperature**
  A temperature at which temperature-sensitive mutants are normal.

- **pernicious**
  Destructive, sometimes fatal.

- **peroneal**
  Relating to the fibula, the outer side of the leg, or the structures located there.

- **peroxisomal enzymes**
  Enzymes localized to the peroxisomes. These enzymes are initially synthesized by the free polyribosomes and then enter the cytoplasm and eventually are localized to the peroxisomes. There are at least 40 enzymes. Some are involved in the production and decomposition of hydrogen peroxide and some are concerned with lipid and amino acid metabolism.

- **peroxisome**
  A subcellular organelle surrounded by a single membrane containing at least 40 enzymes involved in energy production.

- **perspiration**
  Sweat, the salty fluid excreted from the sweat glands of the skin.

- **pest hypothesis**
  The short life-time of a protein is signaled by a region rich in the amino acids proline (P); glutamic acid (E); serine (S); or threonine (T).

- **petechiae**
  Small purplish red spots due to subcutaneous hemorrhages.

- **petit mal**
  A form of epileptic fit beginning in childhood.

- **petite**
  A yeast mutation producing small colonies and altered mitochondrial functions. In cytoplasmic (neutral and suppressive) petites the mutation is a deletion in mitochondrial DNA, while in segregational petites the mutation occurs in nuclear DNA.

- **petite mutation**
  A mutation of yeast that produces small (petite) anaerobic-like colonies.

- **phage**
  A virus for which the natural host is a bacterial cell.

- **phalanges**
  Bones in fingers and toes.

- **phalanx**
  Long bone in the finger or toe.

- **pharmacist**
  A person trained to prepare and distribute medicines and to give information about them.

- **pharmacogenetics**
  The science of how a person's genes affect his or her response to drugs. Research in pharmacogenetics has two goals.One is to identify people whose genetic make-up would make them sick or even die from taking a particular drug.If researchers can identify variations in genes that influence a person's response to a drug, then DNA testing could reveal which patients should avoid the drug.The second goal is to predict who is most likely to benefit from one drug rather than another.The word is used interchangeably with pharmacogenomics.

- **pharmacogenomics**
  The study of the interaction of an individual's genetic makeup and response to a drug; The science of how a person's genome affects his or her response to drugs, in either a positive or negative way.The word is used interchangeably with pharmacogenetics.

- **pharynx**
  Upper portion of the throat; the passageway for air from the nose to the larynx and for food from the mouth to the esophagus.

- **phenocopy**
  A trait not caused by inheritance of a gene but appears to be identical to a genetic trait; A phenotype that is not genetically controlled but looks like a genetically controlled phenotype. An environmentally induced phenotype that resembles the

phenotype produced by a mutation.

- **phenome mapping**
  The conceptual matrix for a comprehensive "phenome" mapping project would be as follows: one axis represents all available knockouts while the other represents a large series of standardized phenotypes that can be screened.

- **phenome maps**
  Can be thought of as lists of similar phenotypes that could be referred to as "pheno- clusters".

- **phenotype**
  The physical characteristics of an organism or the presence of a disease that may or may not be genetic. The clinical features or the observable characteristics of an individual determined by a pair of genes at a given locus (or genotype). The phenotype can vary following interaction with modifying genes or the environment.

- **phenotypic sex determination**
  Sex determination by non-genetic means.

- **phenotypic variance**
  Variance of phenotype due to genotypic and environmental factors combined.

- **phenotyping**
  Diagnostic testing and inference of a particular genotype based on clinical or biochemical presentation (phenotype) of the individual, such as measurement of alpha-1-antitrypsin level, which is greatly reduced in individuals homozygous for the Z allele. With the advent of DNA-based testing, direct mutation analysis (genotyping) is becoming more widely available for many disorders.

- **phenylketonuria (pku)**
  A human metabolic disease caused by a mutation in a gene coding for a phenylalanine processing enzyme (phenylalanine hydroxylase), which leads to accumulation of phenylalanine and mental retardation if not treated; inherited as an autosomal recessive phenotype.

- **pheochromocytoma**
  A tumor (cytoma) of the adrenal gland which causes the adrenal gland to secrete too much adrenalin, potentially causing harm to the heart and blood vessels. Pheos can also occur outside the adrenal glands, and people can have more than two pheos.

- **pheromone**
  A chemical signal, analogous to a hormone, that passes information between individuals.

- **philadelphia chromosome**
  A translocation between the long arms of chromosomes 9 and 22,

often found in the white blood cells of patients with chronic myeloid leukemia.

- **philtrum**
  The vertical groove or dimple in the upper lip.
- **phlegm**
  Thick mucus, especially from the sinuses or respiratory tract.
- **phocomelia**
  Absence of the proximal portion of a limb or limbs; the hands or feet being attached to the trunk by a small, irregularly shaped bone.
- **phosphodiester bond**
  A bond between a two sugar groups and a phosphate group; such bonds form the sugar-phosphate-sugar backbone of DNA and RNA. A diester bond (between phosphoric acid and two sugar molecules) linking two nucleotides together to form the nucleotide polymers DNA and RNA.
- **phosphorylation**
  The addition of phosphate to an organic compound, such as the addition of phosphate to ADP to form ATP (the function of complex V in the electron transport chain) or the addition of phosphate to glucose to produce glucose monophosphate, through the action of enzymes known as phosphotransferases or kinases.
- **photocoagulation**
  Using a special strong beam of light (laser) to seal off bleeding blood vessels such as in the eye. The laser can also burn away blood vessels that should not have grown in the eye. This is the main treatment for diabetic retinopathy.
- **photophobia**
  Unable to tolerate light.
- **photoreactivation**
  The process whereby dimerized pyrimidines (usually thymines) in DNA are restored by an enzyme (deoxyribodipyrimidine photo-lyase) that requires light energy.
- **photosensitivity**
  Abnormal sensitivity to light , especially the eyes.
- **phyletic gradualism**
  The process of gradual evolutionary change over time.
- **phylogenetic**
  Relating to the evolutionary relationships of organisms. A phylogenetic tree, for example, refers to a graphic representation of the evolutionary history of organisms described in a branching pattern. Such trees are made with a variety of information, but for bacteria, a powerful technique is to use the similarity of DNA sequences to deduce relatedness. An assumption is that close relatives share more DNA similarity than

distant ones. However, there are complications with this method, which is described in detail in the last part of the lab.

- **phylogenetic tree**
A diagram showing evolutionary lineages of organisms.

- **physical map**
A map of the locations of identifiable landmarks on DNA (e.g., restriction-enzyme cutting sites, genes), regardless of inheritance. Distance is measured in base pairs. For the human genome, the lowest-resolution physical map is the banding patterns on the 24 different chromosomes; the highest-resolution map is the complete nucleotide sequence of the chromosomes. A chromo-some map of a species that shows the specific physical locations of its genes and/ or markers on each chromosome. Physical maps are particularly important when searching for disease genes by positional cloning strategies and for DNA sequencing; The procedure of physical mapping coarsely divides into two steps First large pieces of DNA (contigs), a library of cloned fragments are ordered according to their position in the genome. Different experimental techniques are used to do that. Roughly, these are clone- probe hybridization mapping, restriction mapping, radiation- hybrid mapping and optical mapping. Second the cloned fragments are cut by restriction enzymes, smaller DNA fragments are obtained which are sequenced in detail (shotgun-sequencing), and the overall sequence in detail is obtained by Sequence Assembly. A physical map consists of a linearly ordered set of DNA fragments encompassing the genome or region of interest. Physical maps are of two types, macro-restriction maps and ordered clone maps. The former consists of an ordered set of large DNA fragments generated by using restriction enzymes whose recognition sequences are infrequently represented in the genome. An ordered clone map consists of an overlapping collection of cloned DNA fragments.

- **physical therapy**
Treatment in which physical agents and methods are used to assist in meeting the specific needs of the individual patient.

- **phytohemagglutinin**
Lectin isolated from the red bean used to agglutinate red blood cells and stimulate lymphocytes to divide; used in preparation of peripheral blood karyotypes.

- **piebald**
A mammalian phenotype in which patches of skin are unpigmented

because of lack of melanocytes; generally inherited as an autosomal dominant.

- **pigment**
  Any coloring matter.
- **pigmentary skin anomalies**
  Cafe-au-lait spots (brown spots in neurofibromatosis), ash leaf spots (depigmented leaf shaped spots in tuberous sclerosis), axillary freckles (freckles under the arms in neurofibromatosis).
- **pigmentation**
  Coloration of the skin and eyes.
- **pilus (plural pili)**
  A conjugation tube; a hollow hair-like appendage of a donor Escherichia coli cell that acts as a bridge for transmission of donor DNA to the recipient cell during conjugation.
- **pineal body**
  A small, cone-shaped structure located in the brain, the function of which is not clearly established.
- **pineal gland**
  A small gland located in the cerebrum.
- **pinna**
  External part of the ear, the portion that is easily visible.
- **pituitary gland**
  A structure in the brain that controls most of the other glands in the body and influences most basic functions through the release of hormones.
- **pituitary gland**
  An endocrine gland in the small, bony cavity at the base of the brain. Often called "the master gland," the pituitary serves the body in many ways- certain sections of the pituitary each secretes important hormones including growth hormone growth (GH) and antidiuretic hormone (ADH).
- **pku**
  Phenylketonuria, an enzyme deficiency condition characterized by the inability to convert one amino acid, phenylalanine, to another, tyrosine, resulting in mental deficiency. plasmid double-stranded, circular, bacterial DNA into which a fragment of DNA from another organism can be inserted.
- **placenta (afterbirth)**
  The organ through which the fetus absorbs oxygen nutrients and other substances; and excretes wastes.
- **placenta abrupto**
  A condition in which the placenta separates prematurely from the uterine wall. This is a serious condition that may result in spontaneous abortion.
- **plagiocephaly**
  Deformation of the skull;usually mild and may disappear.
- **plano-occiput**
  Flat-occipital bone on the back of the head.

- **plano-occiput**
  Flat-occipital bone on the back of the head.

- **plant breeding**
  The application of genetic analysis to development of plant lines better suited for human purposes.

- **plaque**
  An abnormal patch on the skin or other organ or tissue. Plaque of an artery refers to hard formation on the artery walls formed by fat and cholesterol deposits over the years. These lead to hardening of the arteries called "athero-sclerosis"; A clear area on a bacterial lawn, left by lysis of the bacteria through progressive infections by a phage and its descendants. Clear area on a bacterial lawn caused by cell lysis due to viral attack.

- **plasma**
  Protein-rich, cell-free, blood.

- **plasmid**
  Autonomously replicating extra-chromosomal circular DNA molecules, distinct from the normal bacterial genome and nonessential for cell survival under nonselective conditions. Some plasmids are capable of integrating into the host genome. A number of artificially constructed plasmids are used as cloning vectors.

- **plastid**
  A chloroplast prior to the development of chlorophyll.

- **plate**
  (1) A flat dish used to culture microbes. (2) To spread cells over the surface of solid medium in a plate.

- **platelet**
  A part of the blood that causes clotting. Microscopic particles in the blood which stick to one another as part of the mechanism of clotting. Other major blood elements include protein, serum, and red & white blood cells.

- **platelet-derived growth factor (pdgf)**
  A protein, produced by platelets and other cells, that strongly stimulates cell growth and division and is involved in normal wound healing. The gene for PDGF is identical to the proto-oncogene sis.

- **pleiotropic**
  A single gene or gene pair which produces multiple effects, usually because of clinical abnormalities in various organ systems.

- **pleiotropic mutation**
  A mutation that has effects on several different characters.

- **pleiotropy**
  One gene that causes many different physical traits such as multiple disease symptoms. The ability of a gene to affect an

organism in many different ways is called pleiotropy. If one part of an organism's metabolism is affected by a defective gene, there may be many knock-on effects. All the symptoms that result can be wide-ranging and might, initially, seem unconnected.

**Red blood cells**
Normal, healthy red blood cells (**a**) have a characteristic disk shape. They contain hemoglobin (**b**), which is the protein that transports the vital gas oxygen around the body. **Hemoglobin S** The gene for hemoglobin is slightly different in people with sickle-cell anemia. As a result, sufferers have a different type of hemoglobin, called hemoglobin S (**c**). When molecules of hemoglobin S are not carrying oxygen, they have a tendency to form long chains. These chains deform the red blood cells into a sickle shape (**d**).

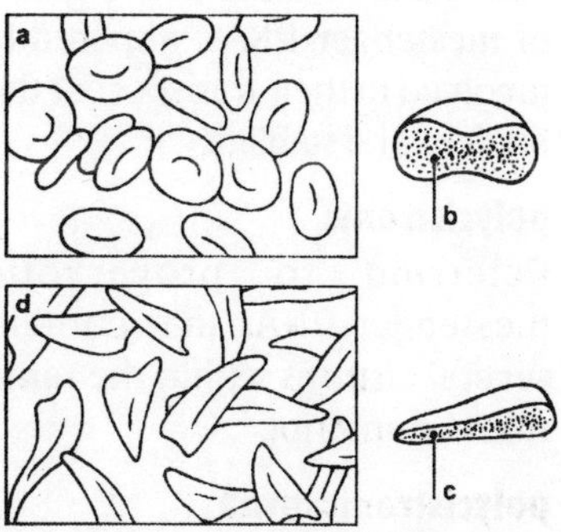


Multiple, often seemingly unrelated, physical effects caused by a single altered gene or pair of altered genes.

- **pleura**
  The membrane that covers the lungs and lines the chest cavity.

- **plexiform**
  Forming an interwoven network of blood vessels, nerves or lymphatics.

- **plexus**
  Network of blood vessels.

- **pluripotency**
  The potential of a cell to develop into more than one type of mature cell, depending on environment.

- **podiatrist**
  A doctor who treats and takes care of people's feet.

- **podiatry**
  The care and treatment of human feet in health and disease.

- **point deletion**
  The deletion of a single nucleotide amino acid on a gene.

- **point mutation**
  A mutation that can be mapped to one specific site within a locus. A small mutation that consists of the replacement (transition or transversion); addition; or deletion (frameshift) of one or a few bases.

- **poisson distribution**
  A mathematical expression giving the probability of observing various numbers of a particular event in a sample when the mean probability of that event on any one trial is very small.

- **poky mutation**
A mutation of Neurospora that produces a petite-like phenotype.

- **polar body**
A small cell (which eventually disintegrates) that is the by-product of meiosis in female animals. One functional ovum and potentially three polar bodies result from meiosis of each primary oocyte.

- **polar gene conversion**
A gradient of conversion frequency along the length of a gene.

- **polar granules**
Cytoplasmic granules localized at the posterior end of a Drosophila oocyte and early embryo. These granules are associated with determinants of the germ-line and posterior structures.

- **polar mutation**
A mutation that affects the transcription or translation of part of the gene or operon downstream of the mutant site. For example, nonsense mutations, frameshift mutations, and insertion sequence(IS)-induced mutations.

- **polarity**
Meaning directionality and referring either to an effect seen in only one direction from a point of origin or to the fact that linear entities (such as a single strand of DNA or RNA or a protein) have ends (5' and 3'; N and C) that differ from each other.

- **polarity gene**
A mitochondrial gene with alleles that are preferentially found in daughter mitochondria after a recombinational event between mitochondria.

- **pollen grain**
The male gametophyte in higher plants.

- **poly(a) tail**
A string of adenine nucleotides added to the 3' end of eukaryotic mRNA after transcription.

- **polyacrylamide**
A material used to make gels for separation of mixtures of macromolecules by electrophoresis.

- **polyadenylation**
The addition of approximately 200 adenosine residues at the 3' end of messenger RNAs, apparently involved in their transport of the nucleus and stability.

- **polycistronic**
Referring to prokaryotic messenger RNAs that contain several cistrons within the same mRNA transcript.

- **polycistronic mrna**
An mRNA that codes for more than one protein.

- **polycystic**
Composed of many cysts.

- **polycystic kidney disease (pkd)**
A group of conditions characterized by fluid filled sacs that slowly develop in both kidneys, eventually resulting in kidney malfunction.

- **poly-da/poly-dt technique**
A method of inserting DNA into a vector by adding poly-dA to the linearised vector and poly-dT to the DNA of interest. Also feasible with poly-dG and poly-dC.

- **polydactyly**
Having more than five fingers on a hand or five toes on a foot; postaxial (on the inner or ulnar side), or preaxial (on the outer or radial side).

- **polydipsia**
A great thirst that lasts for long periods of time; a sign of diabetes.

- **polygenic**
A condition caused by the additive contributions of mutations in multiple genes at different loci.

- **polygenic disorder**
Genetic disorder resulting from the combined action of alleles of more than one gene (e.g., heart disease, diabetes, and some cancers). Although such disorders are inherited, they depend on the simultaneous presence of several alleles; thus the hereditary patterns usually are more complex than those of single-gene disorders.

- **polyhydraminos**
Abnormally large amount of amniotic fluid.

- **polylobulated spleen**
Malformation of the spleen.

- **polymerase**
Polymerase is an enzyme that acts like a molecular assembly line to build new strands of DNA, Any enzyme that catalyzes the formation of DNA or RNA from deoxyribonucleotides or ribonucleotides. Enzymes that catalyze the combining of nucleotides to form RNA or DNA (genetic transcription and DNA replication).

- **polymerase, dna or rna**
Enzyme that catalyzes the synthesis of nucleic acids on preexisting nucleic acid templates, assembling RNA from ribonucleotides or DNA from deoxyribonucleotides.

- **polymerize**
To form a complex compound (polymer) by linking together many smaller elements (residues).

- **polymicrogyria**
Increased number of samll irregular gyri; not necessarily accompanied by mental retardation; commonly seen with the Arnold Chiari Malformation.

- **polymorphism**
Difference in DNA sequence among individuals that may

underlie differences in health. Genetic variations occurring in more than 1% of a population would be considered useful polymorphisms for genetic linkage analysis.

- **polyneuropathy**
  A morbid state in which a number of nerves are affected at the same time.

- **polynucleotide phosphorylase**
  An enzyme that can polymerize nucleotide diphosphates without the need for a primer. The function of this enzyme in vivo is probably in its reverse role as an RNA exonuclease.

- **polyp**
  An abnormal tissue growth arising from a mucous membrane, that develops on the inside wall of a hollow organ, such as the colon.

- **polypeptide**
  A protein or part of a protein made of a chain of amino acids joined by a peptide bond.

- **polyphagia**
  Great hunger; a sign of diabetes. People with this great hunger often lose weight.

- **polyploid**
  A cell or an organism having three or more chromosome sets.

- **polyploidy**
  An increase in the number of haploid sets (23) of chromosomes in a cell. Triploidy refers to three whole sets of chromosomes in a single cell (in humans, a total of 69 chromosomes per cell); tetraploidy refers to four whole sets of chromosomes in a single cell (in humans, a total of 92 chromosomes per cell).

- **polyposis**
  Presence of several polyps.

- **polysaccharide**
  A biological polymer composed of sugar subunits for example, starch or cellulose.

- **polysome**
  The configuration of several ribosomes simultaneously translating the same mRNA. Shortened form of the term polyribosome.

- **polysyndactyly**
  Extra fingers and/or toes (polydactyly) and fusion or webbing of the toes or fingers (syndactyly).

- **polytene chromosome**
  A giant chromosome produced by an endomitotic process in which, following synapsis of the two homologues, multiple rounds of replication produce chromatids that remain synapsed together in a haploid number of chromosomes. Large chromosome consisting of many chromatids formed by rounds of endomitosis following synapsis of the two homologues.

• **polyunsaturated fats**
A type of fat that comes from vegetables.

• **polyuria**
Having to urinate often; a common sign of diabetes.

• **popliteal artery**
Main vessel carrying oxygen-rich blood to the (lower) leg, and running at the back of the knee.

• **population**
A group of organisms of the same species relatively isolated from other groups of the same species.

• **population genetics**
The study of variation in genes among a group of individuals.

• **population risk (synonym background risk)**
The proportion of individuals in the general population who are affected with a particular disorder or who carry a certain gene; often discussed in the genetic counseling process as a comparison to the patient's personal risk given his or her family history or other circumstances.

• **porencephyaly**
Cyst formation in the brain with cerebral cysts that extend from the ventricular system to the subarachnoid space. These are generally caused by destructive, infectious or vascular lesions. A familial type has been described with-dominanat inheritance.

• **porta hepatis**
A horizontal fisssure in the liver, containing blood and lymph vessels, nerves and the hepatic ducts.

• **position effect**
Used to describe a situation in which the phenotype expressed by a gene is altered by changes in the position of the gene within the genome. For instance genes translocated to regions of heterochromatin are often not expressed.

• **positional cloning**
A technique used to identify genes, usually those that are associated with diseases, based on their location on a chromosome. Requires a genetic map with a large number of markers (especially in the region of interest), and the use of physical mapping and DNA sequencing technologies to isolate and sequence the targeted gene, Cloning or identification of a gene for a particular disease based on its location in the genome, determined by a collection of methods including linkage analysis, genomic (physical) mapping, and bioinformatics, when no information about the biochemical basis of the disease is known; distinguished from the more common strategy of gene cloning beginning with a known protein product, determining its

amino acid sequence, and using that information to isolate the gene

- **position-effect variegation**
  Variegation caused by the inactivation of a gene in some cells through its abnormal juxtaposition with heterochromatin.

- **positive assortative mating**
  A situation in which like phenotypes mate more commonly than expected by chance.

- **positive control**
  Regulation mediated by a protein that is required for the activation of a transcription unit.

- **positive interference**
  When the occurrence of one crossover reduces the probability that a second will occur in the same region.

- **positive predictive value(synonym ppv)**
  The likelihood that an individual with a positive test result actually has the particular gene in question, is affected, or will develop the disease.

- **post**
  Prefix denoting after or behind.

- **post mortem**
  Examination of a body after death.

- **postaxial**
  On the back side, behind the axis or center line.

- **posterior**
  The back surface.

- **posterior angulation of auricle**
  Ears slightly rotated on the head.

- **posterior triangle**
  An anatomical area bounded in the front by the back border of the sternocleidomastoid (strap) muscle of the neck, in the back by the front border of the trapezius (shoulder) muscle, and at the base by the collarbone.

- **posteriorly angulated ears**
  Backward angled ears.

- **postnasal**
  At or from the back of the nose.

- **postnatal**
  The time period after birth.

- **postpartum period**
  The period of time shortly after childbirth.

- **postreplicative repair**
  A DNA repair process initiated when DNA polymerase bypasses a damaged area. enzymes in the rec system are used.

- **post-term pregnancy**
  A pregnancy that lasts longer than 42 weeks.

- **post-transcriptional modification**
  Changes in eukaryotic mRNA, tRNA or other RNAs made after transcription has been completed. The changes to mRNA include

addition of a 5'cap and 3' polyA tail and removal of introns, and to tRNA include modification of bases and removal of introns.

- **post-zygotic event**
  A mutational event or abnormality in chromosome replication/segregation that occurs after fertilization of the ovum by the sperm, often leading to mosaicism (two or more genetically distinct cell lines within the same organism).

- **prader-willi syndrome**
  A condition characterized by obesity and insatiable appetite, mental deficiency, small genitals, and short stature. May be deletion of 15 chromosome.

- **preauricular**
  Area in front of the ear, between the tragus and cheek.

- **preauricular pits**
  An indentation situated in front of the auricle of the ear.

- **preauricular tags**
  An appendage situated in front of the auricle of the ear.

- **precancerous polyps**
  Growths in the colon that often become cancerous.

- **predictive gene tests**
  It tests to identify gene abnormalities that may make a person susceptible to certain diseases or disorders.

- **predictive testing**
  Testing offered to asymptomatic individuals with a family history of a genetic disorder and a potential risk of eventually developing the disorder

- **predisposing mutation (synonym susceptibility gene)**
  A gene mutation that increases an individual's susceptibility or predisposition to a certain disease or disorder. When such a mutation is inherited, development of symptoms is more likely but not certain.

- **predisposition**
  To have a tendency or inclination towards something in advance.

- **predispositional testing**
  Testing of an asymptomatic individual in whom the discovery of a gene mutation indicates that eventual development of findings related to a specific diagnosis is likely but not certain. A negative result may not exclude the possibility of future development of the disease from other causes.

- **preeclampsia**
  A condition that some women with diabetes have during the late stages of pregnancy. Two signs of this condition are high blood pressure and swelling because the body cells are holding extra water.

- **preemptor stem**
A configuration of leader transcript mRNA that allows transcription in attenuator-controlled amino acid operons.

- **preimplantation diagnosis (synonym preimplantation testing)**
A procedure used to decrease the chance of a particular genetic condition for which the fetus is specifically at risk by testing one cell removed from early embryos conceived by in vitro fertilization and transferring to the mother's uterus only those embryos determined not to have inherited the mutation in question.

- **premature chromosome condensation (pcc)**
A method of studying chromosomes in the interphase stage of the cell cycle.

- **premature labor or delivery**
Onset of labour or delivery/birth before 37 completed weeks since the last normal menstrual period of a pregnancy. Current terminology is "Preterm".

- **prematurity**
Underdevelopment; the condition of an infant born too soon. Refers to infants delivered before 37 weeks from the first day of the last menstrual period.

- **pre-mrna**
The first (primary) transcript from a protein coding gene is often called a pre-mRNA and contains both introns and exons. Pre-mRNA requires splicing (removal) of introns to produce the final mRNA molecule containing only exons.

- **prenatal**
The time before birth, while a baby is developing during pregnancy. The period of time between the conception and birth of an infant.

- **prenatal diagnosis (synonym prenatal testing)**
Testing performed during pregnancy to determine if a fetus is affected with a particular disorder. Chorionic villus sampling (CVS), amniocentesis, periumbilical blood sampling (PUBS), ultrasound, and fetoscopy are examples of procedures used either to obtain a sample for testing or to evaluate fetal anatomy. The examining fetal cells taken from the amniotic fluid, the primitive placenta (chorion), or the umbilical cord for biochemical, chromosomal, or gene alterations. Examining fetal cells taken from the amniotic fluid, the primitive placenta (chorion), or the umbilical cord for biochemical, chromosomal, or gene alterations.

- **presymptomatic diagnosis**
Diagnosis of a genetic condition before the appearance or onset of clinical symptoms.

- **presymptomatic testing**
  Testing of an asymptomatic individual in whom the discovery of a gene mutation indicates certain development of findings related to a specific diagnosis at some future point. A negative result excludes the diagnosis.

- **preterm**
  Delivered/born before 37 completed weeks since the last normal menstrual period of a pregnancy.

- **preterm labor**
  Contractions that start opening the cervix before week 37 of pregnancy; also called premature labor.

- **prevalence**
  The number of people in a given group or population who are reported to have a disease.

- **pribnow box**
  Relatively invariant sequence of six nucleotides (concensus TATAAT) in prokaryotic promoters centred at the position minus 10 (10 base pairs upstream from the transcription start site).

- **primary oocyte**
  A cell that undergoes meiosis in female animals.

- **primary spermatocyte**
  A cell that undergoes the first meiotic division in male animals. See secondary spermatocyte.

- **primary structure**
  The sequence of polymerized amino acids in a protein.

- **primary transcript**
  The product of eukaryotic transcription before post-transcriptional modifications take place.

- **primase**
  An enzyme that creates an RNA primer for initiation of DNA replication.

- **primer**
  Short preexisting polynucleotide chain to which new deoxyribonucleotides can be added by DNA polymerase, Nucleotides used in the polymerase chain reaction to initiate DNA synthesis at a particular location. Primers used in PCR are usually approximately 20 base pairs in length, Oligonucleotides that have been designed and manufactured to bind to a specific part of a known segment of DNA. DNA polymerase can then extend the oligonucleotide and replicate the DNA. The process allows replication of the specific known segment of DNA, particularly in conjunction with PCR.

- **primosome**
  A complex of two proteins, a primase and a helicase, that initiates RNA primers on the lagging DNA strand during DNA replication.

- **prion**
  Protein infectious agent associated with several neurological diseases (scrapie; kuru; Creutzfeld-Jakob syndrome; Alzheimer's disease). Each disease has a different prion.

- **privacy**
  In genetics, the right of people to restrict access to their genetic information.

- **private mutation (synonym unique mutation)**
  A rare disease-causing mutation observed in a few families.

- **probability**
  The long term frequency of an event relative to all alternative events, and usually expressed as decimal fraction. The expectation of the occurrence of a particular event.

- **probability theory**
  The conceptual framework concerned with quantification of probabilities.

- **proband (synonym index case, propositus)**
  The affected individual through whom a family with a genetic disorder is ascertained; may or may not be the consultand (the individual presenting for genetic counseling).

- **proband**
  The affected subject who led to the research done on their family.

- **probe**
  Single-stranded DNA or RNA molecules of specific base sequence, labeled either radioactively or immunologically, that are used to detect the complementary base sequence by hybridization. A specific, pre-fabricated sequence of DNA or RNA, labeled by one of several methods, used to detect the presence of a complimentary sequence by binding (hybridizing) to it. Defined nucleic acid (DNA or RNA) that can be used to identify, usually through autoradiography, specific DNA or RNA molecules bearing the complementary sequence. A labeled (radioactive; antigen; enzyme; fluorescent) nucleic acid complementary to the sequence being searched for in a restriction digest, genome library, northern blot or in situ hybridization.

- **processivity**
  The ability of an enzyme to repetitively continue its catalytic function without dissociating from its substrate.

- **product of meiosis**
  One of the (usually four) cells formed by the two meiotic divisions.

- **product rule**
  The probability of two independent events occurring simultaneously is the product of the individual probabilities. The

rule stating that the probability of the occurrence of independent events is the product of their separate probabilities.

- **productive cough**
  A cough in which phlegm or mucus is dislodged, enabling a person to clear mucus from the lungs.
- **proflavin**
  A mutagen that tends to produce frameshift mutations.
- **progeny testing**
  Breeding of offspring to determine their genotypes and that of their parents.
- **prognasthism**
  Marked (obvious) protrusion of the jaw.
- **prognosis**
  The forecast of the course and probable outcome of a disease; Telling a person now what is likely to happen in the future because of having a disease.
- **prognostic**
  Relating to a forecast of probable course or outcome.
- **progressive**
  Advancing, especially in an unfavorable course.
- **prokaryote**
  Cell or organism lacking a membrane-bound, structurally discrete nucleus and other subcellular compartments. Bacteria are examples of prokaryotes; An organism lacking a true nucleus, such as a bacterium or a blue-green alga.
- **prokaryotic cell**
  A cell having no nuclear membrane and hence no separate nucleus.
- **proliferative retinopathy**
  A disease of the small blood vessels of the retina of the eye.
- **prolonged labor**
  A difficult labor that does not accomplish a vaginal birth within 18 to 24 hours.
- **prolonged rupture of membranes**
  Greater than 24 hours between spontaneous or artificial breach in the amnion and chorion, releasing amniotic fluid or liquor, and the delivery of the fetus; its significance is an increasing liability to health- and life-threatening infection of the fetus, and to a lesser extent maternal infection.
- **prominent**
  Obvious, or projecting beyond the surface.
- **promoter**
  A regulatory region a short distance upstream from the 5' end of a transcription start site that acts as the binding site for RNA polymerase. A region of DNA to which RNA polymerase binds in order to initiate transcription.

- **promoter region**
  A specific region just upstream from a gene that acts as a binding site for transcription factors and RNA polymerase during the initiation of transcription

- **pronucleus**
  The nucleus of a sperm or egg prior to fertilization; Either of the two haploid gamete nuclei just prior to their fusion in the fertilized ovum. Transgenic lines are often generated by microinjection of the transgene into the pronuclear region of these haploid gametes.

- **proofread**
  Literally to read for the purpose of detecting errors for later correction. DNA polymerase has 3' to 5' exonuclease activity which is used during polymerization to remove nucleotides it has recently added if they are incorrectly paired, and is a correcting ability to remove errors in replication. The correction of errors in the nucleotide sequence that can occur during replication, transcription, or translation.

- **proofreader genes**
  DNA repair genes. Certain genes that are part of a DNA repair pathway; when altered, they permit mutations to pile up throughout the DNA.

- **prophage**
  A phage chromosome inserted as part of the linear structure of the DNA chromosome of a bacterium. A temperate phage integrated into the host chromosome.

- **prophase**
  The early stage of nuclear division during which chromosomes condense and become visible. The initial stage of mitosis or meiosis in which chromosomes become visible and the spindle apparatus forms.

- **prophylactic surgery**
  It is surgery to remove tissue that is in danger of becoming cancerous, before cancer has the chance to develop. Surgery to remove the breasts of women at high risk of developing breast cancer is known as prophylactic mastectomy.

- **proplastid**
  Mutant plastids that do not grow and develop into chloroplasts.

- **propositus**
  The person through whom a pedigree was discovered.

- **prosthesis**
  A man-made substitute for a missing body part such as an arm or a leg; also an implant such as for the hip.

- **protease**
  A protein that digests other proteins.

- **protein**
  A large molecule composed of one or more chains of amino acids

in a specific order; the order is determined by the base sequence of nucleotides in the gene that codes for the protein. Proteins are required for the structure, function, and regulation of the body's cells, tissues, and organs; and each protein has unique functions. Examples are hormones, enzymes, and antibodies. A molecule that carries out the business of cells.Enzymes and hormones are types of proteins.Most proteins have folds and bends, and their three-dimensional structures allow them to interact with other proteins, forming dynamic networks. One of the three main classes of food. Proteins are large, complex molecules made of amino acids, which are called the building blocks of the cells. The cells need proteins to grow and to mend themselves. Protein is found in many foods such as meat, fish, poultry, and eggs. The sequence of the amino acids, and thus the function of the protein, is determined by the sequence of the base pairs in the gene that encodes it. Proteins are essential to the structure, function, and regulation of the body. Examples are hormones, enzymes, and antibodies. A molecule composed of amino acids linked together in a particular order specified by a gene's DNA sequence. Proteins perform a wide variety of functions including serving as enzymes, structural components or signaling molecules.

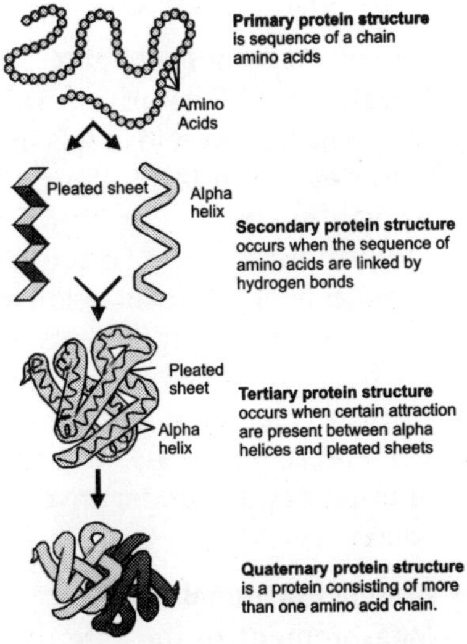


- **protein analysis**

  One of several different testing methods that reveals either the structure or function of a particular protein product

- **protein expression map**

  Since 2D Electrophoresis gel patterns reveal not only the amounts of protein, but is unrivaled in its ability to detect post- translational modifications, the 2DE protein map provides much more relevant information about cellular dynamics than the corresponding expression map at the mRNA level. By comparing the 2DE gel patterns of samples exposed to different physiological conditions or different drug treatments it is possible to identify groups of proteins with related functions or whose expression is interdependent.

- **protein expression mapping**
  Details the distribution and abundance of protein in specific samples, under defined physiological conditions. Quantitative study of global changes in protein expression in tissues, cells or body fluids using 2D gels and image analysis. Currently carried out by 2D gel electrophoresis, though alternatives are under investigation.

- **protein functional assay**
  Measurement of the rate of a chemical reaction that takes place in the presence of an enzyme contained in a sample taken from an individual. Reduced enzymatic activity may indicate carrier status or the diagnosis of a particular genetic disease

- **protein interaction maps**
  Hybrigenics comprehensive protein interaction maps using automated yeast- two- hybrid methodology in pathogens and in cDNA of normal and diseased tissues.

- **protein linkage maps**
  With respect to a genome- wide use of the two- hybrid assay in the case of yeast, the goal is to find which proteins in the yeast genome interact with every other protein. This process would generate protein linkage maps, delineating large networks of interacting proteins. The approximately 6,000 yeast proteins can potentially interact in 18 million pair wise combinations.

- **protein product**
  The protein molecule assembled under the direction of a gene.

- **protein suicide mechanism**
  In dominant disorders, one mutant subunit leads to the loss of function of an entire multimeric protein, e.g., collagen.

- **protein truncation testing (synonym ptt)**
  Means of identifying the shortened (truncated) proteins that result from mutations which specifically cause premature termination of mRNA translation.

- **proteinuria**
  Too much protein in the urine. This may be a sign of kidney damage.

- **proteome**
  Proteins expressed by a cell or organ at a particular time and under specific conditions; A collection of proteins.The human proteome is the collection of proteins found in the human body. A proteome can also refer to the set of proteins in a particular cell.

- **proteome map**

A number of organizations have announced plans to produce a map of the proteome, including Myriad Genetics, Large Scale Biology, CuraGen and others.

- **proteomics**

The study of the set of proteins produced (expressed) by an organism, tissue or cell, and the changes in protein expression patterns in different environments and conditions.

- **proteus syndrome**

A condition characterized by distorted asymmetric growth of the body and enlarged head, enlarged feet, multiple nevi on the skin; mode of inheritance is unknown.

- **prothrombin**

A substance found in circulating blood that interacts with calcium salts to form thrombin, necessary for blood clotting.

- **proto-oncogene**

The normal, pre-cancerous equivalent of the oncogene.

- **proto-oncogene**

The non-activated form of a cellular oncogene in an untransformed cell. A gene that, when mutated or otherwise affected, becomes an oncogene. Normal genes that are found in normal eukaryotic cells concerned with various aspects of cell division. If amplified, mutated, rearranged, or picked up by a retrovirus, they may give rise to oncogenes that can cause cancer.

- **protoplast**

A plant cell whose wall has been removed.

- **prototroph**

A strain of organisms that will proliferate on minimal medium.

- **provirus**

A virus chromosome integrated into the DNA of the host cell.

- **proximal**

Situated towards the centre of the body; opposite of distal.

- **pseudo**

False, appearing similar or identical to something it is not.

- **pseudoallele**

Allele that is functionally but not structurally allelic, that is wild-type recombinants can be recovered by intragenic recombination from heterozygotes containing two different pseudoalleles.

- **pseudoautosomal gene**

A gene that occurs on both sex-determining heteromorphic chromosomes.

- **pseudoautosomal region**

The distal tip of the Y chromosome short arm, which undergoes crossover with the distal tip of the

X chromosome short arm during meiosis in the male.

- **pseudodominance**
The sudden appearance of a recessive phenotype in a pedigree, due to deletion of a masking dominant gene. The phenomenon in which a recessive allele shows itself in the phenotype when only one copy of the allele is present, as in hemizygous alleles or in deletion heterozygotes .

- **pseudodominant inheritance**
An autosomal recessive condition present in individuals in two or more generations of a family, thereby appearing to follow a dominant inheritance pattern. Common explanations include 1) a high carrier frequency; 2) birth of an affected child to an affected individual and a genetically related (consanguineous) reproductive partner

- **pseudogene**
A sequence of DNA similar to a gene but nonfunctional; probably the remnant of a once-functional gene that accumulated mutations; A copy of a gene that usually lacks introns and other essential DNA sequences necessary for function; pseudogenes, though genetically similar to the original functional gene, are not expressed and often contain numerous mutations.

- **pseudohypertrophic**
Enlarged organ or part caused by over-growth of fatty or fibrous tissue.

- **psoriasis**
Chronic, recurrent skin disease characterized by patches of flaking skin with discoloration.

- **psychogenic**
Originating in the mind; also pertaining to the development of the mind.

- **psychomotor**
Movement of muscles under the direction of the brain.

- **psychosis**
Mental disturbance of serious magnitude that may be characterized by loss of contact with reality. Delusions and hallucinations are often present.

- **pterygium colli**
Redundant skin folds in the neck.

- **ptosis**
Drooping of an organ, but usually in reference to the eyelid.

- **puberty**
The time when body changes particular to the sex occur and when reproduction becomes possible.

- **public policy**
A set of action guidelines or rules that result from the actions or lack of actions of governmental entities.

- **pulmonary hypertension**
High pressure in pulmonary circulation.

- **pulmonary hypoplasia**
Underdeveloped lungs.

- **pulse-chase experiment**
An experiment in which cells are grown in radioactive medium for a brief period (the pulse) and then transferred to nonradioactive medium for a longer period (the chase).

- **pulsed field electrophoresis**
An electrophoretic technique that allows the separation of relatively long (>5,000 kb) sequences of DNA.

- **pulsed-field gel electrophoresis**
An electrophoretic technique in which the gel is subjected to electrical fields alternating between different angles, allowing very large DNA fragments to snake through the gel, and hence permitting efficient separation of mixtures of such large fragments.

- **punctuated equilibrium**
The evolutionary process involving long periods without change (stasis) punctuated by short periods of rapid speciation.

- **punnett square**
A diagrammatic representation of a particular cross used to predict the progeny of the cross. A grid used as a graphic representation of the progeny zygotes resulting from different gamete fusions in a specific cross.

- **pupil**
The circular opening in the center of the iris through which light passes into the eye.

- **pure-breeding line or strain**
A group of identical individuals that always produce offspring of the same phenotype when intercrossed.

- **purine**
A nitrogen-containing, double-ring, basic compound that occurs in nucleic acids. The purines in DNA and RNA are adenine and guanine. A type of nitrogen base; the purine bases in DNA and RNA are adenine and guanine.

- **purpura**
Purple spots and patches caused by leakage of blood into the tissues under the skin.

- **pyloric**
Relating to the pylorus, a muscular device to an orifice or lumen of an organ, as the muscular tissue around the aboreal outlet of the stomach.

- **pyloric stenosis**
Obstruction at the outlet of the stomach.

- **pyloromyotomy**
Surgical procedure which cuts the muscle of the pylorus to allow

easier passage of the food from the stomach to the small intestine.

- **pyloroplasty**
  Surgical procedure to increase the size of the valve from the stomach to the small intestine.

- **pylorus**
  The lower part of the stomach opening into the duodenum.

- **pyrimidine**
  A nitrogen-containing, single-ring, basic compound that occurs in nucleic acids. The pyrimidines in DNA are cytosine and thymine; in RNA, cytosine and uracil; Nitrogenous bases of which thymine is found in DNA; uridine in RNA; and cytosine in both.

- **qtl mapping quantitative trait loci mapping**
  A phenotype driven approach to gene function. As such it permits the discovery of new genes and can be contrasted with gene-driven approaches such knock-out and knock-in mice which allow for the study of known genes. QTL reflect natural genetic variations as they exist in the mouse strains under study. We are limited to detecting those genes that vary among the available strains. However the natural variations among mouse strains are vast and largely untapped.

- **quadriparesis**
  Incomplete paralysis of all four limbs; tetraparesis.

- **quadriplegia**
  Paralysis of all four limbs.

- **quantitative inheritance**
  The mechanism of genetic control of traits showing continuous variation.

- **quantitative pcr (synonym kinetic quantitative pcr, real time quantitative pcr)**
  The use of PCR to determine the amount of DNA or RNA in a sample; commonly used to detect heterozygous deletion mutations and duplication mutations

- **quantitative variation**
  Variation measured on a continuum (eg height in human beings) rather than in discrete units or categories. See continuous variation. The existence of a range of phenotypes for a specific character, differing by degree rather than by distinct qualitative differences.

- **quasidominance**
  The pattern of inheritance produced by the mating of an affected homozygote with an individual heterozygous for the same recessive trait so that homozygous affected members appear in two or more successive generations.

- **quaternary structure**
  The association of polypeptide subunits to form the final structure of a protein.

- **r plasmid**
  A plasmid containing one or several transposons with resistance genes. Plasmids carrying genes controlling resistance to various drugs.
- **r.e.m. sleep**
  The period of sleep known as Rapid Eye Movement sleep, when dreaming seems to occur.
- **radial**
  Relating to the radius, a bone in the forearm.
- **radial artery**
  One of the main arteries of the arm, running down its full length into the hand. Arteries carry blood away from the heart.
- **radiation hybrid**
  A hybrid cell containing small fragments of irradiated human chromosomes. Maps of irradiation sites on chromosomes for the human, rat, mouse, and other genomes provide important markers, allowing the construction of very precise STS maps indispensable to studying multifactorial diseases.
- **radiation hybrid mapping**
  A method for ordering genetic loci along CHROMOSOMES. The method involves fusing irradiated donor cells with host cells from another species. Following cell fusion, fragments of DNA from the irradiated cells become integrated into the chromosomes of the host cells. Molecular probing of DNA obtained from the fused cells is used to determine if two or more genetic loci are located within the same fragment of donor cell DNA.
- **radiation hybrid rh maps**
  Chromosome maps that are calculated from RH score vectors. An RH score vector is the pattern of assay results of a particular STS (marker) on a particular panel. The vector consists of 1's (did amplify) and 0's (did not amplify). Simplistically speaking, the more similar two score vectors are, the closer the markers are on the chromosome.
- **radiologist**
  A physician specializing in diagnostic techniques for viewing internal organs and tissues without surgery. Radiological methods include X-ray, MRI, computed tomography (CT) scan, ultrasound, angiography, and nuclear isotopes.
- **radiosensitivity testing (synonym colony survival essay, CSA)**
  Testing specific to ataxia-telangiectasia (A-T) and other disorders in which cells are particularly sensitive to ionizing radiation; demonstrates colony formation of a blood lymphocyte cell line following irradiation, which is abnormal in approxi-

mately 99% of patients with clinically diagnosed A-T, though the sensitivity of such testing in light of a suspected but unsure diagnosis of A-T has not yet been documented

- **radioulnar**
  Relating to both the radius and ulna, the two bones in the lower arm between the elbow and wrist.

- **radius**
  Smaller of the two bones in lower arm.

- **rales**
  Abnormal breathing sounds, sometimes indicating fluid in the air sacs of the lung.

- **ram mutation**
  Ribosomal ambiguity mutation that allows incorrect tRNAs to be incorporated into the translation process.

- **rami**
  Dividing of a nevus or blood vessel.

- **random genetic drift**
  Changes in allelic frequency due to sampling error. Changes in allele frequency that result because the genes appearing in offspring are not a perfectly representative sampling of the parental genes. (eg. in small populations).

- **random mating**
  Mating between individuals where the choice of partner is not influenced by the genotypes (with respect to specific genes under study). The mating of individuals in a population such that the union of individuals with the trait under study occurs according to the product rule of probability.

- **random strand analysis**
  Mapping studies in organisms that do not keep together all the products of meiosis.

- **rarefaction**
  Become lighter or less dense.

- **rash**
  A group of spots on an area of inflamed skin.

- **r-banding**
  A chromosome banding technique in which chromosomes are heated in a phosphate buffer; produces dark and light bands in patterns that are the reverse of those produced by G-banding.

- **reading frame (synonym exon)**
  A sequence of messenger RNA that is translated into an amino acid chain, three bases at a time, each triplet sequence coding for a single amino acid; The succession of codons determined by reading nucleotides in groups of three from a specific initiation codon.

- **readthrough**
  Transcription or translation beyond the normal termination

signals in DNA or mRNA respectively.

- **realized heritability**
  Heritability measured by a response to selection. The ratio of the single-generation progress of selection to the selection differential of the parents.

- **reannealing**
  Spontaneous realignment of two single DNA strands to re-form a DNA double helix.

- **rearrangement**
  A structural alteration in a chromosome, usually involving breakage and reattachment of a segment of chromosome material, resulting in an abnormal configuration; examples include inversion and translocation

- **rec system**
  Several loci controlling genes (recA; recB; recC and others) involved in postreplicative DNA repair.

- **receptor**
  A transmembrane or intracellular protein involved in transmission of a cell signal.

- **receptor element**
  A controlling element in maize that can insert into a gene (making it mutant) and that can also excise (thus making the mutation unstable); both of these functions are nonautonomous, being under the influence of a regulator element.

- **receptors**
  Areas on the outer part of a cell that allow the cell to join or bind with a substance.

- **recessive**
  A trait or disorder that appears only in a child who has received two copies of the same mutant gene, one from each parent; A mode of inheritance in which a gene must be present from both parents for the trait to become manifest in an offspring; A gene that is phenotypically manifest in the homozygous state but is masked in the presence of a dominant allele.

- **recessive allele**
  A gene that is expressed only when its counterpart allele on the matching chromosome is also recessive (not dominant). Autosomal recessive disorders develop in persons who receive two copies of the mutant gene, one from each parent who is a carrier.

- **recessive gene**
  A gene which will be expressed only if there are two identical copies or, for a male, if one copy is present on the X chromosome.

- **recessive phenotype**
  The phenotype of a homozygote for the recessive allele; the parental phenotype that is not expressed in a heterozygote.

- **reciprocal altruism**
  An apparently altruistic behavior performed with the understanding that the recipient will reciprocate at some future date.

- **reciprocal cross**
  A cross, with the phenotype of each sex reversed as compared with the original cross, to test the role of parental sex on inheritance pattern. A pair of crosses of the type genotype A(female) X genotype B(male) and genotype B(female) X genotype A(male).

- **reciprocal translocation**
  When a pair of chromosomes exchange exactly the same length and area of DNA. Results in a shuffling of genes; A chromosomal configuration in which (usually) the ends of two non-homologous chromosomes have become exchanged. A translocation in which part of one chromosome is exchanged with a part of a separate non-homologous chromosome.

- **recombinant**
  In genetic mapping studies an offspring having a non-parental allele combination. An individual or cell with a genotype produced by recombination.

- **recombinant chromosome**
  A chromosome in an offspring that has a genotype not found in either parent, due to crossing over in meiosis.

- **recombinant clone**
  Clone containing recombinant DNA molecules.

- **recombinant dna**
  A form of DNA produced by splicing together segments of DNA from two or more organisms.

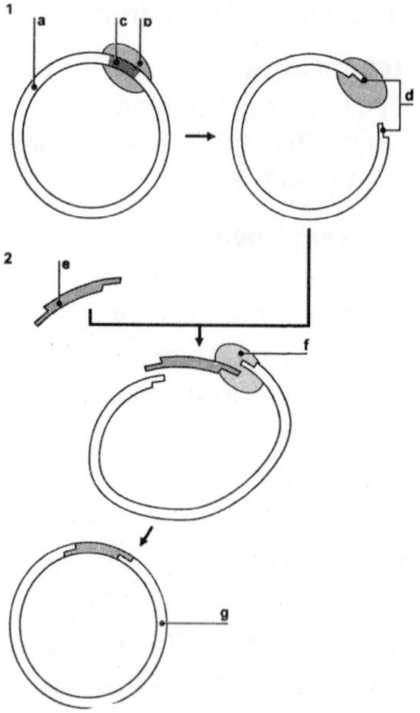


1. First, Boyer and Cohen cut an E. coli plasmid (circular DNA that is separate from the cell's own chromosome) called pSC101 (a) with EcoRI (b). This plasmid has a single recognition site (c) for EcoRI, and it was cut into a linear molecule with sticky (overhanging) ends (d).
2. Another DNA molecule was also cut with EcoRI. This foreign DNA (e) was then

mixed with the linearized pSC101 plasmid and the molecules joined together with enzyme DNA ligase (f). The hybrid DNA molecule produced (g) was a recombinant DNA.

- **recombinant dna molecules**

A combination of DNA molecules of different origin that are joined using recombinant DNA technologies.

- **recombinant dna technology**

Procedure used to join together DNA segments in a cell-free system (an environment outside a cell or organism). Under appropriate conditions, a recombinant DNA molecule can enter a cell and replicate there, either autonomously or after it has become integrated into a cellular chromosome.

- **recombinant frequency (rf)**

The proportion (or percentage) of recombinant cells or individuals.

- **recombination**

The process by which progeny derive a combination of genes different from that of either parent. In higher organisms, this can occur by crossing over; The exchange of a segment of DNA between two homologous chromosomes during meiosis leading to a novel combination of genetic material in the gamete; A phenomenon, also known as recombination, that sometimes occurs during the formation of sperm and egg cells (meiosis); a pair of chromosomes (one from the mother and the other from the father) break and trade segments with one another.

- **recombination fraction**

In linkage analysis, the fraction of meiotic events that show a recombination between two loci.

- **recombinational repair**

The repair of a DNA lesion through a process, similar to recombination, that uses recombination enzymes.

- **recon**

A term coined by Seymour Benzer for the smallest recombinable unit within a cistron. A region of a gene within which there can be no crossing-over; now known to be a single nucleotide pair.

- **rectum**

The reservoir for feces located between the last (sigmoid) part of the large bowel and the anus.

- **recurrence risk**

The likelihood that a trait or disorder present in one family member will occur again in other family members in the same or subsequent generations

- **red blood cells**

A hemoglobin-containing blood cell, red blood cells (RBC) carry oxygen in the blood, and supply oxygen from the lungs to tissues throughout the body.. They are also called red corpuscles.

- **redivac**

A device for continuously draining fluid via a tube (catheter) from body cavities.

- **reduced penetrance**

When the effect of a mutated gene for a dominant disease is somehow modified or reduced and does not always cause disease when present.

- **reduced penetrance allele (synonym intermediate allele)**

In autosomal dominant disorders caused by nucleotide repeat expansion, an abnormally large allele that may or may not result in an abnormal phenotype in a normal life span. The abnormal phenotype may be very-late-onset disease and/or a different phenotype. Reduced penetrance alleles are larger than mutable normal alleles and smaller than full penetrance alleles.

- **reduction division**

A nuclear division that produces daughter nuclei each having one-half as many centromeres as the parental nucleus. The first meiotic division reduces the number of chromosomes and centromeres to half that of the original cell.

- **redundant**

Repeated or duplicated unnecessarily.

- **reflex**

An involuntary response to a stimulus.

- **reflex testing**

Follow-up testing automatically initiated when certain test results are observed in the laboratory; used to clarify or elaborate on primary test results.

- **reflex, deep tendon**

Contraction of a muscle in response to tapping the tendon or guider with a reflex hammer; it requires intact sensory nerve supply to transmit the stretching of receptors in the muscle, and intact motor nerve supply for the muscle to contract.

- **refractory**

Not yielding, as in a condition that resists treatment or a nerve or muscle that resists stimulation.

- **regression**

A term coined by Galton for the tendency of the quantitative traits of offspring to be closer to the population mean than are their parents' traits. It arises from a combination of factors - dominance, gene interactions, and environmental influences on traits.

- **regression coefficient**

The slope of the straight line that most closely relates two correlated variables.

- **regulator gene**
A gene primarily involved in controlling another (structural) gene. Genes that are involved in turning on or off the transcription of structural genes.

- **regulatory dna**
DNA that controls the activity of genes.In the human genome, regulatory DNA sequences tend to be short and located near the genes they control.

- **regulatory gene**
A gene coding for a protein that regulates other genes.

- **regulatory region or sequence**
A DNA base sequence that controls gene expression.

- **rejection**
Refusal to accept, as with a transplanted organ.

- **relapse**
Recurrence of disease or symptoms after apparent recovery.

- **relaxed mutant**
A mutant that does not exhibit the stringent response under amino acid starvation.

- **release factors (rfi and rf2)**
Proteins in prokaryotes responsible for termination of translation and release of the newly synthesized polypeptide when a nonsense codon appears in the A site of the ribosome. Replaced by eRF in eukaryotes.

- **remission**
Lessening or disappearance of symptoms of a disease for a time.

- **renal**
A term that means having something to do with the kidneys.

- **renal capsule**
The fibrous connective tissue that surrounds each kidney.

- **renal cell cancer**
A type of kidney cancer.

- **renal failure**
The inability of the kidneys to excrete wastes, concentrate urine and maintain electrolyte balance.

- **renal pelvis**
The area at the center of the kidney. Urine collects here and is funneled into the ureter.

- **renner complex**
Specific gametic chromosome combination in Oenothera the evening primrose.

- **repeat sequences**
The length of a nucleotide sequence that is repeated in a tandem cluster.

- **repetitive dna**
Sequences of varying lengths that occur in multiple copies in the genome; it represents much of the human genome; DNA made up of copies of the same or nearly the same nucleotide sequence. DNA sequences that are present in

many copies per chromosome set. Repetitive DNA sequences may be closely linked (eg satellite DNA or VNTR loci) or dispersed throughout the genome or parts of the genome (e.g., alu family).

- **replica plating**
  A technique to rapidly transfer microorganism colonies from a master plate, in an exact spatial pattern, to a number of further plates.

- **replication**
  DNA synthesis. The process of copying. The identical duplication of DNA.

- **replication analysis (synonym replication banding, X-chromosome inactivation study, XCI)**
  A cytogenetic technique that uses specialized banding procedures (replication banding) to identify the late-replicating (inactive) X chromosome in cells. Because it is less complicated, less expensive, and less subjective, molecular testing is now used more commonly than replication analysis for X-chromosome inactivation studies.

- **replication fork**
  The point at which the two strands of DNA are separated to allow replication of each strand.

- **replication fork**
  The unwound region of the DNA double helix in which replication takes place.

- **replication segregation**
  Refers to changes in the proportions of mitochondrial DNA alleles as the mitochondria reproduce.

- **replicative transposition**
  The transposition of a transposable element to a new location without it being lost from the original location.

- **replicon**
  A chromosomal region whose replication is controlled by a single adjacent DNA replication initiation site. A genetic unit of replication including a length of DNA and its site for initiation of replication.

- **replisome**
  The DNA-replicating structure at the replication fork consisting of two DNA polymerase III enzymes and a primosome (primase and DNA helicase).

- **reporter gene**
  A gene whose phenotypic expression is easy to monitor; used to study promoter activity in different tissues or developmental stages. Recombinant DNA constructs are made in which the reporter gene is attached to a promoter region of particular interest and the construct transfected into a cell or organism.

- **repressible operon**
  Synthesis of a coordinated group of enzymes, involved in a single

synthetic (anabolic) pathway, is repressible if excess quantities of (usually) the end product of the pathway leads to cessation of transcription of the genes encoding the enzymes of the pathway.

- **repression**
  The condition of an inactive gene. Lack of activity (transcription) due to presence of repressor.

- **repressor**
  A protein that regulates a gene by turning it off; The protein product of a regulator gene that acts to control transcription of inducible and repressible operons. A molecule that binds to the operator and prevents transcription of an operon. Generally any molecule that can reversibly inactivate a gene.

- **reproductive cells**
  Egg and sperm cells. Each mature reproductive cell carries a single set of 23 chromosomes. The creation of gametes is called gametogenesis, in which gametocytes divide by meiosis into various gametes.

- **reproductive isolating mechanism**
  Any environmental; behavioural; mechanical; and physiological barrier that prevents two individuals of different populations producing viable progeny.

- **reproductive success**
  The relative production of offspring by a particular genotype.

- **reproductive system**
  In women, the organs that are directly involved in producing eggs and in conceiving and carrying babies.

- **repulsion**
  Allelic arrangement of two linked heterozygous loci, in which each homologous chromosome has one mutant (a or b) and one wild-type (A or B) allele (i.e., Ab/aB). Two linked heterozygous gene pairs in the arrangement, Ab/aB.

- **resection**
  A term used to describe the removal of a tumor from an organ such as a kidney, while retaining (sparing) the organ itself.

- **resolution**
  Degree of molecular detail on a physical map of DNA, ranging from low to high.

- **resolving power**
  The ability of an experimental technique to distinguish between two genetic conditions (typically discussed when one condition is rare (eg. recombination between very closely linked loci) and of particular interest).

- **respiratory distress**
  Pathological increase in the effort and frequency of breathing movements.

- **respiratory failure**
  Inability to maintain normal tensions of oxygen and carbon dioxide in the blood.

- **respiratory system**
  The organs that are involved in breathing. These include the nose, throat, larynx, trachea, bronchi, and lungs.

- **restriction digest**
  The result of the action of a restriction endonuclease on a DNA sample; The process in which DNA is exposed to restriction enzymes (restriction endonuclease), causing it to be cleaved into fragments of DNA called restriction fragments.

- **restriction endonuclease**
  Endonuclease that recognizes a particular short DNA sequence which they cleave. They help to protect cells from viral infection and are used in work with DNA; Naturally occurring enzymes which can cut DNA at specific sites, or base sequences. Each enzyme recognizes a specific sequence of base pairs and will only cut the DNA at these sites.

- **restriction enzyme**
  An endonuclease that will recognize a specific target nucleotide sequence in DNA and break the DNA chain at the target; a variety of these enzymes are known, and they are extensively used in genetic engineering.

- **restriction enzyme cutting site**
  A specific sequence of DNA at which a particular restriction enzyme cuts the DN A.

- **restriction enzyme, endonuclease**
  A protein that recognizes specific, short nucleotide sequences and cuts DNA at those sites. Bacteria contain over 400 such enzymes that recognize and cut more than 100 different DNA sequences, It is enzymes that can cut strands of DNA at specific base sequences; Enzymes that recognize specific double stranded DNA sequences and cleave the DNA at or near the recognition site. Restriction enzymes are derived and named after bacterial strains.

- **restriction fragment length polymorphism**
  Natural (polymorphic) variation in DNA sequence between individuals which abolishes or creates endonuclease restriction (cutting) sites, resulting in DNA fragments of different lengths when DNA is digested by an endonuclease; Variation between individuals in DNA fragment sizes cut by specific restriction enzymes; polymorphic sequences that result in RFLPs are used as markers on both physical maps and genetic linkage maps. RFLPs usually are caused by mutation at a cutting site.

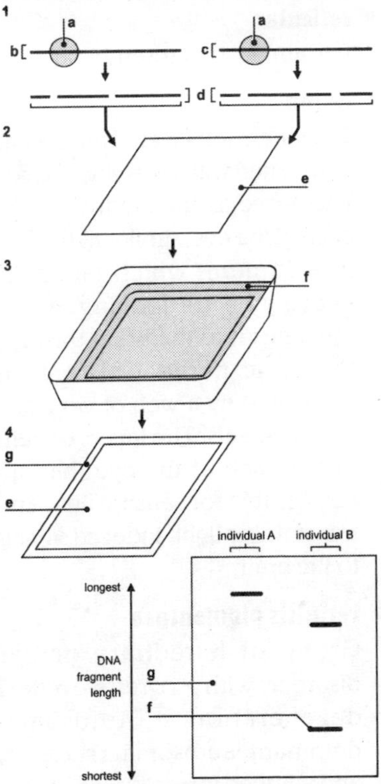


1. Cutting the DNA The same restriction enzyme (a) is used to cut the DNA (b and c) from different individuals, digesting the DNA into fragments (d).
2. Southern blotting These fragments are separated, according to their length, into invisible bands by gel electrophoresis and then transferred to a nitrocellulose membrane (e). This process is known as Southern blotting.
3. DNA probe The membrane is then soaked with a radioactive DNA probe solution (f). This probe will bind to any DNA on the membrane that has a complementary base sequence. Unbound probes are washed off.
4. Results The membrane is placed against a photographic film (g), which darkens wherever radioactivity is present. Therefore, the bands (f) on the photographic film indicate where on the membrane the radioactive probe bound.

   Because the DNA in the region that binds the probe is cut a different number of times when comparing the two individuals, different fragment lengths are shown up by the probe. These are the RFLPs.

- **restriction fragment length polymorphism analysis (synonym RFLP analysis, RFLP testing)**

Fragment of DNA of predictable size resulting from digestion (cutting) of a strand of DNA by a given restriction enzyme. DNA sequence alterations (mutations) that destroy or create the sites at which a restriction enzyme cuts DNA change the size (and number) of DNA fragments resulting from digestion by a given restriction enzyme.

- **restriction map**

A description of restriction endonuclease cleavage sites within a piece of DNA. Generating such a map is usually the first step in characterizing an unknown DNA, and a prerequisite to manipulating it for other purposes. Typically, restriction enzymes that cleave DNA infrequently (e.g. those with 6 bp recognition sites) and are relatively inexpensive are used to produce at a map.

- **restriction mapping**
  Use of restriction endonucleases to analyze and generate a physical map of genomes, genes, or other segments of DNA.

- **restriction site**
  A sequence of DNA that is recognized by an endonuclease (a protein that cuts DNA) as a site at which the DNA is to be cut

- **restriction-enzyme cutting site**
  A specific nucleotide sequence of DNA at which a particular restriction enzyme cuts the DNA. Some sites occur frequently in DNA (e.g., every several hundred base pairs); others much less frequently (rare-cutter; e.g., every 10,000 base pairs).

- **restrictive condition**
  An environmental condition under which a conditional mutant shows the mutant phenotype.

- **restrictive temperature**
  A temperature at which temperature-sensitive mutants display the mutant phenotype.

- **resuscitation**
  Revival of breathing or heartbeat after cessation or apparent death.

- **reticular**
  Pertaining to or resembling a net.

- **retina**
  The innermost layer of the eyeball concerned with receiving images, The nerve tissue that lives at the back of the eye, similar to the film in a camera, which takes the image you are looking at and transmits it to the brain through the optic nerve. This area is nourished by a web of very fine blood vessels. The layers of cells in the back of the eye that are responsible for sensing light and transmitting light- induced signals to the brain.

- **retinitis pigmentosa**
  Group of hereditary ocular disorders with progressive retinal degeneration. Autosomal dominant, autosomal recessive, and x-linked forms.

- **retinoblastoma**
  An eye cancer caused by the loss of a pair of tumor-suppressor genes; the inherited form typically appears in childhood, since one gene is missing from the time of birth; A childhood malignant cancer of the retina of the eye. reverse transcriptase viral enzyme used to make cDNA, A cancer of the human retina. Predisposition to retinoblastoma is inherited as an autosomal dominant. A childhood cancer of retinoblast cells caused by the inactivation of an anti-oncogene.

- **retinopathy**
  Diseased condition of the retina usually associated with visual impairment.

- **retrognathia**
  Backwards displacement of the lower jaw.

- **retroperitoneal space**
  The potential space just behind the visceral peritoneum.

- **retrotransposon (retroposon)**
  A class of genetic elements that includes retroviruses and transposons that have an intermediate RNA stage. A transposon that was created by reverse transcription of an RNA molecule.

- **retroviral infection**
  The presence of retroviral vectors, such as some viruses, which use their recombinant DNA to insert their genetic material into the chromosomes of the host's cells. The virus is then propogated by the host cell.

- **retrovirus**
  An RNA virus that replicates by first being converted into double-stranded DNA by reverse transcriptase.

- **reverse genetics**
  A molecular approach to identify genes on the basis of their location within a genome, without prior knowledge of the gene product. Also known as positional cloning.

- **reverse genetics**
  The experimental procedure that begins with a cloned segment of DNA, or a protein sequence, and uses this knowledge to introduce programmed mutations (through directed mutagenesis) back into the genome in order to investigate gene and protein function.

- **reverse transcriptase**
  An enzyme used by retroviruses to form a complementary DNA sequence (cDNA) from their RNA. The resulting DNA is then inserted into the chromosome of the host cell.

- **reversion**
  The production of a wild-type gene from a mutant gene. The return of a mutant to the wild-type phenotype by way of a second mutational event.

- **rflp mapping**
  A technique in which DNA restriction fragment length polymorphisms (RFLPs) are used as reference markers for mapping in relation to known genes or other RFLP loci.

- **rh factor**
  A blood factor located in red blood cells. Eighty-five percent of the population carry the blood factor and are Rh positive. Fifteen percent are missing the factor from their blood cells and are Rh negative.

- **rhabdomyomas**
  A benign (non-cancerous) neoplasm (tumor) derived from striated muscle occuring in the heart in children.

- **rhinitis**
  Inflammation of the nasal mucous membrane usually resulting in thick catarrhal discharge.

- **rhinoplasty**
  A procedure using plastic surgery in which the structure of the nose is changed.

- **rhizomelic rna**
  A chemical similar to DNA. The several classes of RNA molecules play important roles in protein synthesis and other cell activities.

- **rho**
  A protein factor required to recognize certain transcription termination signals in Escherichia coli.

- **rho-dependent terminator**
  A DNA sequence signaling the termination of transcription; termination requires the presence of the rho protein.

- **rho-independent terminator**
  A DNA sequence signaling the termination of transcription; the rho protein is not required for termination.

- **ribonucleic acid (rna)**
  A chemical that is very similar to one strand of the DNA double helix. RNA delivers important genetic messages to the cytoplasm of cells, where proteins are made. In RNA, the letter "U" replaces the letter "T" in DNA ("U" stands for Uracil).

- **ribose**
  The five-carbon sugar that serves as a component of RNA.

- **ribosomal protein**
  One of the ribonucleoprotein particles that are the sites of translation.

- **ribosomal rna (rrna)**
  A class of RNA found in the ribosomes of cells.

- **ribosome**
  The small cellular structure in which RNA translates the genetic code into proteins. A complex organelle (composed of proteins plus rRNA) that catalyzes translation of messenger RNA into an amino acid sequence. Ribosomes are made up of two non-identical subunits each consisting of a different rRNA and a different set of proteins.

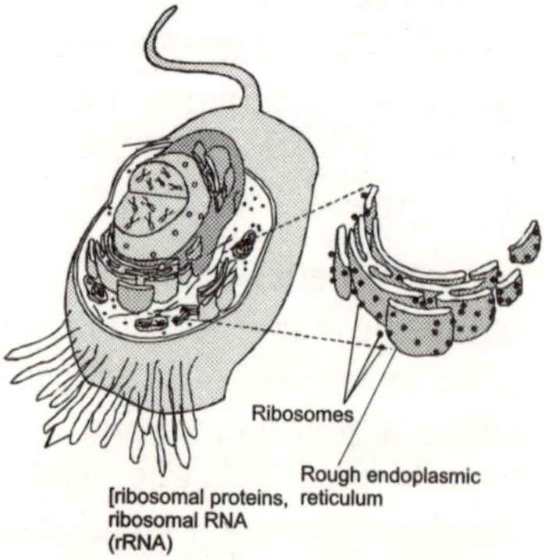

Ribosomes consist of two subunits that fit together and work as one to translate the mRNA into a polypeptide chain during protein synthesis. Prokaryotic subunits consist of one or two and eukaryotic of one or three very large RNA molecules (known as ribosomal RNA or rRNA) and multiple smaller protein molecules.

- **ribozyme**

Catalytic or autocatalytic RNA. RNA with enzymatic activity, for instance, self-splicing RNA molecules in Tetrahymena.

- **ring chromosome**

A structurally abnormal chromosome in which the end of each chromosome arm has been deleted and the broken arms have reunited to form a ring.

- **risk assessment**

Calculation of an individual's risk, employing appropriate mathematical equations, of having inherited a certain gene mutation, of developing a particular disorder, or of having a child with a certain disorder based upon analysis of multiple factors including family medical history and ethnic background

- **risk assessment modification**

Alteration of the assessment of an individual's genetic risk based upon previously unknown information about the family history or upon the results of genetic testing; depending on the nature of the new information, risk may be either increased or decreased.

- **risk communication**

In genetics, a process in which a genetic counselor or other medical professional interprets genetic test results and advises patients of the consequences for them and their offspring.

- **rna editing**

The insertion of uridines into mRNAs after transcription is completed; controlled by guide RNA (gRNA). May also sometimes involve insertion of cytidines and possible deletions of bases.

- **rna in situ hybridization**

A technique that is used to identify the spatial pattern of expression of a particular transcript (usually an mRNA). In this technique, the probe is labeled, either radioactively or by chemically attaching a fluorochrome visualised by fluorescence or an enzyme that can convert a substrate to a visible dye. A tissue or organism is soaked in a solution of single-stranded probe under conditions that allow the probe to hybridize to complementary RNA sequences in the cells; unhybridized probe is then removed. Radioactive probe is detected by autoradiography. Fluorochrome is detected by fluorescence microscopy. Enzyme labeled probe is detected by soaking the tissue in the substrate; the dye develops in sites where the transcript of interest was expressed.

- **rna interference, or rnai**

A system in cells for "turning off," or silencing, genes.Some plants use RNAi to silence the genes of invading pathogens, and some animals may as well.In the laboratory, scientists mimic RNAi to test the functions of individual genes.The system has potential as a therapy if scientists can figure out how to trigger the silencing of "overactive" genes in people, such as those involved in cancer.

- **rna phage**

Phage whose genetic material is RNA. They are the simplest known phages.

- **rna polymerase**

An enzyme that catalyzes the synthesis of an RNA strand from a DNA template. The enzyme that polymerizes RNA by using DNA as a template. It can also act as a primase initiating DNA replication. (Also known as transcriptase or RNA transcriptase).

- **rna replicase**

A polymerase enzyme that catalyzes the self-replication of single-stranded RNA.

- **robertsonian fusion**

Fusion of two acrocentric chromosomes at the centromere.

- **robertsonian translocation**

The joining of two acrocentric chromosomes at the centromeres with loss of their short arms to form a single abnormal chromosome; in acrocentric chromosomes the centromere is located near the end of the chromosome; acrocentric chromosomes are the Y chromosome and chromosome numbers 13, 14, 15, 21, and 22

- **rocker-bottom feet**

The plantar surface (bottom surface) of the foot is shaped like the rocker of a rocking chair.

- **rods**

Long, slender structures within the retina that perceive faint light. Also, rod-shaped bacteria (bacilli).

- **rolling-circle replication**

A model of DNA replication that accounts for a circular DNA molecule producing linear daughter double helices.

- **rrna (ribosomal rna)**

A class of RNA molecules, coded in the nucleolar organizer, that have an integral (but poorly understood) role in ribosome structure and function. RNA components of the subunits of the ribosomes.

- **rt-pcr**

Abbreviation for reverse transcriptase polymerase chain reaction.

- **rubinstein-taybi syndrome**

Condition with multiple congenital anomalies including: mental deficiency, broad thumbs, small head, broad nasal bridge and beaked nose.

- **rupture**
  Tearing of tissue (as in a hernia) or disruption of an organ.

- **sacroiliac**
  Relating to the sacrum and iliac in the lower back.

- **sacroiliac joint**
  The juncture between the sacrum and the ilium.

- **sacrum**
  Triangular bone at the base of the spinal column.

- **sampling distribution**
  The distribution of frequencies with which various possible events could occur or a probability distribution defined by a particular mathematical expression .

- **sanger method**
  The enzymatic method for determining the exact nucleotide sequence of a cloned fragment of DNA.

- **sanger sequence**
  "Plus and minus" or "primed synthesis" method; DNA is synthesized so it is radioactively labeled and the reaction terminates specifically at the position corresponding to a given base.

- **sanger sequencing**
  A widely used method of determining the order of bases in DNA.

- **sar - scaffold attachment region**
  The position along eukaryotic DNA where it is anchored to the central scaffold of the chromosome.

- **sarcoma**
  A type of cancer that starts in bone or muscle.

- **satellite**
  A chromosomal segment that branches off from the rest of the chromosome but is still connected by a thin filament or stalk.

- **satellite chromosome**
  Chromosome that seems to be an addition to the normal genome.

- **satellite dna**
  DNA that forms a separate band in a bouyant density gradient because of its different nucleotide composition (A:T rich DNAs are less dense than G:C rich DNAs). Highly repetitive eukaryotic DNA primarily located around centromeres. Satellite DNA usually has a different buoyant density than the rest of the cell's DNA. A portion of the DNA that differs enough in base composition so that it forms a distinct band on cesium chloride gradient centrifugation; usually contains highly repetitive DNA sequences.

- **saturation mutagenesis**
  Induction and recovery of large numbers of mutations in one area

of a genome, or in one biological function, in the hope of identifying all the genes in that area, or affecting that function.

- **scad**
  Short-Chain Acyl-CoA Dehydrogenase Deficiency.

- **scaffold**
  In genomic mapping, a series of contigs that are in the right order but not necessarily connected in one continuous stretch of sequence, The eukaryotic chromosome structure remaining when DNA and histones have been removed; made from nonhistone proteins. The central framework of a chromosome to which the DNA solenoid is attached as loops; composed largely of topoisomerase.

- **scanning hypothesis**
  Proposed mechanism by which the eukaryotic ribosome recognizes the initiation region of an mRNA after binding the 5' capped end of it. The ribosome scans the mRNA for the initiation codon.

- **scapulohumeral**
  Relating to the scapula (shoulder blade) and the humerus (bone of the upper arm).

- **scar tissue**
  A mark left on damaged tissue after it has healed. It can form on the skin or on internal wounds.

- **sciatic nerve**
  The largest nerve in the body provides sensory and motor function to the lower extremeties.

- **scientific method**
  A procedure used by scientists to test hypotheses by making predictions about the outcome of an experiment before the experiment is performed. The results provide support or refutation of the hypothesis.

- **sclera**
  The white, fibrous outer membrane of the eyeball.

- **sclerae**
  The outer envelope or covering of the eye.

- **sclerodermatous**
  Resembling or marked by scleroderma, a thickening of the skin.

- **sclerosis**
  A induration or hardening, especially hardening of a part from inflammation and in diseases of the interstitial substance. The term is used chiefly for such a hardening of the nervous system due to hyperplasia of the connective tissue or to designate hardening of the blood vessels.

- **scoliosis**
  Abnormal curvature of the spine.

- **screening**
  Testing designed to identify individuals in a given population

who are at higher risk of having or developing a particular disorder, or having a gene mutation for a particular disorder. It is looking for evidence of a particular disease such as cancer in persons with no symptoms of disease.

- **screening technique**
  A technique to determine the genotype or phenotype of an organism.

- **scrotum**
  The pouch that holds the testicles.

- **seborrhea**
  A accumulation of scales of greasy skin, often on the scalp. Dandruff.
  second division segregation (sds)
  The allele arrangement (2+2+2+2) in the spores of Ascomycetes with ordered spores that indicates a crossover between a locus and its centromere. A pattern of ascospore genotypes for a gene pair showing that the two alleles segregate into different nuclei only at the second meiotic division, as a result of a single crossover between that gene pair and its centromere; can only be detected in a ordered ascus.

- **secondary diabetes**
  When a person gets diabetes because of another disease or because of taking certain drugs or chemicals.

- **secondary oocyte**
  A cell formed by meiosis I in female animals.

- **secondary sexual character**
  The sex-associated phenotype of somatic tissues in sexually dimorphic animals.

- **secondary spermatocyte**
  The product of the first meiotic division in male animals.

- **secondary structure**
  The alpha-helical or beta-sheet configuration of the polypeptide backbone of a protein.

- **second-degree relative**
  Any relative who is two meioses away from a particular individual in a pedigree; a relative with whom one quarter of an individual's genes is shared (i.e., grandparent, grandchild, uncle, aunt, nephew, niece, half-sibling).

- **second-site mutation**
  The second mutation of a double mutation within a gene. In many cases, the second-site mutation suppresses the first mutation, so that the double mutant has the wild-type phenotype.

- **secrete**
  To make and give off such as when the beta cells make insulin and then release it into the blood so that the other cells in the body can use it to turn glucose (sugar) into energy.

- **secretion**
  Fluid formed by a gland, containing enzymes, hormones or waste products.

- **sector**
  An area of tissue or colony whose phenotype is detectably different from the surrounding tissue or colony phenotype.

- **sedimentation**
  The sinking of a molecule under the opposing forces of gravitation and buoyancy.

- **segmental transplantation**
  A surgical procedure in which a part of a pancreas that contains insulin-producing cells is placed in a person whose pancreas has stopped making insulin.

- **segmentation**
  The process by which the correct number of segments are established in a developing segmented animal.

- **segregation**
  The normal biological process whereby the two pieces of a chromosome pair are separated during meiosis and randomly distributed to the germ cells.

- **segregation, rule of**
  Mendel's first principle describing how genes are passed from one generation to the next.

- **segregational load**
  Genetic load caused when a population is segregating less fit homozygotes because of heterozygote advantage.

- **segregational petite**
  A petite that in a cross with wild-type produces 50% petite and 50% wild-type progeny; caused by a nuclear mutation.

- **seizure**
  A seizure is a sudden attack of epileptic convulsion. It is a result of involuntary electrical activity in the brain. It can be associated with uncontrolled motor (movement) or sensory system action. Accordingly, a patient suffering a seizure may experience uncontrollable body movements, unusual smells or tastes and have loss of consciousness (awareness of surroundings).

- **selection**
  The process of determining the relative share allotted individuals of different genotypes in the propagation of a population; the selective effect of a gene can be defined by the probability that carriers of the gene will reproduce.

- **selection coefficient(s)**
  The proportional excess or deficiency of fitness of one genotype in relation to another genotype.

- **selection differential**
  The difference between the mean of a population and the mean of the individuals selected to be parents of the next generation.

- **selection progress**
The difference between the mean of a population and the mean of the offspring in the next generation born to selected parents.

- **selection-mutation equilibrium**
An equilibrium allele frequency resulting from the balance between selection against the allele and mutation recreating this allele.

- **selective medium**
A culture medium that is enriched with a particular substance to allow the growth of particular strains of organisms.

- **selective neutrality**
A situation in which different alleles of a certain gene confer equal fitness.

- **selective system**
An experimental technique that enhances the recovery of specific (usually rare) genotypes.

- **self**
The fusion of male and female gametes from the same individual.

- **self-assembly**
The ability of certain multimeric biological structures to assemble from their component parts through random movements of the molecules and formation of weak chemical bonds between surfaces with complementary shapes.

- **self-fertilization**
Fertilization in which the two gametes are from the same individual.

- **selfish dna**
A segment of the genome with no apparent function other than to ensure its own replication.

- **semiconservative replication**
The mode by which DNA replicates. Each strand acts as a template for a new double helix. The established model of DNA replication in which each double-stranded molecule is composed of one parental strand and one newly polymerized strand.

- **semisterility (half sterility)**
The phenotype of individuals heterozygotic for certain types of chromosome aberration; expressed as a reduced number of viable gametes and hence reduced fertility. Nonviability of a proportion of gametes or zygotes.

- **sensitivity**
The frequency with which a test yields a positive result when the individual being tested is actually affected and/or has the gene mutation in question, Tendency to be acutely affected by a stimulus or substance.

- **sensorimotor**
A term applied to the combination of the input of sensations and the output of motor activity. The motor activity reflects what is

happening to the sensory organs such as the visual, auditory, tactual and kinesthetic sensations. Also referred to as "perceptual motor".

- **sensorineural deafness**
  Deafness caused from a central nervous system defect.

- **septal**
  Referring to a septum, a thin wall separating two cavities or masses of softer tissue.

- **septal defect**
  Hole in the wall separating the two atria or the two ventricles.

- **septum**
  Thin partition within or between anatomical structures or organs.

- **sequelae**
  A condition following as a consequence of a disease.

- **sequence (n.)**
  The sequence of genetic "letters" in a piece of DNA.A short DNA sequence might be: ACGTAC-GTACGT

- **sequence (v.)**
  To determine the sequence of genetic "letters" in a piece of DNA or an entire human genome.

- **sequence alteration (synonym mutation)**
  Any alteration in a gene from its natural state; may be benign (commonly referred to as a "polymorphism"), pathogenic, or of unknown significance.

- **sequence assembly**
  A process whereby the order of multiple sequenced DNA fragments is determined.

- **sequence tagged site (sts)**
  Short (200 to 500 base pairs) DNA sequence that has a single occurrence in the human genome and whose location and base sequence are known. Detectable by polymerase chain reaction, STSs are useful for localizing and orienting the mapping and sequence data reported from many different laboratories and serve as landmarks on the developing physical map of the human genome. Expressed sequence tags (ESTs) are STSs derived from cDNAs.

- **sequencer**
  An apparatus used for deciphering the order of bases in a strand of DNA.

- **sequencing**
  The process of identifying the order in which chains of repeating units of base pairs appear in DNA and identifying the order of amino acids in proteins. Researchers label copies of a DNA sequence with fluorescent markers, then run them through a sequencing machine. In proteins, amino acids are removed one at a time from the end of a protein and identified with an automated system.

Determination of the order of base sequences in either DNA or RNA molecules or proteins.

- **sequencing technology**

The instrumentation and procedures used to determine the order of nucleotides in DNA.

- **sequential**

Occurring in order of arrangement.

- **serotonin**

A neurotransmitter involved in the processes of sleep and memory, as well as other neurological functions.

- **serous microcystic adenomas**

Grapelike clusters of cysts which may occur in the pancreas. Cysts are composed of epithelium-lined collections of serous fluid that vary in size from several millimeters to over 10 cm. (over three inches).

- **serum**

Clear fluid which remains after the corpuscles and fibrin have been removed from the blood.

- **sex chromosome**

The X or Y chromosome in human beings that determines the sex of an individual. Females have two X chromosomes in diploid cells; males have an X and a Y chromosome. The sex chromosomes comprise the 23rd chromosome pair in a karyotype.

- **sex determination**

The mechanism in a given species by which sex is determined; in many species sex is determined at fertilization by the nature of the sperm that fertilizes the egg.

**Sex chromosomes**

In humans, one of the pairs of homologous chromosomes – the sex chromosomes – is responsible for determining the sex of an individual. The sex chromosomes exist in two forms, *X* and *Y*, so called because of their characteristic shape during cell division.

1. Female sex chromosomes Female sex chromosomes are both X, giving the individual the genetic constitution (genotype) XX.
2. Male sex chromosomes One male sex chromosome is an X (a) and the other is a Y (b), giving the individual the genotype XY.

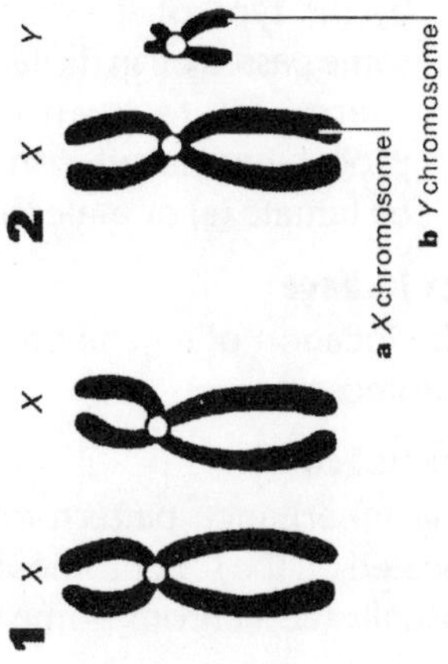

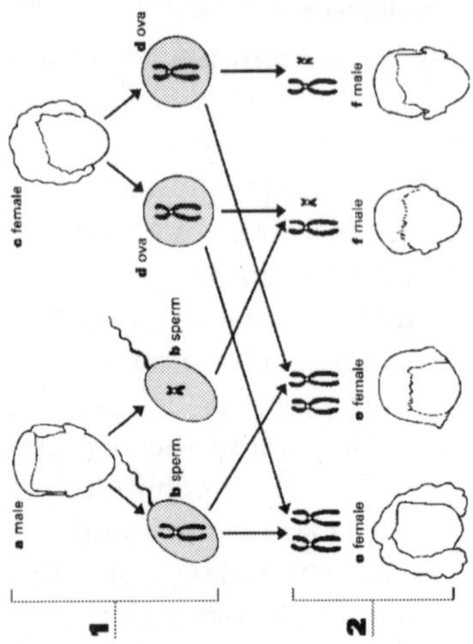


**How sex is determined**

1. A male (a) produces sperm (b) which may contain, with equal probability, either an *X* or a *Y* chromosome. A female (c) produces ova (d) which always carry an *X* chromosome.
2. When a sperm and ovum fuse at fertilization, the sex of the resulting child is determined by the type of sex chromosome passed on in the father's sperm. There is an equal probability that offspring will be female (e) or male (f).

- **sex linkage**

The location of a gene on a sex chromosome.

- **sex linked**

The inheritance pattern of loci located on the sex chromosomes (usually the X chromosome in XY species); also refers to the loci themselves.

- **sex reversal**

A syndrome known in humans and mice in which chromosomally XX individuals develop as males. In some cases, sex reversal is now known to be due to the translocation of the testis-determining region of the Y chromosome to the tip of the X chromosome in such individuals.

- **sex switch**

A gene, normally found on the Y chromosome in mammals, that directs the indeterminate gonads toward development as testes.

- **sex-controlled trait**

Traits that appear more of time in one sex than in the other.

- **sex-determining region y (sry)**

The sex switch or testis-determining factor in human beings located on the Y chromosome. (Sry in mice.)

- **sexduction**

Sexual transmission of donor Escherichia coli chromosomal genes on the fertility factor. A process whereby a bacterium gains access to and incorporates foreign DNA brought in by a modified F factor during conjugation.

- **sex-lethal**

A gene in Drosophila, located on the X chromosome, that is a sex switch directing development toward femaleness when it is in the on state. It is regulated by numerator and denominator elements that act to influence the genic balance equation (X/A).

- **sex-limited trait**
  Trait expressed in only one sex. It may be controlled by sex linked or autosomal loci.

- **sex-ratio phenotype**
  A trait in Drosophila whereby females produce mostly if not only daughters.

- **sexual selection**
  The forces determined by mate choice acting to cause one genotype to mate more frequently than another genotype.

- **shine-delgarno hypothesis**
  A proposal that prokaryotic mRNA is aligned at the ribosome by complementarity between the mRNA upstream from the initiation codon and the 3' end of the 16S rRNA.

- **shock**
  A severe condition that disturbs the body. A person with diabetes can go into shock when the level of blood glucose (sugar) drops suddenly.

- **short stature**
  Height/length less than the 5th percentile for age.

- **shotgun method**
  Sequencing method that involves randomly sequenced cloned pieces of the genome, with no foreknowledge of where the piece originally came from. This can be contrasted with "directed" strategies, in which pieces of DNA from known chromosomal locations are sequenced. Because there are advantages to both strategies, researchers use both random (or shotgun) and directed strategies in combination to sequence the human genome.

- **shotgun sequencing**
  A method of determining the DNA sequence of a genome..The first step in shotgun sequencing is to copy a genome many times, then shred the copies into fragments of DNA that can be "read" by machines.Next, computers identify the fragments that belong next to each other in the genome and assemble them into a complete genome sequence.

- **shotgun technique**
  Cloning a large population of different DNA fragments, known to contain a fragment of interest, as a prelude to selecting or screening for that one particular clone containing the fragment of interest for intensive study.

- **shunt**
  1. A passage that diverts blood flow from one route to another. May occur naturally or be created surgically. 2. A catheter (tube) that carries cerebrospinal fluid from a

ventricle in the brain to another area of the body.

- **shuttle vector**
  A vector (e.g. a plasmid) constructed in such a way that it can replicate in at least two different host species (eg a prokaryote and a eukaryote). A DNA recombined into such a vector can be tested or manipulated in several cell types.

- **siblings or sibs**
  A person's brothers and sisters.

- **sibship**
  The group comprising all the siblings (brothers and sisters) in a family.

- **sickle cell anemia**
  An hereditary, chronic form of hemolytic anemia characterized by breakdown of the red blood cells; red blood cells undergo a reversible alteration in shape when the oxygen tension of the plasma falls slightly and a sickle-like shape forms. An inherited, potentially lethal disease in which a defect in hemoglobin, the oxygen-carrying pigment in the blood, causes distortion (sickling) and loss of red blood cells, producing damage to organs throughout the body.

- **sickled cells**
  In children with sickle cell disease, hemoglobin molecules in red blood cells stick to one another and cause the red cells to become crescent or sickle shaped. Sickled cells cannot pass easily through tiny blood vessels.

- **sigma factor**
  The protein that gives promoter-recognition specificity to the RNA polymerase core enzyme of bacteria.

- **sign**
  Physical evidence of the existence of something which can be demonstrated by a medical doctor.

- **signal hypothesis**
  The major mechanism whereby proteins that insert into or cross a membrane are synthesized by a membrane-bound ribosome. The first thirteen to thirty-six amino acids synthesized, termed a signal peptide, are recognized by a signal recognition particle that draws the ribosome to the membrane surface by interaction with a docking protein. The signal peptide may later be removed from the protein.

- **signal sequence**
  The N-terminal sequence of a secreted protein, which is required for transport through the cell membrane.

- **signal transduction cascade**
  Refers to a series of sequential events, such as protein phosphorylations, consequent upon binding of ligand by a transmembrane receptor, that

transfer a signal through a series of intermediate molecules until final regulatory molecules, such as transcription factors, are modified in response to the signal.

- **silencer**
  The cis regulatory element that reduces transcription of a gene.

- **silent carriers**
  When both parents carry defective, recessive genes (genes determine hereditary characteristics).

- **silent gene**
  A mutant gene that has no detectable phenotypic effect.

- **silent mutation**
  Mutation in which the function of the protein product of the gene is unaltered.

- **simian crease**
  Single transverse palbral flexian crease in hand.

- **simian crease or simian line**
  Single transverse (crosswise) palbral flexian crease in the hand, common in Down syndrome.

- **simplex case**
  A single occurrence of a disorder in a family.

- **sine**
  Short interspersed element. A type of small dispersed repetitive DNA sequence (eg Alu family in the human genome) found throughout a eukaryotic genome.

- **single nucleotide polymorphism (also called snp, pronounced "snip")**
  A single "letter" of DNA that may vary from one person to the next.At a particular location in the genome, one person may have an "A" while another has a "T." In the human genome, a SNP occurs on average about once every thousand DNA "letters."

- **single strand**
  One half of a DNA double helix.

- **single-gene disorder**
  Hereditary disorder caused by a mutant allele of a single gene (e.g., Duchenne muscular dystrophy, retinoblastoma, sickle cell disease).

- **single-gene disorder (also called mendelian disorder)**
  A disease caused by a single gene that is inherited in a straightforward manner from parent or parents to child.Huntington's disease and cystic fibrosis are examples.The term "Mendelian" refers to Gregor Mendel, the Austrian who did pioneering work on genes and traits in ordinary garden peas by showing that a ingle trait, such as color, can be determined by a single gene.Compared to "complex diseases," Mendelian disorders are relatively rare.

- **single-strand binding protein**
  Protein that binds to single-stranded DNA usually near the replication fork to stabilize the single strands.

- **single-stranded conformational polymorphism (synonym SSCP)**
  A type of mutation scanning; the identification of abnormally migrating single-stranded DNA segments on gel electrophoresis.

- **sinuses**
  Empty spaces or cavities usually within a bony structure.

- **sister chromatid exchange (synonym sce)**
  Exchange of genetic material between the two chromatids of a single chromosome during the cell division process; similar to crossing-over (recombination), except that the exchange involves the two sister chromatids of a single chromosome, whereas crossing-over refers to exchange of genetic material between the two homologous chromosomes of a chromosome pair.

- **site-directed mutagenesis**
  The process of creating mutations at specific locations, in contrast to naturally occurring random mutations.

- **site-specific recombination**
  A crossover event, such as the integration of phage lambda, that requires homology of only a very short region and uses an enzyme specific for that recombination. Recombination occurring between two specific sequences that need not be homologous; mediated by a specific recombination system.

- **skeletal anomalies of the spine**
  Lordosis (swayback), kyphosis (hunchback), scoliosis, (s-shaped curve).

- **skeleton**
  The skeleton is composed of bones and is the framework of the body.

- **skew**
  A distortion of the shape of the normal distribution toward one side or the other.

- **skewed x-inactivation**
  A nonrandom pattern of inactivation of one of the X chromosomes in a female that can arise through a variety of mechanisms. When this occurs, the active X chromosome may bear the mutant allele and the female will show signs and symptoms of the disease. The female is called a manifesting heterozygote or a carrier.

- **sky (spectral karyotyping)**
  A visualization of all of the chromosomes in the genome all together with each chromosome labeled with a different color. The SKY technique is useful for

identifying chromosome abnormalities.

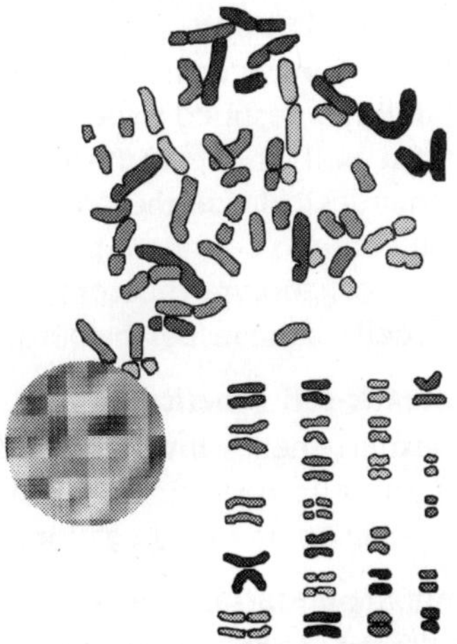

- **smaf(sub malleolar ankle foot orthodontic)**
  Plastic foot braces worn as inserts in the shoes.

- **small intestine**
  The part of the digestive tube connecting the stomach to the colon. The small intestine is divided into the duodenum, jejunum, and ileum.

- **sne**
  Subacute Necrotizing Encephalomyelopathy, or Leigh Disease or Syndrome.

- **snp maps**
  A collection of SNPs that can be superimposed over the existing genome map, creating greater detail and facilitating further genetic studies. Current estimates indicate that a very dense marker map (30,000 - 1,000,000 variants) would be required to perform haplotype - based association studies. We have constructed a SNP map of the human genome with sufficient density to study human haplotype structure, enabling future study of human medical and population genetics.

- **snrnp**
  Small nuclear ribonucleoprotein (RNA plus protein) particle. Component of the spliceosome, the intron-removing apparatus in eukaryotic nuclei .

- **sociobiology**
  The study of the evolution of social behavior in animals.

- **solenoid structure**
  The supercoiled arrangement of DNA in eukaryotic nuclear chromosomes produced by coiling the continuous string of nucleosomes (about 7 nucleosomes per turn).

- **somatic**
  Relating to the trunk, the wall of a body cavity, or the body in general.

- **somatic cell**
  A cell that is not destined to become a gamete; a cell whose genes will cannot be passed on to future generations.

- **somatic cell gene therapy**
  Incorporating new genetic material into cells for therapeutic

purposes. The new genetic material cannot be passed to offspring; The insertion of new DNA material into a particular tissue of an affected individual in such a way that the inserted DNA does not enter the germline.

- **somatic cell genetic mutation**
A change in the genetic structure that is neither inherited nor passed to offspring. Also called acquired mutations.

- **somatic cell hybrid**
Hybrid cell line derived from two different species; contains a complete chromosomal complement of one species and a partial chromosomal complement of the other; human/hamster hybrids grow and divide, losing human chromosomes with each generation until they finally stabilize, the hybrid cell line established is then utilized to detect the presence of genes on the remaining human chromosome.

- **somatic doubling**
A disruption of the mitotic process that produces a cell with twice the normal chromosome number.

- **somatic hypermutation**
The occurrence of a high level of mutation in the variable regions of immunoglobulin genes.

- **somatic mosaicism**
Two or more genetic or cytogenetic cell lines within the cells of the body (may or may not include the germline cells).

- **somatic mutation**
A mutation occurring in any cell that is not destined to become a germ cell; if the mutant cell continues to divide, the individual will come to contain a patch of tissue of genotype different from the cells of the rest of the body.

- **somatic-cell genetics**
Asexual genetics, involving study of somatic mutation, mitotic crossing-overand segregation.

- **somatic-mutation theory**
A theory to account for the high degree of antibody variability. It suggests that mutation of a basic immunoglobulin gene accounts for all the different types of immunoglobulins produced by B lymphocytes.

- **somatostatin**
A human growth hormone.

- **sonogram**
The image produced by ultrasound.

- **sos box**
The region in the promoter of various genes that is recognized by the LexA repressor. Release of repression results in the induction of the SOS response.

- **sos repair**
The error-prone process whereby gross structural DNA damage is circumvented by allowing

replication to proceed past the damage through imprecise polymerization.

- **sos response**

Repair systems (recA; uvr) induced by the presence of single-stranded DNA that usually occurs from postreplicative gaps caused by various types of DNA damage. The RecA protein, stimulated by single-stranded DNA, is involved in the inactivation of the LexA repressor thereby inducing the response.

- **southern blot (synonym Southern analysis, Southern blot analysis, Southern blotting, Southern blotting analysis)**

Molecular genetic testing technique used to detect differences in the lengths of DNA fragments following restriction enzyme digestion (commonly known as RFLPs restriction fragment length polymorphisms). The lengths of restriction fragments can vary due to mutations occurring between two restriction sites (e.g., large insertions, large deletions, and highly expanded trinucleotide repeats) or within a restriction site (e.g., single base pair changes). Transfer of electrophoretically separated fragments of DNA, after denaturation, from the gel to an absorbent sheet of material, such as nitrocellulose, to which the DNA binds. The sheet is immersed in a solution containing a labeled probe that will hybridize to fragment(s) of interest. The method was first devised by E. M. Southern to transfer DNA fragments from an agarose gel to a nitrocellulose paper for hybridization, but similar transfer methods are now also used for transfering RNA or protein to papers of a variety of types followed by hybridization (RNA) or labeled antibody treatment (protein) to identify specific molecules.

- **southern blotting**

A technique for transferring resolved DNA segments to a nitrocellulose filter, usually after restriction enzyme digestion and gel electrophoresis. The DNA segment of interest is then probed with a labeled complimentary nucleic acid and its position determined by audioradiography.

- **spacer dna**

Regions of non-transcribed DNA between transcribed repeated genes such as ribosomal RNA genes in eukaryotes. Its function is probably to do with ensuring the high rates of transcription associated with these genes.

- **spasm**

A sudden powerful, involuntary contraction of the muscle.

- **spasticity**

Increased muscle tone (hypertonic), involuntary resistance of weak muscle caused by passive range of motion followed by sudden relaxation of muscle, associated with exaggeration of reflexes. Causes stiffness, awkward movements, and loss of voluntary muscle control.

- **spasticity**
  Increased muscular tone with exaggeration of the tendon reflexes.

- **specialized (restricted) transduction**
  The situation in which a particular phage will transduce only specific regions of the bacterial chromosome. Form of transduction based on faulty looping out by a temperate phage. Only loci neighbouring the attachment site can be transduced.

- **speciation**
  A process whereby over time one species evolves into a different species (anagenesis) or whereby one species diverges to become two or more species (cladogenesis).

- **species**
  A group of organisms belong to the same biological species if they are capable of interbreeding to produce fertile offspring. However the biological test of a species is not always available, and so there is also a morphological species concept based on anatomical similarities.

- **specificity**
  The frequency with which a test yields a negative result when the individual being tested is actually unaffected and/or does not have the gene mutation in question

- **specific-locus test**
  A system for detecting recessive mutations in diploids. Normal individuals treated with mutagen are mated to testers that are homozygous for the recessive alleles at a number of specific loci; the progeny are then screened for recessive phenotypes.

- **spectral karyotype (sky)**
  A graphic of all an organism's chromosomes, each labeled with a different color. Useful for identifying chromosomal abnormalities.

- **speech therapy**
  Treatment in which speech and language needs of an individual patient are addressed, may also include oral/motor therapy.

- **spermatid**
  The four products of meiosis in males that develop into sperm.

- **spermatocyte**
  (1) (Zoological) A cell which undergoes meiosis and thereby produces spermatids. See primary spermatocyte and secondary spermatocyte. (2) (Botanical) A cell that becomes converted to a spermatozoid (a small motile male gamete with

flagella) without intervention of cell division.

- **spermatogenesis**
  The process of sperm production.
- **spermatogonium**
  A cell type in the testes of male vertebrates that gives rise to primary spermatocytes by mitosis.
- **spermiogenesis**
  The process by which spermatids mature into sperm cells.
- **sphincter**
  A circular band of muscle fibers that constricts or closes a passage or opening.
- **spina bifida**
  A congenital condition that results from altered fetal development of the spinal cord, part of the neural plate fails to join together and bone and muscle are unable to grow over this open section.
- **spinal canal**
  The channel in the spinal column that contains the spinal cord.
- **spinal column**
  The skeletal structure composed of the vertebrae that encloses the spinal cord.
- **spinal cord**
  That part of the central nervous system contained within the vertebral column.
- **spindle**
  The set of tubulin fibers that appear to move eukaryotic chromosomes during division. The microtubule apparatus that controls chromosome movement during mitosis and meiosis.
- **spine**
  A column of bones and cartilage in the back which begin at the base of the skull and continue to the pelvis.
- **spiral cleavage**
  The cleavage process in molluscs and some invertebrates whereby orientation of the spindle at mitosis is at an angle to the original egg axis.
- **spirillum**
  A spiral bacterium.
- **splayed labia majora**
  A minor malformation of the outer area of the female genitalia.
- **spleen**
  An organ that produces lymphocytes, filters the blood, stores blood cells, and destroys those that are aging. It is located on the left side of the abdomen near the stomach. An organ which is part of the lymphatic system aiding in the red blood cell development.
- **splice site**
  Location in the DNA sequence where RNA removes the noncoding areas to form a continuous gene transcript for translation into a protein.

- **spliceosome**
Protein-RNA complex that removes introns from eukaryotic nuclear RNAs.

- **splice-site mutation**
A mutation that alters or abolishes the specific sequence denoting the site at which the splicing of an intron takes place. Such mutations result in one or more introns remaining in the mature messenger RNA and can disrupt the generation of the protein product

- **splicing (synonym splicing mutation)**
The process by which introns, non-coding regions, are excised out of the primary messenger RNA transcript and exons (i.e., coding regions) are joined together to generate mature messenger RNA.

- **spondylolisthesis**
Forward movement of the body on one of the lower lumbar vertabra or the vertbra below it or on the sacrum.

- **spontaneous mutation**
A mutation occurring in the absence of mutagens, usually due to errors in the normal functioning of cellular enzymes.

- **sporadic**
The chance occurrence of a disorder or abnormality that is not likely to recur in a family, Occurring in isolated cases.

- **sporadic cancer**
Cancer that occurs randomly and is not inherited from parents. Caused by DNA changes in one cell that grows and divides, spreading throughout the body.

- **spore**
(1) In plants and fungi, sexual spores are the haploid cells produced by meiosis. (2) In fungi, asexual spores are somatic cells that are cast off to act either as gametes or as the initial cells for new haploid individuals.

- **sporophyte**
The diploid sexual-spore-producing generation in the life cycle of plants. The stage in which meiosis occurs. The stage of a plant life cycle that produces spores by meiosis and alternates with the gametophyte stage.

- **sputum**
The fluid produced by the lungs and lower airway and ejected by coughing.

- **sscp (synonym single-stranded conformational polymorphism)**
A type of mutation scanning; the identification of abnormally migrating single-stranded DNA segments on gel electrophoresis.

- **stabilizing selection**
A type of selection that removes individuals from both ends of a phenotypic distribution thus

maintaining the same distribution mean. Natural selection that maintains a high incidence of optimal (most successful) forms in a population is called stabilizing selection. It occurs in all populations, but is particularly apparent when an environment stays reasonably constant over time. In such cases, natural selection:

- tends to eliminate extreme forms from the population (1 to 2), and
- results in an optimum phenotype (such as birth weight) that is close to the mean value of the characteristic for that population (3).

In this way, stabilizing selection tends to promote the best fit of a population to its stable environment

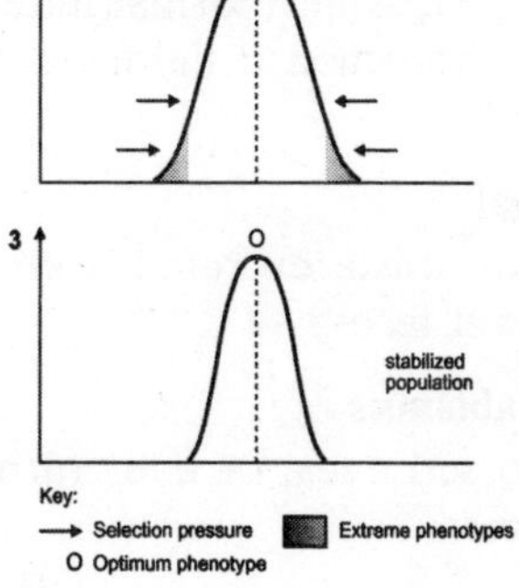


- **stacking**
The packing of the flattish nitrogen base-pairs at the centre of the DNA double helix.

- **staggered cuts**
The cleavage of two opposite strands of duplex DNA at points near one another.

- **standard deviation**
The square root of the variance.

- **standard error of the mean**
The standard deviation divided by the square root of the sample size. It is the standard deviation of a sample of means.

- **stasipatric speciation**
Instantaneous speciation caused by polyploidy.

- **statistic**
A computed quantity characteristic of a population, such as the mean. Measurements of attributes of a sample from a population.

- **statistical distribution**
The array of frequencies of different quantitative or qualitative classes in a population.

- **status epilepticus**
A situation in which two major epileptic seizures occur, one right after the other. In such a case, immediate emergency room attention is required. Status epilepticus happens rarely.

- **stem cell**

  Undifferentiated, primitive cells in the bone marrow that have the ability both to multiply and to differentiate into specific blood cells; An "immature" cell that can become any type of cell in the body.Scientists are investigating ways to coax human stem cells into becoming replacement cells for people with diseases.

- **stem-loop structure**

  A lollipop-shaped structure formed when a single-stranded nucleic acid molecule loops back on itself to form a complementary double helix (stem) topped by a loop.

- **stenosis**

  Unnatural narrowing of a passage or opening in the body.

- **stenosis, aortic**

  Narrowing of the valve opening between the left ventricle and the aorta.

- **stenosis, mitral**

  Narrowing of the valve between the left atrium and ventricle.

- **sternum**

  A narrow flat bone in the middle of the chest-breastbone.

- **steroid receptor**

  A family of related proteins that act as transcription factors when bound to their cognate hormone ligands. Not all members of this family actually bind to steroids; the name derives from the first family member that was discovered, which was a steroid hormone receptor.

- **stiff hand syndrome**

  Thickening of the skin of the palm that results in loss of ability to hold hand straight. This condition occurs only in people with diabetes.

- **stochastic**

  A process with an indeterminate or random element as opposed to a deterministic process that has no random element.

- **stoma**

  Artificially created opening between two passages or body cavities - often found where a G-Tube is inserted.

- **stomach**

  A muscular pouch that helps in the digestion of food by mixing it with digestive juices and churning it into a thin liquid; The complex organ of the body between the esophagus and the small intestine which functions in the digestion of food.

- **stool**

  Body waste excreted from the bowel; feces.

- **strabismus**

  Crossed eyes, or eyes turning inward.

• **strabismus**
Lack of parallelism of the visual axis of the eyes.(crossed eyes, cross-eyed, etc). A deviation of one or both eyes so that both cannot be directed at the same object at the same time.

• **strain**
A pure-breeding lineage, usually of haploid organisms, bacteria, or viruses.

• **stridor**
Unusual noise during respiration - mostly inhalation.

• **stringent factor**
A protein catalyzing the formation of an unusual nucleotide (guanosine tetraphosphate, ppGpp) during the stringent response under amino acid starvation conditions.

• **stringent response**
A translational control mechanism of prokaryotes that represses tRNA and rRNA synthesis during amino acid starvation.

• **stroke**
Sudden, severe attack that results in brain damage. Usually sudden paralysis or speech difficulty results from injury to the brain or spinal cord by a blood clot, hemorrhage or occlusion of blood supply to the brain from a narrowed or blocked artery.

• **stroke**
Disease caused by damage to blood vessels in the brain. Depending on the part of the brain affected, a stroke can cause a person to lose the ability to speak or move a part of the body such as an arm or a leg. Usually only one side of the body is affected.

• **structural gene**
A gene encoding the amino acid sequence of a protein.

• **structural genomics**
The effort to determine the 3D structures of large numbers of proteins using both experimental techniques and computer simulation.

• **subglottic stenosis**
Narrow throat below the vocal cords.

• **subglottis**
The lowest part of the larynx; the area from just below the vocal cords down to the top of the trachea.

• **subluxatin**
Incomplete dislocation-relationship is altered but contact remains between the joint surfaces remains.

• **submetacentric chromosome**
A chromosome whose centromere lies between its middle and its end but closer to the middle.

• **substitution**
In genetics, a type of mutation due to replacement of one nucleotide in a DNA sequence by another nucleotide or replacement of one

amino acid in a protein by another amino acid.

- **subtelomeric fish screen**
  Uses DNA probes that are specific for the subtelomeric areas on the long arm and short arm of each chromosome, allowing for the detection of cryptic and submicroscopic subtelomeric deletions and translocations, a significant cause of moderate to severe mental retardation.

- **subtelomeric region**
  The chromosomal region just proximal to the telomere (end of the chromosome) composed of highly polymorphic repetitive DNA sequences that are typically situated adjacent to gene-rich areas. Microdeletions and subtle rearrangements that disrupt genes in the subtelomeric regions can cause mental retardation; use of fluorescent in situ hybridization (FISH) to evaluate subtelomeric regions is usually required for detection of these abnormalities.

- **subvital gene**
  A gene that causes the death of some proportion (but not all) of the individuals that express it.

- **sulciform**
  A groove, especially of the brain.

- **sum rule**
  The probability that one or the other of two mutually exclusive events will occur is the sum of their individual probabilities. The rule that states that the probability of the occurrence of mutually exclusive events is the sum of the probabilities of the individual events.

- **supercoil**
  A closed double-stranded DNA molecule that is twisted on itself; Negative (tending to unwind the helix) or positive (tending to wind the helix) coiling of double-stranded DNA that differs from the relaxed state.

- **supergene**
  Several loci, which usually control related aspects of the phenotype, in close physical association.

- **superinfection**
  Phage infection of a cell that already harbours a prophage.

- **supernatant**
  Supernatant is the remaining solution suspended with the remaining components that is left behind after a mixture is centrifuged, such as in subcellular fractionation, or precipitated. The concentrated material left at the bottom of the centrifuged supernatant is known as a pellet.

- **supernumary chromosome**
  A small chromosome containing a centromere occasionally seen in tissue culture, often in a mosaic state (present in some cells but not in others). A marker chromosome may be of little clinical significance or, if it contains material from one or both arms of another chromosome, may

create an imbalance for whatever genes are present; assessment to establish the clinical significance, particularly if found in a fetal karyotype, is often difficult.

- **supersuppressor**

A mutation that can suppress a variety of other mutations; typically a nonsense suppressor.

- **supportive care**

Treatment given to prevent, control, or relieve complications and side effects and to improve the patient's comfort and quality of life.

- **suppressive petite**

A petite that in a cross with wild-type produces progeny of which variable non-Mendelian proportions are petite.

- **suppressor gene**

A gene that can suppress the action of another gene, A gene that, when mutated, apparently restores the wild-type phenotype to a mutation at another locus.

- **suppressor mutation**

A mutation that counteracts the effects of another mutation. A suppressor maps at a different site than the mutation it counteracts, either within the same gene or at a more distant locus. Different suppressors act in different ways.

- **supraglottis**

The upper part of the larynx, including the epiglottis; the area above the vocal cords.

- **supravalvar**

Above aortic or pulmonary valve.

- **surfactant**

A substance lining the air sacs in the lungs which enhances expansion of the lungs during inspiration.

- **survival of the fittest**

In evolutionary theory the survival of only those organisms best able (fittest) to obtain and utilize resources. This phenomenon is the cornerstone of Darwin's theory of evolution by natural selection.

- **susceptibility gene**

A gene mutation that increases the likelihood that an individual will develop a certain disease or disorder. When such a mutation is inherited, development of symptoms is more likely but not certain.

- **suture**

The process of joining two surfaces by stitching; or, the surgical stitch itself, A form of fibrous joint as binds the parts of the skull, or a sewing to unite two surfaces.

- **svedberg unit**

A unit of sedimentation rate during centrifugation. Abbr. is S as in 50S.

- **sympatric speciation**

Speciation in which the evolution of reproductive isolating

mechanisms occurs within the range and habitat of the parent species. This form of speciation may be common in parasites.

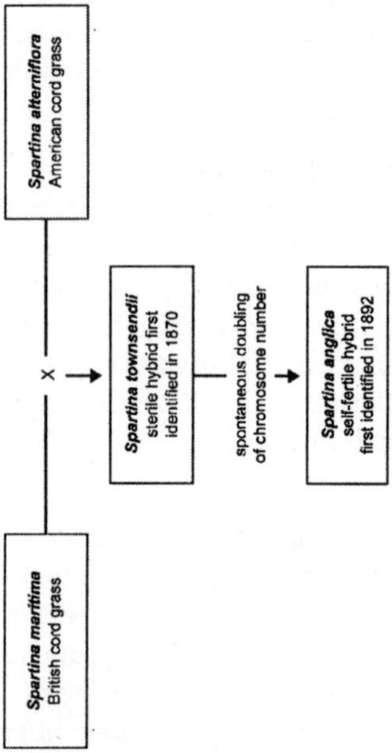


- **symphysis pubis**
  A cartilaginous joint between two pubic joints.

- **symptom**
  A sign of disease. A feeling or other subjective complaint suggestive of a medical condition. (Having to urinate often is a symptom of diabetes.).

- **symptomatic**
  The patient is experiencing symptoms.

- **synapse**
  The junction of two nerve cells (neurons).

- **synapsis**
  The point-by-point pairing of homologous chromosomes during zygotene or in certain Dipteran tissues (eg Drosophila salivary glands) that undergo endomitosis. Close pairing of homologs at meiosis.

- **synaptonemal complex**
  A proteinaceous complex that apparently mediates synapsis during zygotene stage and then disintegrates. A complex structure that unites homologous chromosomes during the prophase of meiosis.

- **syncytial blastoderm**
  In insects, the syncytial stage of blastoderm preceding the formation of cell membranes around the individual nuclei of the early embryo.

- **syncytium**
  A single cell with many nuclei.

- **syndactyly**
  A webbing or fusion of adjacent fingers or toes, usually between the 3rd and 4th fingers and the 2nd and 3rd toes.

- **syndrome**
  The group or recognizable pattern of symptoms or abnormalities that indicate a particular trait or disease, Group of symptoms or features occurring together often enough to constitute a disorder to which a particular name is given.

- **syngeneic**
  Genetically identical members of the same species.

- **synophrys**
  Hypertrophy (general increase in bulk) and fusion (joining) of the eyebrows in the midline.

- **synostosis**
  Knitting together of bony material where normally the bones would be separate.

- **synovial fluid**
  The fluid found in a joint.

- **synteny**
  Genes occurring in the same order on chromosomes of different species; All loci on one chromosome are said to be syntenic (literally on the same ribbon). Loci may appear to be unlinked by conventional genetic tests for linkage but still be syntenic.

- **synteny test**
  A test that determines whether two loci belong to the same linkage group (ie are syntenic) by observing concordance (occurence of markers together) in hybrid cell lines.

- **syrinx**
  A fluid-filled sac, like a cyst, but occurring inside the spinal cord where it has the shape of an elongated tube lying inside the spinal cord and the bony spinal column.

- **systemic**
  Pertaining to a whole body. A word used to describe conditions that affect the entire body rather than one of its parts. Diabetes is a systemic disease because it involves many parts of the body such as the pancreas, eyes, kidneys, heart, and nerves.; Relating to a whole system or group of organs

- **systemic treatment**
  Treatment that reaches cells all over the body by traveling through the bloodstream.

- **t cell**
  A type of white blood cell (lymphocyte) that is part of the body's immune system.

- **tachycardia**
  Abnormally rapid heart rate (more than 100 beats per minute).

- **tactaac box**
  A consensus sequence surrounding the lariat branch point of eukaryotic pre-mRNA introns and used during splicing.

- **tandem duplication**
  Adjacent identical chromosome segments.

- **tandem repeat sequences**
  Multiple copies of the same base sequence on a chromosome; used as markers in physical mapping.

- **target theory**

A theory that predicts response curves based on the number of events required to cause the phenomenon. Used to determine whether point mutations are single events.

- **targeted gene knockout**

The introduction of a null mutation in a gene by a designed alteration in a cloned DNA sequence that is then introduced into the genome by homologous recombination and replacement of the normal allele.

- **targeted mutagenesis**

Deliberate change in the genetic structure directed at a specific site on the chromosome. Used in research to determine the targeted region's function.

- **targeted mutation analysis (synonym mutation analysis)**

Testing for the presence of a specific mutation (e.g., Glu6Val for sickle cell anemia), a specific type of mutation (e.g., the trinucleotide repeat expansion associated with spinocerebellar ataxia type 1, deletions associated with Duchenne muscular dystropy), or set of mutations (e.g., a panel of mutations for cystic fibrosis), as opposed to complete gene sequencing or mutation scanning, which detect most mutations in the tested region.

- **tata box**

A DNA sequence (concensus TATAAA) at about minus 25 (ie. 25 nucleotides upstream of the transcription start site) in the promoter region of many eukaryotic genes involved in binding RNA polymerase via a TATA binding protein. Analogous to the Pribnow box in prokaryotes.

- **tautomeric shift**

The spontaneous isomerization of a nitrogen base to an alternative hydrogen-bonding form, possibly resulting in a mutation. Reversible shifts of proton position in a molecule. Bases in nucleic acids shift between keto and enol forms or between amino and imino forms.

- **tay-sachs**

An incurable recessive genetic disorder that usually develops within the first year of a child's life, causing the build-up of fat deposits in the brain. Children born with Tay-Sachs die before the age of ten.

- **tay-sachs disease**

An inherited disease of infancy characterized by profound mental retardation and early death; it is caused by a recessive gene mutation; a fatal degenerative disease of the nervous system due to a deficiency of hexosamidase A, causing mental deficiency, paralysis, mental deterioration, and blindness; found primarily but not exclusively among Ashkenazi Jews. Autosomal recessive.

- **t-cell receptor**
  Surface protein of T lymphocyte cells that allow the T cells to recognize infected host cells.

- **t-dna**
  A portion of the Ti plasmid that is inserted into the genome of the host plant cell.

- **technology transfer**
  The process of transferring scientific findings from research laboratories to the commercial sector.

- **telangiectasia**
  A condition of dilated capillary blood vessels, often multiple in character and forming simple tumours composed of blood.

- **telecanthus**
  Wide-set eyelid openings, may be synonymous with hypertelorism.

- **telecanthus**
  Wide-set eye openings (may be synonymous with hypertelorism). Increased distance between the inner corners of the eyes.

- **telocentric chromosome**
  A chromosome whose centromere lies at one end.

- **telomerase**
  The enzyme that directs the replication of telomeres. An enzyme that adds telomeric sequences to the ends of eukaryotic chromosomes. No template is necessary.

- **telomere**
  The end of a chromosome. This specialized structure is involved in the replication and stability of linear DNA molecules. The segment at the end of each chromosome arm which consists of a series of repeated DNA sequences that regulate chromosomal replication at each cell division. Some of the telomere is lost each time a cell divides, and eventually, when the telomere is gone, the cell dies.

- **telomere maps**
  Telomeres are the tips of the chromosomes. They are crucial in maintaining the chromosomes' stability and are important in the cell cycle and ageing. Because of the way the physical maps are constructed, many telomeres of chromosomes are left out.

- **telophase**
  The terminal stage of mitosis or meiosis in which chromosomes uncoil; the spindle breaks down; and cytokinesis usually occurs. The late stage of nuclear division when daughter nuclei re-form.

- **temperate phage**
  A phage that can enter into lysogeny with its host. A phage that can become a prophage.

- **temperature**
  The temperature is the specific degree of hotness or coldness of the body. It is usually measured with a thermometer.

- **temperature-sensitive mutant**
  An organism that has a wild-type phenotype at a permissive temperature but a mutant phenotype at a restrictive (non-permissive) temperature.

- **template**
  (1) A pattern serving as a mechanical guide. (2) In DNA replication each strand of the duplex acts as a template for the synthesis of a new double helix. (3) A molecular mold that shapes the structure or sequence of another molecule. For example, the nucleotide sequence of DNA acts as a template to control the nucleotide sequence of RNA during transcription.

- **temporal**
  Relating to the temporal or temple region of the head.

- **temporomandibular joint**
  The joint between the lower jaw and the temporal bone of the skull.

- **tempral lobes**
  Areas located on each side of the brain that are important in processing memory information as well as hearing and some language function.

- **tendon**
  A tough, inelastic connective tissue that joins muscle to another structure, usually bone. When a tendon becomes inflamed, the condition is referred to as tendinitis or tendonitis.

- **teratogen**
  An agent capable of causing congenital malformation(s), (e.g., environmental agents, recreational drugs, medications, infectious diseases, etc.); Any agent that may cause a change in the form (ie. birth defect) or function (ie. mental retardation) when the fetus is exposed during pregnancy.

- **teratogenic**
  Substances such as chemicals or radiation that cause abnormal development of a embryo.

- **terminator sequence**
  A sequence in DNA that signals termination of transcription to RNA polymerase.

- **tertiary structure**
  The further folding of a protein bringing alpha-helices and beta-sheets into three-dimensional arrangements. The folding or coiling of the secondary structure to form a three-dimensional molecule.

- **test-cross**
  The crossing of an organism, with an unkown genotype, to a homozygous recessive organism (tester). A cross between an individual of unknown genotype or a heterozygote (or a multiple

heterozygote) to a homozygous recessive individual.

- **tester**

An individual homozygous for one or more recessive alleles and used in a test-cross.

- **testes**

The testicles (singular testicle), are the male generative glands in animals. Male mammals have two testicles, which are often contained within an extension of the abdomen called the scrotum.

- **testicular feminization syndrome**

A human condition, inherited as an X-linked recessive, caused by a mutation in a gene coding for the androgen (testosterone) receptor, in which genetical (XY) males develop female secondary sexual characters.

- **testing of hypotheses**

The determination of whether to accept or reject a proposed hypothesis based on the likelihood of the experimental results.

- **testis-determining factor (tdf)**

General term for the gene determining maleness in human beings (Tdf in mice).

- **tetrad**

(1) Four homologous chromatids in a bundle in the first meiotic prophase and metaphase. The meiotic configuration of four chromatids first seen in pachytene. There is one tetrad per pair (bivalent) of homologous chromosomes. (2) The four haploid product cells from a single meiosis.

- **tetrad analysis**

The use of tetrads (definition 2) to study the segregation of chromosomes and genes during meiosis.

- **tetraparental mouse**

A mouse that develops from an embryo created by the experimental fusion of two separate embryos (blastulas) from matings of different parents.

- **tetraplegia**

Paralysis of all four limbs.

- **tetraploid**

(1) A cell having four chromosome sets. (2) an organism composed of such cells.

- **tetratype (t)**

A tetrad containing four different genotypes, two parental and two recombinant. A spore arrangement in Ascomycetes that consists of two parental and two recombinant spores indicating a single crossover between two linked loci.

- **thalamus**

Part of the brain through which nearly all sensory input passes to the cerebral cortex.

- **thalassemia**

Inherited anemias (includes alpha thalassemia, beta thalassemia, etc.) found predominantly among people of Mediterranean descent.

- **thermocycler**
A device with an incubation well whose temperature can be programmed to change very rapidly, accurately, and in repetitive cycles. An incubation well is a metal block into which special sample tubes fit perfectly.

- **theta structure**
An intermediate structure formed during the replication of a circular DNA molecule.

- **thorax**
The portion of the anatomy below the neck and above the diaphragm; the chest.

- **three-point cross**
A cross involving three loci.

- **three-point testcross**
A testcross involving one parent with three heterozygous gene pairs and another (tester) with three homozygous recessive gene pairs.

- **thrombocytopeniz**
Condition in which there is an abnormally small number of platelets in the blood.

- **thrush**
An infection of the mouth. Patches of whitish-colored skin in the mouth are signs of this disease.

- **thymidine**
The nucleoside having thymine as its base.

- **thymine**
One of the four bases that make up the letters ATGC in DNA. Thymine ("T") always pairs with adenine ("A"); A base; one of the molecular components of DNA and RNA. Always bonds with adenine (T-A).

- **thymine dimer**
A pair of abnormally chemically bonded adjacent thymine bases in DNA, resulting from damage by ultra-violet irradiation. The cellular processes that repair this lesion often make errors that create mutations.

- **thyroid gland**
Endocrine gland in the neck that produces thyroxine and calcitonin, hormones involved in the regulation of growth and metabolic rate.

- **ti plasmid**
A circular plasmid of Agrobacterium tumefaciens that enables the bacterium to infect plant cells and produce a tumour (crown gall tumour).

- **tibia**
The larger of the two bones in the lower leg; the shin bone.

- **tibialis anterior muscle**
A shin muscle which pulls up the great toe.

- **tic**
An involuntary muscular contraction; a twitch or movement.

- **tinnitus**
  A ringing in one or both ears. It may also be a roaring or hissing sound.

- **tissue**
  A group or layer of cells that together perform a specific function.

- **titubation**
  The appearance of staggering or stumble.

- **tonic**
  The phase of a grand mal seizure that is marked by prolonged muscular contraction (rigidity).

- **topical**
  Pertaining to the surface of the body.

- **topoisomer**
  Topological form of DNA with the same sequence as another but differing in linking number (supercoiling).

- **topoisomerase**
  Enzymes of two types that can remove (or create) supercoiling in duplex DNA by creating transitory breaks in one (type I) or both (type II) strands of the sugar-phosphate backbone.

- **totipotency**
  The ability of a cell to proceed through all the stages of development and thus produce a normal adult.

- **totipotent**
  The state of a cell that can give rise to any and all adult cell types as compared with a differentiated cell whose fate is determined.

- **toxic**
  Harmful; having to do with poison.

- **toxicogenomics**
  The study of how genomes respond to environmental stressors or toxicants. Combines genome-wide mRNA expression profiling with protein expression patterns using bioinformatics to understand the role of gene-environment interactions in disease and dysfunction; The science of how a person's genome affects his or her response to potentially toxic substances in the environment, such as pollutants.A goal of research in toxico-genomics is to identify the genes that predispose some people to become sick when they encounter toxins in their daily lives.

- **toxin**
  A poisonous substance.

- **trachea**
  The windpipe, which leads from the back of the throat to the lungs. Trachea is a common biological term for an airway through which respiratory air transport takes place in organisms.

- **tracheoesophageal fistula**
  An abnormal connection between the windpipe and upper digestive tract.

- **tracheostomy**
  Surgery to create an opening (stoma) into the windpipe. The opening itself may also be called a tracheostomy.

- **tracheostomy button**
  A 1/2- to 1-1/2-inch-long plastic tube placed in the stoma to keep it open.

- **tracheostomy tube**
  A 2- to 3-inch metal or plastic tube that keeps the stoma and trachea open. Also called a trach ("trake") tube.

- **tracheotomy**
  Surgical opening into the windpipe to provide an artificial airway.

- **trait**
  A physical characteristic, such as red hair, that has a genetic component.

- **trans**
  Meaning across and referring usually to the geometric configuration of two mutant alleles (ab) across from each other on a pair of homologous chromosomes (Ab/aB).

- **trans configuration (synonym repulsion)**
  Term which indicates that an individual who is heterozygous at two neighboring loci has the two mutations in question on each of the two homologous chromosomes.

- **trans conformation**
  In a heterozygote involving two mutant sites (ab) within a gene or gene cluster, the arrangement, Ab/aB.

- **trans-acting**
  Referring to mutations of, for example a repressor gene, that act through a diffusable protein product and can therefore act at a distance not simply on the DNA molecule in which they occur.

- **transcript map**
  A genetic map in which expressed sequences, e.g., mRNAs, mRNA transcripts, corresponding to genes are mapped; a functional blueprint of the genome, In only a year or two, most human genes will be sequence- tagged and placed on various physical maps. Such a 'transcript map' (or 'expression map') of the genome will be an important part of the sequencing infrastructure, as well as a critical resource for the positional candidate approach to gene cloning. One of the specific goals of the US Human Genome Project is the construction of a high resolution STS map of the genome. One of the early problems with gene- based STSs was that there simply were not

enough unique human gene sequences to bother with. But all of that changed with the advent of EST sequencing, at which time several groups began mapping ESTs albeit on a limited scale and only to the resolution of a chromosome assignment.

- **transcription**

The synthesis of an RNA copy from a sequence of DNA (a gene); the first step in gene expression; The process of copying information from DNA into new strands of messenger RNA (mRNA). The mRNA then carries this information to the cytoplasm, where it serves as the blueprint for the manufacture of a specific protein; The process by which DNA passes genetic information to RNA. Transcription is the first step in producing proteins; The formation of an RNA molecule from a DNA template through complementary base pairing reactions. Transcription occurs in the nucleus.

- **transcription factor (synonym zinc finger protein)**

A protein that aids in the activation and regulation of transcription, in which messenger RNA is synthesized from the DNA template; zinc finger proteins are one type of transcription factor; A protein that binds to a cis-regulatory element (eg. an enhancer, a TATA box) and thereby, directly or indirectly, affects the initiation of transcription. Eukaryotic proteins that aid RNA polymerase to recognize promoters. Analogous to prokaryotic sigma factors.

- **transcriptome**

The full complement of activated genes, mRNAs, or transcripts in a particular tissue at a particular time

- **transcriptome maps**

Consist of "expression clusters" of co-regulated genes. Challenges ahead for computational biology include the integration of clusters obtained for the transcriptome, the interactome, the phenome, and the localizome.

- **transducing particle**

A defective phage carrying part of the host genome in place of part of the phage genome.

- **transduction**

The transfer of bacterial genetic material from one bacterium to another using a phage as a vector; The movement of genes from a bacterial donor to a bacterial recipient using a phage as the vector. A process whereby a cell can gain access to and incorporate foreign DNA brought in by a viral particle.

- **transfection**

The introduction of foreign DNA into a host cell; The process by which exogenous DNA in solution is introduced into cells. The introduction of foreign DNA into eukaryotic or prokaryotic cells.

- **transfer operon (tra)**
  Operon containing genes that produce the male (F-pili producing) bacterial phenotype. The F+(plus) cell (male cell) can transfer the fertility factor (F plasmid) to an F-(minus) (female) cell.

- **transfer rna (trna)**
  A class of RNA having structures with triplet nucleotide sequences that are complementary to the triplet nucleotide coding sequences of mRNA.

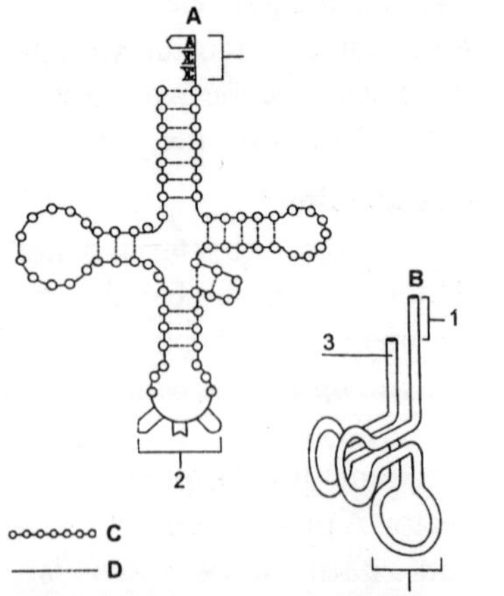


A Cloverleaf model of tyrosine transfer RNA (tRNA)
B Three dimensional representation of tRNA
C Nucleotide chain
D Hydrogen bond

1 Amino acid binding site
2 Anticodon (mRNA) binding site)
3 Nucleotide chain

The role of tRNAs in protein synthesis is to bond with amino acids and transfer them to the ribosomes, where proteins are assembled according to the genetic code carried by mRNA.

- **transform**
  (1) In microbiology and genetics the modification of one genotype by the external application of DNA from a cell of another genotype. (2)In oncology (the study of cancer formation) the conversion of a normal cell into a cancerous one by mutation or transfection.

- **transformation**

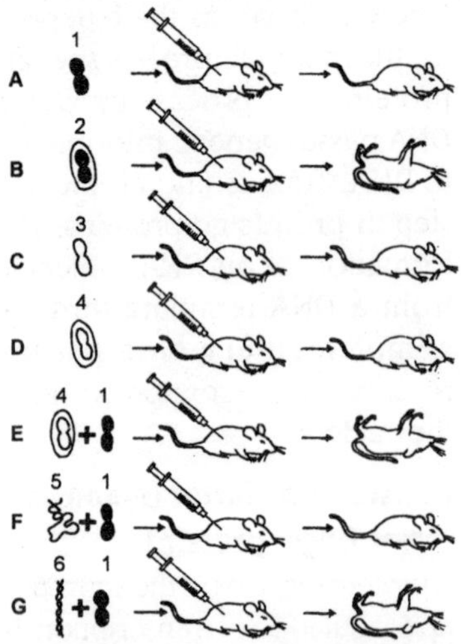


Genetic transformation of pneumonia bacteria. The dead mice (B, E, G) had living S-type pneumococcus in the bloodstream.
A - E Experiments of Griffiths, 1928
F & G Experiments of Avery etal 1944

1 Rough (R-type) non-virulent Pneumococcus
2 Smooth (S-type) virulent Pneumococcus
3 Heat-killed R-type Pneumococcus
4 Heat-killed S-type pneumococcus
5 Protein from S-type Pneumococcus
6 DNA from S-type Pneumococcus

A process by which the genetic material carried by an individual cell is altered by incorporation of exogenous DNA into its genome. (1) The modification of a genome by the external application of DNA from a cell of different genotype. (2) Conversion of normal eukaryotic cells to a cancer-like state of uncontrolled division.

- **transformer**
  An allele in fruit flies (Drosophila) that converts chromosomal females into sterile males.

- **transforming retrovirus**
  A retrovirus carrying an additional DNA sequence (often an oncogene) that confers the ability to transform infected cells to malignant phenotype.

- **transfusion**
  Delivery of blood or a blood component into the bloodstream.

- **transgene**
  A foreign gene; typically, a gene produced by recombinant DNA techniques.

- **transgenic**
  An experimentally produced organism in which DNA has been artificially introduced and incorporated into the organism's germ line.

- **transgenic organism**
  one into which a cloned genetic material has been experimentally transferred, a subset of these foreign gene express themselves in their offspring. Turner syndrome a chromosomal condition in females (usually 45,XO) due to monosomy of the X- chromosome; characterized by short stature, failure to develop secondary sex characteristics, and infertility.

- **transient diploid**
  The stage of the life cycle of predominantly haploid fungi (and algae) during which meiosis occurs.

- **transition**
  A type of nucleotide-pair substitution involving the replacement of a purine with another purine, or of a pyrimidine with another pyrimidine for example GC with AT.

- **transition mutation**
  A mutation in which a purine/ pyrimidine base pair is replaced with a base pair in the same purine/pyrimidine relationship eg. GC with AT.

- **translation**
  The process of turning instructions from mRNA, base by base, into chains of amino acids that then fold into proteins. This process takes place in the cytoplasm, on structures called ribosomes, The process in which a genetic code carried by messenger RNA directs the synthesis of proteins from amino acids. Translocation occurs in the cytoplasm.

- **translocase (ef-g)**
  Elongation factor in prokaryotes necessary for proper translocation at the ribosome during the translation process.

- **translocation (synonym chromosome rearrangement)**
  A chromosome alteration in which a whole chromosome or segment of a chromosome becomes attached to or interchanged with another whole chromosome or segment, the resulting hybrid segregating together at meiosis; balanced translocations (in which there is no net loss or gain of chromosome material) are usually not associated with phenotypic abnormalities, although gene disruptions at the breakpoints of the translocation can, in some cases, cause adverse effects, including some known genetic disorders; unbalanced translocations (in which there is loss or gain of chromosome material) nearly always yield an abnormal phenotype. A rearrangement occurring when a piece of one chromosome is broken off and joined to another chromosome. An individual with a balanced translocation has the normal amount of chromosomal material. A person with an unbalanced translocation will have a loss or gain of chromosomal material.

- **translucent**
  Partially transparent, allowing some light to pass through.

- **transmembrane receptor**
  A protein that spans the plasma membrane of a cell, with the extracellular domain of the protein having the ability to bind to a ligand and the intracellular domain having an activity (such as a protein kinase) that can be altered (either increased or decreased) upon ligand binding.

- **transmission genetics**
  The study of the mechanisms involved in the passage of genes from one generation to the next.

- **transplantation**
  The surgical transfer of an organ or tissue from one position (or person) to another.

- **transposable element**
  A class of DNA sequences that can move from one chromosomal site to another.

- **transposable genetic element**
  A general term for any genetic unit that can insert into a chromosome, exit, and relocate; includes insertion sequences, transposons, some bacterio-phages, and controlling element. A region of the genome, flanked by inverted repeats, a copy of which can be inserted at another place; also called a transposon or a jumping gene.

- **transposon**
A mobile piece of DNA that is flanked by terminal repeat sequences and typically bears genes coding for transposition functions.

- **transverse colon**
The part of the large bowel between the ascending and descending colon, lying in the upper abdomen.

- **transversion**
A type of nucleotide-pair substitution involving the replacement of a purine with a pyrimidine, or vice versa for example GC with TA, A mutation in which purine is substituted for pyrimidine or vice versa.

- **transversion mutation**
A mutation in which a purine/ pyrimidine replaces a pyrimidine/ purine base pair or vice versa eg. GC with TA.

- **trauma**
Injury or damage, A wound, hurt, or injury to the body. Trauma can also be mental such as when a person feels great stress.

- **tremor**
Involuntary trembling.

- **tremor**
Repetative, often irregular oscillatory (back & forth) movements caused by alternating, or synchronous but irregular, contractions of opposing muscle groups.

- **triceps**
Muscle in the upper arm that extends the forearm.

- **tricuspid valve**
Heart valve between the right atrium and the right ventricle.

- **trigeminal nerve**
The nerve that delivers sensory stimuli to the brain from the face, teeth and tongue.

- **trihybrid**
An organism heterozygous at three loci.

- **trimester**
A term used to define a period of three months. In pregnancy, the first trimester is 1-12 weeks; the second trimester is 13-26 weeks, and the third or last trimester is 27- delivery.

- **trinucleotide repeat**
Sequences of three nucleotides repeated a number of times in tandem within a gene.. Normal polymorphic variation in repeat number with no clinical significance commonly occurs between individuals. Abnormally large alleles are classified in increasing order of size as mutable normal alleles, reduced penetrance alleles, and full penetrance alleles, respectively.

- **trinucleotide repeat testing**
Quantification of the number of trinucleotide repeats (sets of three nucleotides of identical sequence) in a segment of DNA.

- **triphalangeal thumb**
  The presence of three phalanges (bones in the fingers or toes) in the thumb, normally composed of only two.

- **triple screen te**
  Also referred to as a "Multiple Markers Screen". A prenatal diagnostic test for fetal abnormalities performed between the 16th and 18th week of pregnancy. The test measures the levels of three substances circulating in the mother's blood: alpha-fetoprotein (AFP), human chorionic gonadotrophin (hCG) and unconjugated oestriol (uE3). Changes in the levels of these three substances are associated with the presence of Down syndrome or other fetal disorders.

- **triplegia**
  Paralysis that involves three appendages, usually both legs and one arm.

- **triplet**
  The three nucleotide pairs that compose a codon; A sequence of 3 nucleotides comprising a codon of a nucleic acid and representing the code for an amino acid (triplet code, codon).

- **triplet code**
  A code in which a given amino acid is specified by a set of three nucleotides.

- **triplet repeat**
  A unit of three DNA bases (e.g., CAG, CTG, CGG) that is present in multiple copies, scattered throughout the genome. A number of neurogenetic conditions have been ascribed to expansion of triplet repeat size.

- **triploid**
  A cell having three chromosome sets, or an organism composed of such cells.

- **trisomic**
  A diploid cell with an extra chromosome. Basically a diploid with an extra chromosome of one type, producing a chromosome number of the form 2n + 1.

- **trisomy**
  Possessing three copies of a particular chromosome instead of the normal two copies; The presence of a single extra chromosome, yielding a total of three chromosomes of that particular type instead of a pair. Partial trisomy refers to the presence of an extra copy of a segment of a chromosome.

- **trisomy 13**
  Caused by an extra copy of chromosome 13, which results in multiple internal and external physical defects and severe mental retardation.

- **trisomy 18**
  A congenital disease caused by an extra copy of chromosome 18. Infants with trisomy 18 rarely survive past six months of age due

to multiple internal and external physical defects.

- **trisomy rescue**
The phenomenon in which a fertilized ovum initially contains 47 chromosomes (i.e., is trisomic), but loses one of the trisomic chromosomes in the process of cell division such that the resulting daughter cells and their descendants contain 46 chromosomes, the normal number.

- **tritium**
A radioactive isotope of hydrogen.

- **trna (transfer rna)**
Transfer RNA. Small RNA molecules that carry amino acids to the ribosome for polymerization into a polypeptide. During translation the amino acid is inserted into the growing polypeptide chain when the anticodon of the tRNA pairs with a codon on the mRNA being translated.

- **truncal obesity**
Fat deposited in the thorax and abdomen, instead of the hips and thighs.

- **truncation selection**
A breeding technique in which individuals in whom quantitative expression of a phenotype is above or below a certain value (the truncation point) are selected as parents for the next generation.

- **truss**
A device used to hold a hernia or organ in position.

- **tubular**
Resembling a tube.

- **tubule**
A small tube or canal, especially in the kidneys.

- **tumor**
A mass of excess tissue. An abnormal growth that is solid and may be benign or malignant.

- **tumor-suppresser gene**
A gene thought to suppress formation of tumors; loss of suppression leads to malignant transformation. P53 is an example of a tumor-suppresser gene, Genes that normally restrain cell growth but, when missing or inactivated by mutation, allow cells to grow uncontrolled.

- **tumour**
Abnormal growth of tissue, literally means a swelling.

- **tumour suppressor gene**
A gene encoding a protein that suppresses tumour formation. A gene that normally prevents unlimited cell division. When both copies of the gene are lost or mutated the cell is transformed to a cancer phenotype. Examples are the P53, retinoblastoma and Wilm's tumour.

- **tumour virus**
A virus that is capable of inducing a cancer.

- **turner syndrome**
  A congenital condition in females designated by a 45,X genotype. Turner syndrome is a genetic abnormality caused by the complete or partial absence of one of the two X sex chromosomes found. An abnormal human female phenotype produced by the presence of only one X chromosome (XO).

- **twin spot**
  A pair of mutant sectors within wild-type tissue, produced by a mitotic crossover in an individual of appropriate heterozygous genotype.

- **two-point cross**
  A cross involving two loci.

- **two-strand double crossover**
  A double crossover that involves only two of the four chromatids of a tetrad.

- **tympanoplasty**
  Repair or reconstruction of a damaged eardrum.

- **type i diabetes mellitus**
  See: Insulin-dependent diabetes mellitus.

- **type i error**
  In statistics the rejection of a true hypothesis.

- **typological thinking**
  The concept that organisms of a species conform to a specific norm. In this view variation is considered abnormal.

- **tyrosyluria**
  Enhanced urinary excretion of certain metabolites or tyrosine.

- **ulcer**
  A break in the skin; a deep sore. People with diabetes may get ulcers from minor scrapes on the feet or legs, from cuts that heal slowly, or from the rubbing of shoes that do not fit well. Ulcers can become infected.

- **ulna**
  Larger of the two bones in the forearm.

- **ultralente insulin**
  A type of insulin that is long acting.

- **ultrasound**
  A diagnostic procedure that projects high-frequency sound waves into the body and changes the echoes into pictures (sonograms) shown on a monitor. Different types of tissue reflect sound waves differently. This makes it possible to find abnormal growths, A non-invasive diagnostic technique which provides pictures of organs and structures inside the body. It works like the sonar used by submarines, bouncing sound waves off an object and using a computer to interpret the sound returned. The interpretation of an ultrasound is very dependent upon body structure, the amount of body fat and the skill of the operator. The test is used to monitor a baby's

growth and development during pregnancy and to identify any physical abnormalities.

- **ultraviolet radiation**
Invisible rays that are part of the energy that comes from the sun. Ultraviolet radiation can burn the skin and cause skin cancer. It is made up of two types of rays, UVA and UVB. UVB rays are more likely than UVA rays to cause sunburn, but UVA rays pass further into the skin. Scientists have long thought that UVB radiation can cause melamona and other types of skin cancer. They now think that UVA radiation also may add to skin damage that can lead to cancer. For this reason, skin specialists recommend that people use sunscreens that block both kinds of radiation.

- **umbilical artery**
One of (normally) two high-pressure, narrow-calibre, blood vessels carrying oxygen-poor blood from the fetus to the placenta, and accompanying a single umbilical vein.

- **umbilical cord**
The fibrous cord-like structure containing two arteries and a vein and connecting the fetus to the placenta. Oxygen and nutrients from the mother's circulation pass through the umbilical cord to the fetus.

- **umbilical hernia**
A bulge caused by stretched tissue around the umbilicus.

- **umbilicus**
The scar formed at the site of attachment of the umbilical cord to the fetus; the navel.

- **unaffected**
An individual who does not manifest any symptoms of a particular condition

- **underdominance**
A condition in which the phenotypic expression of the heterozygote is less than that of either homozygote.

- **undescended testicle**
Failure of a testicle to enter the scrotum.

- **unequal crossing over**
Mispairing and exchange of DNA between genetically similar, nonhomologous chromosome regions that results in duplication or deletion of DNA in each daughter cell; Crossing over between similar DNA sequences that are misaligned, resulting in sequences with deletion or duplication of DNA segments. A cause of a number of genetic variants, e.g., -thalassemia and Lepore hemoglobin.

- **unequal crossover**
A crossover between homologs that are not perfectly aligned.

- **unilateral**
Involving one side only.

- **uninemic chromosome**
A chromosome consisting of one double helix of DNA.

- **uniparent disomy**
A pair of homologous chromosomes inherited from one parent with no contribution from the other parent.

- **uniparental disomy (synonym upd)**
The situation in which both members of a chromosome pair or segments of a chromosome pair are inherited from one parent and neither is inherited from the other parent; uniparental disomy can result in an abnormal phenotype in some cases.

- **uniparental disomy study (synonym UPD analysis, UPD study)**
Testing used to identify if specific chromosomes or chromosomal segments are maternally or paternally derived; can aid in confirming the clinical diagnosis of certain disorders for which UPD is a possible underlying etiology.

- **uniparental inheritance**
The transmission of certain phenotypes from one parental type to all the progeny; such inheritance is generally produced by organelle (mitochondria, chloroplast) genes.

- **unique dna**
A length of DNA with no repetitive DNA sequences.

- **unmixed codon family**
Group of four codons sharing their first two bases and coding for the same amino acid.

- **unproven methods**
Treatments that use substances or methods of treating disease that have not been shown effective by accepted scientific methods.

- **unstable diabetes**
A type of diabetes when a person's blood glucose (sugar) level often swings quickly from high to low and from low to high. Also called "brittle diabetes" or "labile diabetes.

- **unstable mutation**
A mutation that has a high frequency of reversion; a mutation caused by the insertion of a controlling element, whose subsequent exit produces a reversion.

- **unusual bases**
Other bases in addition to the normal adenine; cytosine; guanine; and uracil. Found primarily in tRNAs and produced by post transcription modification of one of the normal bases.

- **upstream**
A convention on DNA related to the position and direction of transcription by RNA polymerase (5'>3'). Downstream (or 3' to) is in the direction of transcription whereas upstream (5' to) is in the direction from which the polymerase has come.

- **uracil**
A nitrogenous base normally found in RNA but not DNA; uraci

is capable of forming a base pair with adenine.

- **urea**
  One of the chief waste products of the body. When the body breaks down food, it uses what it needs and throws the rest away as waste. The kidneys flush the waste from the body in the form of urea, which is in the urine.

- **ureters**
  Long tubes, one leading from each kidney, which convey the urine to the bladder.

- **urethra**
  Hollow tube through which urine (and semen in men) is transported from the bladder to outside the body.

- **urethral stenosis**
  Narrowing of the anatomical tube which drains the urinary bladder.

- **urf**
  Unassigned reading frame. An open reading frame (ORF) whose function has not yet been determined.

- **uridine**
  The nucleoside having uracil as its base.

- **urinary**
  Referring to the urinary system which removes urine from the body (kidneys, bladder, and the connecting tubes).

- **urination**
  Act of voiding urine.

- **urine**
  Fluid waste produced in the kidneys, stored in the bladder, and released through the urethra.

- **urological**
  Concerned with the urinary system.

- **urologist**
  A doctor who sees men and women for treatment of the urinary tract and men for treatment of the genital organs.

- **uterus**
  Often called the womb, this is the organ in which a fetus develops. During pregnancy, the uterus expands. But when a woman is not pregnant, the uterus is small, hollow, and shaped like a flattened pear.

- **uvea**
  Layer of the eye beneath the sclera, consisting of the iris, ciliary body and choroid. The visible pigments in the eye are seen in the uvea.

- **uvula**
  The prominent anatomic structure dangling downward visibly at the back of the mouth (pharynx).

- **vagina**
  The passage (birth canal) connecting the female external genitalia with the uterus.

- **vaginal birth or delivery**
  Birth of a baby through the birth canal (vagina).

- **vagus nerve**

Nerve that serves the esophagus, larynx, stomach, intestines, lungs and heart.

- **valvular**

Relating to an anatomical valve, in this case a valve of the heart.

- **variable**

A property that may have different values in various cases.

- **variable expressivity**

Variation in clinical features (type and severity) of a genetic disorder between affected individuals, even within the same family, Refers to the variable severity of a genetic trait. Individuals with the same mutant gene with pleiotropic effects frequently show variable expressivity due to either environmental effects or effects of other genes modifying the expression of the mutant gene.

- **variable number of tandem repeat polymorphism (vntr)**

A series of allelic fragment lengths related to each other by a variable number of tandemly repeated DNA sequences, in an interval between two restriction enzyme sites. Because many allele sizes are possible, these loci are useful to distinguish between individuals, as in DNA fingerprinting.

- **variable number tandem repeats**

Linear arrangement of multiple copies of short repeated DNA sequences that vary in length and are highly polymorphic, making them useful as markers in linkage analysis.

- **variable region**

A region in an immunoglobin molecule that shows many sequence differences between antibodies of different specificities; the part of the antibody that binds to the antigen.

- **variable-number-of-tandem-repeats (vntr) locus**

Locus that is hypervariable because of tandemly repeated DNA sequences. Presumably variability is generated by unequal crossing over or slippage during replication. A chromosomal locus at which a particular repetitive sequence is present in different numbers in different individuals of a population or in the two different chromosome homologues in one diploid individual.

- **variance**

The average squared deviation about the mean of a set of data. A measure of the variation around the central class of a distribution; the average squared deviation of the observations from their mean value.

- **variant**

An individual organism that is recognizably different from an arbitrary standard type in that species.

- **variate**
  A specific numerical value of a variable.

- **variation**
  The differences among parents and their offspring or among individuals in a population.

- **varicose veins**
  Veins that are twisted and swollen just below the skin. Veins carry blood back to the heart.

- **variegation**
  The occurrence within a tissue of sectors or clones with differing phenotypes. Patchiness; a type of position effect that results when particular loci are contiguous with heterochromatin.

- **varus**
  Angulation of a bone towards the midline.

- **vas deferens**
  Duct that transports sperm from the testes to the ejaculatory duct.

- **vascular**
  The conducting tissues (phloem, xylem) of plants. Term applied to a plant tissue or region consisting of conductive tissue (phloem and xylem); also, to a pathogen that grows primarily in the conductive tissues of a plant, and in animals pertaining to or having many blood vessels.

- **vector**
  A "carrier." In gene therapy, for example, the method of carrying and inserting the desired gene into the target cell.

- **vein**
  Blood vessel that returns blood to the heart. a vein is a blood vessel which carries blood toward the heart. Veins form part of the circulatory system. The vessels that carry blood away from the heart are known as arteries.

- **venereal**
  Involving the genital organs.

- **ventilation**
  Exchange of air in and out of the lungs.

- **ventilator**
  A machine that assists or controls breathing; a respirator.

- **ventricle**
  A small cavity or chamber.

- **ventricular**
  Relating to the ventricle (a normal cavity), as in the heart or brain.

- **ventricular septal defect (vsd)**
  Congenital heart defect; hole in the wall between ventricles.

- **vermilion**
  Red part of the lip.

- **vermis**
  Worm-like structure; usually refers to the vermis of the cerebellum, which is part of the brain.

- **vernix caseosa**
  A slippery, white, fatty substance covering the skin of a fetus.

- **vertebra**
One of 33 bony segments that form the spinal column. There are 7 cervical, 12 thoracic, 5 lumbar, 5 sacral (fused into one sacrum bone) and 4 coccygeal (fused into one coccyx bone).

- **vertebral body**
The cylindrical expansion of the front of each bony ring (vertebra) of the spinal column.

- **verterbral artery**
One of a pair of arteries carrying oxygen-rich blood from the aorta, up the back of the neck, contributing to the Circle of Willis and supplying predominantly the back of the head and brain, including the cerebellum.

- **vertigo**
A sensation of dizziness or loss of balance, inability to walk a straight line, or "walking into walls".

- **vesicle**
A small sac containing liquid.

- **vestibular system**
Pertaining to the sensory system located in the inner ear that allows the body to maintain balance.

- **vestubular stimulation**
Activities that stimulate the structures of the inner ear that provide and maintain a sense of balance.

- **viability**
The probability that a fertilized egg will survive and develop into an adult organism.

- **viroid**
RNA molecule that is a plant pathogen.

- **virulent phage**
A phage that cannot become a prophage; infection by such a phage always leads to lysis of the host cell.

- **virus**
A noncellular biological entity that can reproduce only within a host cell. Viruses consist of nucleic acid covered by protein; some animal viruses are also surrounded by membrane. Inside the infected cell, the virus uses the synthetic capability of the host to produce progeny virus; A particle consisting of a nucleic acid (RNA or DNA) genome surrounded by a protein coat (capsid) and sometimes also a membrane, which can replicate only after infecting a host cell. A virus particle may exist free of its host cell but is incapable of replicating on its own.

- **viscera**
Internal body organs in the abdominal area, including the kidney, liver, pancreas, stomach, intestines, and adrenal glands.

- **visceral**
The internal organs, especially those located within the abdominal cavity.

- **visceral**
Pertaining to the internal body organs.

• **vital**
Necessary to maintain life. Breathing is a vital function.

• **vital signs**
Respiration, heart rate and body temperature.

• **vitiligo**
Nonpigmented white patches.

• **vitrectomy**
Removing the gel from the center of the eyeball because it has blood and scar tissue in it that blocks sight. An eye surgeon replaces the clouded gel with a clear fluid.

• **vitreous fluid**
A jellylike substance that fills most of the interior of the eye.

• **vitreous humor**
Gelatinous substance found within the eye.

• **v-j joining**
The joining of a variable (V) gene segment and a joining (J) gene segment in the first step of the formation of a functioning immunoglobulin gene.

• **vntr**
Variable number tandem repeats; any gene whose alleles contain different numbers of tandemly repeated oligonucleotide sequences.

• **vocal cords**
Two small bands of muscle within the larynx. They close to prevent food from getting into the lungs, and they vibrate to produce the voice.

• **void**
To empty the bladder in order to obtain a urine sample for testing.

• **vomit**
The ejection of contents of the stomach through the mouth; or, the material itself.

• **von hippel-lindau syndrome**
An autosomal dominant condition characterized by the anomalous growth and proliferation of blood vessels on the retina of the eye and the cerebellum of the brain; cysts and cancers in the kidneys, pancreas, and adrenal glands.

• **vsd (ventricular septal defect)**
Congenital heart defect; hole in the wall between ventricles.

• **vulva**
External genitalia of the female including the clitoris and labia.

• **wahlund effect**
A subdivided population contains fewer heterozygotes than predicted despite the fact that all subdivisions are in Hardy-Weinberg equilibrium.

• **webbing**
Congenital condition when adjacent structures (as fingers or toes) are joined by a broad band of tissue not normally present to such a degree.

• **western blot**
A technique used to identify and locate proteins based on their

ability to bind to specific antibodies; The separation of proteins on an electrophoretic gel for identification by immunological techniques. A technique for identifying specific antibodies or proteins in which proteins are separated by electrophoresis, transferred to nitrocellulose, and reacted with antibody.

- **western blotting**

  A technique for identifying a particular protein using antibodies after electrophoretic separation in a gel and transfer to a membrane.

- **western blotting analysis**

  A technique used to identify a specific protein; the probe is a radioactively labeled antibody raised against the protein in question.

- **wheezing**

  A whistling noise in the chest which occurs during breathing when the airways are compressed.

- **white blood cell count**

  Number of infection-fighting cells in a unit (conventionally 1 litre) of blood.

- **white blood cells**

  Any of a group of blood cells that have no hemoglobin and migrate into tissues to fight infection and digest cell debris. White blood cells (WBC) circulate in the blood and lymphatic system and harbor in the lymph glands and spleen. They are part of the immune system responsible for both directly (T cells and macrophages) and indirectly (B cells producing antibodies) attacking foreign invaders of the body.

- **white matter (of the brain)**

  Parts of the brain, notably the cortex (shell) of the cerebral hemispheres, composed of nerve cells "insulated" with a coating of myelin. White matter is one of the two main solid components of the central nervous system. It is composed of myelinated nerve cell processes, or axons, which connect various grey matter areas (the locations of nerve cell bodies) of the brain to each other and carry nerve impulses between neurons. Cerebral and spinal white matter do not contain dendrites, which can only be found in grey matter along with neural cell bodies and shorter axons.

- **whole genome clone- based maps**

  The International Human Genome Mapping Consortium describe how they constructed the first whole-genome physical map, how they created the templates from which the genome was sequenced and demonstrated how the map was essential for the accurate assembly of the human genome by the publicly funded effort.

- **widow's peak**

  Hairline which comes to a point in the center.

- **wild type**
  The genotype or phenotype that is found in nature or in the standard laboratory stock for a given organism. The phenotype of a particular organism when first seen in nature.

- **wild type allele**
  The normal, as opposed to the mutant, gene or allele

- **wilms' tumor**
  A kidney cancer (tumor) that occurs in children, usually before age 5.

- **wobble**
  The ability of certain bases at the third position of an anticodon in tRNA to form hydrogen bonds in various ways, causing alignment with several possible codons. Referring to the reduced constraint of the third base of an anticodon as compared with the other bases thus allowing additional complementary base pairings.

- **womb**
  The common term for uterus, a muscular organ inside which the baby grows during pregnancy.

- **x chromosome**
  A sex chromosome; normal females carry two X chromosomes.

- **x chromosome inactivation**
  In female mammalian embryos, the early random inactivation of the genes on one of the X chromosomes, leading to mosaicism for functions coded by heterozygous X-linked genes.

- **x hyperactivation**
  In Drosophila the process by which the structural genes of the male X chromosome are transcribed at the same rate as the two X chromosomes of the female combined.

- **x linkage**
  The inheritance pattern of genes found on the X chromosome but not on the Y.

- **x:a ratio**
  The ratio between the X chromosome and the number of sets of autosomes.

- **x-and-y linkage**
  The inheritance pattern of genes found on both the X and Y chromosomes (rare).

- **xanthomatosis**
  An accumulation of an excess of lipids in the body due to disturbance of lipid metabolism and marked by the formation of foam cells in skin lesions.

- **x-autosome translocation**
  The reciprocal translocation between the X chromosome and one of the autosomes.

- **x-chromosome inactivation**
  In females, the phenomenon by which one X chromosome (either maternally or paternally derived) is randomly inactivated in early

embryonic cells, with fixed inactivation in all descendant cells; first described by the geneticist Mary Lyon.

- **x-chromosome inactivation study**
  Molecular genetic testing to assess the relative proportion of methylated (inactive) X chromosomes to unmethylated (active) X chromosomes; used to determine if X-chromosome inactivation is random or skewed.

- **xenograft**
  Tissue or organs from an individual of one species transplanted into or grafted onto an organism of another species, genus, or family. A common example is the use of pig heart valves in humans.

- **xeroderma pigmentosum**
  A disease in human beings caused by a defect in the UV mutation repair system.

- **x-inactivation**
  The repression of one of the two X-chromosomes in the somatic cells of females as a method of dosage compensation; at an early embryonic stage in the normal female, one of the two X-chromosomes undergoes inactivation, apparently at random, from this point on all descendent cells will have the same X-chromosome inactivated as the cell from which they arose, thus a female is a mosaic composed of two types of cells, one which expresses only the paternal X-chromosome, and another which expresses only the maternal X-chromosome.

- **x-inactivation centre (xic)**
  locus on the X chromosome in mammals at which inactivation is initiated.

- **x-linked**
  Everyone gets one chromosome from their mother and one from their father. The mother always gives an "X" chromosome, and the father gives either an "X" (which causes a female child) or a "Y" (which causes a male child). If a disorder is x-linked it is only found on the x chromosome. So in the case of a male child, if that child has an x-linked disorder, it was passed on by the mother. In the case of a female child, the defective gene could have come from either parent.

- **x-linked dominant**
  Describes a dominant trait or disorder caused by a mutation in a gene on the X chromosome. The phenotype is expressed in heterozygous females as well as in hemizygous males (having only one X chromosome); affected males tend to have a more severe phenotype than affected females.

- **x-linked lethal**
  A disorder caused by a dominant mutation in a gene on the X

chromosome that is observed almost exclusively in females because it is almost always lethal in males who inherit the gene mutation

- **x-linked recessive**

A mode of inheritance in which a mutation in a gene on the X chromosome causes the phenotype to be expressed in males who are hemizygous for the gene mutation (i.e., they have only one X chromosome) and in females who are homozygous for the gene mutation (i.e., they have a copy of the gene mutation on each of their two X chromosomes). Carrier females who have only one copy of the mutation do not usually express the phenotype, although differences in X-chromosome inactivation can lead to varying degrees of clinical expression in carrier females

- **x-ray crystallography**

A technique, using X rays, to determine the atomic structure of molecules that have been crystallized. A technique for deducing molecular structure by aiming a beam of X rays at a crystal of the test compound and measuring the scatter of rays.

**Principle**

- The short wavelength of X rays allows them to penetrate substances that do not transmit light.
- The atoms (**a**) in crystals and crystalline (crystal-like) structures are arranged in planes (**b**) that have regular spaces between them. X rays passing through the crystal are diffracted (spread out) in a regular pattern by the atoms of these planes, which act as minute mirrors.
- Different crystalline structures produce unique diffraction patterns and these patterns can be used to determine the atomic structure of the substance.

**How it Works**

1 Accelerated electrons (**a**) are aimed at a solid tungsten target (**b**). When they strike the target, X rays (**c**) are produced.

2 A parallel beam of X rays is directed toward the sample (**d**).

3 The X-ray beam penetrates the sample and is diffracted by its atomic structure. These diffracted X rays (**e**) are recorded on a photographic plate (**f**). Where X rays have reinforced each other, a spot (**g**) is exposed. The sample is rotated a few degrees and exposed to another burst of X rays. This is repeated until the sample has been rotated through a full 360°.

4 Analysis of the final pattern allows the atomic structure of

the sample to be inferred. Powerful computers are used n to analyze complex patterns.

**DNA STRUCTURE**

In 1953, Francis Crick (born 1916) and James Watson (born 1928) used the work of Maurice Wilkins (born 1916) and Rosalind Franklin (1920–58) to determine the structure of DNA (deoxyribonucleic acid). DNA samples were prepared that were enough like crystals to be able to diffract X rays. This picture, taken by Franklin in 1952, had a very regular pattern that indicated DNA is coiled.

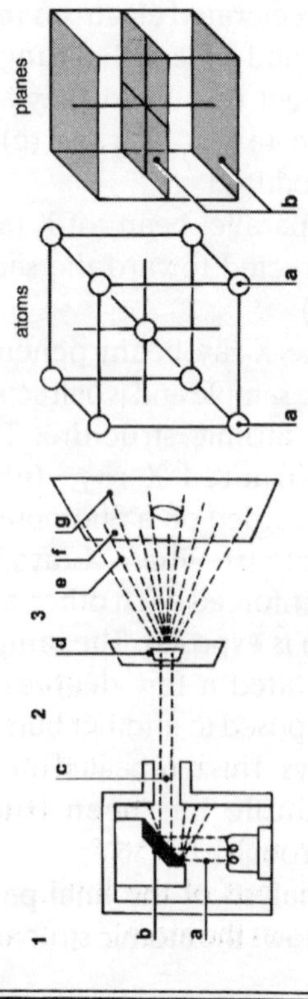


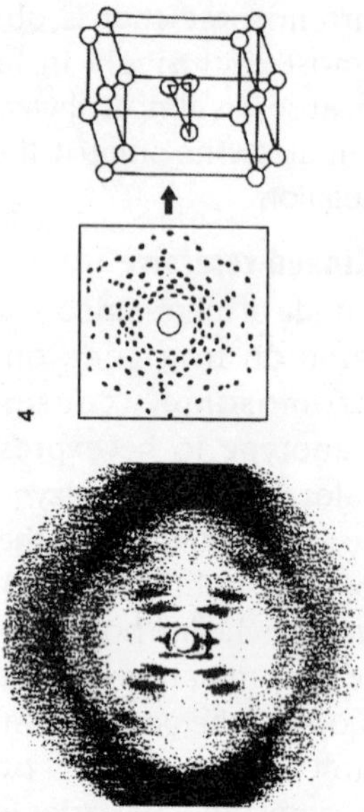

- **x-rays**

  A diagnostic imaging technique used to diagnose disease or injury where high-energy radiation in low doses passes through the body to create images of hard tissues (like bones and solid tumors) onto photographic film. Also high-energy radiation is used in high doses to treat cancer.

- **xx**

  The two chromosomes that determine sex - one chromozome from mother and one from father. The mother always gives an "X" chromozome, and if the father gives an "X" as well, you get a female child.

- **xy**

  The two chromosomes that determine sex - one chromozome

from mother and one from father. The mother always gives an "X" chromozome, and if the father gives a "Y", you get a male child.

- **xyy syndrome**
Genetic condition in males with extra Y chromosome (in 1 in 1000 male births). Symptoms: tall stature (over 6'), may including sterility, developmental delay, learning problems.

- **y chromosome**
A sex chromosome; normal males carry one Y and one X chromosome.

- **y linkage**
The inheritance pattern of genes found on the Y chromosome but not on the X (rare).

- **y linked**
Inheritance pattern of loci located on the Y chromosome only. Also refers to the loci themselves.

- **yac**
Yeast artificial chromosome; a linear vector into which a large fragment of DNA can be inserted; the development of YAC's in 1987 has increased the number of nucleotides which can be cloned. Originating from a bacterial plasmid; a YAC contains additionally a yeast centromeric region (CEN); a yeast origin of DNA replication (ARS); and two telomere regions (TEL). YACs are capable of cloning very large pieces of DNA.

- **yac maps**
Yeast artificial chromosome maps, a type of physical map.

- **y-junction**
The point of active DNA replication where the double helix opens up so that each strand can serve as a template.

- **z dna**
A left-handed form of DNA found under physiological conditions in short GC segments that are methylated. It may be important in regulating gene expression in eukaryotes.

- **zfy gene**
Originally believed to be the human male sex switch gene located on the short arm of the Y chromosome. ZFY stands for zinc finger protein on the Y chromo-some.

- **zinc finger**
Configuration of a DNA-binding protein that resembles a finger with a base, usually cysteines and histidines, binding a zinc ion. Discovered in a transcription factor in Xenopus but present in a large number of different proteins.

- **zinc finger proteins**
Transcription-activator proteins containing finger-like structures containing zinc atoms.

- **zoo blot**
A Southern blot containing conserved DNA sequences from

related genes of different species. It is taken as evidence that the sequences are coding sequences from a specific gene.

- **zygonema (zygotene stage)**
  The stage of prophase I of meiosis in which synapsis occurs.

- **zygosity testing**
  The process through which DNA sequences are compared to assess whether individuals born from a multiple gestation (twins, triplets, etc.) are monozygotic (identical) or dizygotic (fraternal); often used to identify a suitable donor for organ transplantation or to estimate disease susceptibility risk if one sibling is affected.

- **zygote**
  The diploid cell formed by the fusion of the haploid male and female gametes, and having the potential of developing into a new organism.

- **zygote**
  The unique diploid cell formed by the fusion of two haploid cells (often an egg and a sperm) that will divide mitotically to create a differentiated diploid organism.

- **zygotic induction**
  When a prophage is passed into an F- cell during conjugation it may begin vegetative growth. The sudden release of a lysogenic phage from an Hfr chromosome when the prophage enters the F- (minus) cell, and the subsequent lysis of the recipient cell.

- **zygotic selection**
  The forces acting to cause differential mortality of an organism at any stage (other than gametes) in its life cycle.